Fat-Burning FOODS

Fat-Burning FOODS

Originally published as *Fat Burning Foods*, *More Fat Burning Foods*, and *The Fat Burning Foods Cookbook*.

Judy Jameson and Porter Shimer
with recipes edited by Betty Bianconi, R.D.

BARNES & NOBLE BOOKS
NEW YORK

This edition published by Barnes & Noble, Inc.,
by arrangement with Publishing Properties LLC.

2004 Barnes & Noble Books

ISBN 0-7607-5831-X

Printed and bound in the United States of America

04 05 06 07 08 09 MC 9 8 7 6 5 4 3 2 1

CONTENTS

Book One
Fat-Burning Foods
and Other Weight-Loss Secrets
1

Book Two
More Fat-Burning Foods
and Other Weight-Loss Secrets
189

Book Three
Fat-Burning Foods Cookbook
381

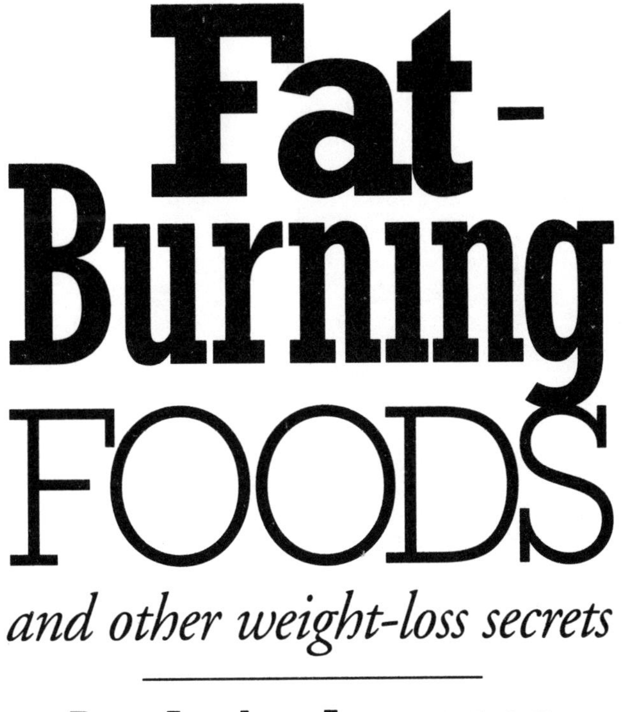

By Judy Jameson

5 Park Center Court, Suite 300
Owings Mills, Maryland 21117, USA

Cover design by Carla Frank
Printed in the United States of America
HE003U

CONTENTS

INTRODUCTION
5

CHAPTER 1
THE SECRET OF PERMANENT WEIGHT LOSS
11

CHAPTER 2
STEP-BY-STEP TO A SLIMMER YOU
71

CHAPTER 3
KEEPING IT OFF—YOU CAN DO IT!
107

CHAPTER 4
MENUS AND RECIPES FOR FAT-BURNING SUCCESS
129

INTRODUCTION

CONGRATULATIONS! You've just taken the first step towards easy, permanent weight loss. Being concerned about those extra pounds will be a thing of the past after you discover fat-burning foods and learn other weight-loss secrets. The following new discoveries in weight loss can make you more slender and energetic than ever before!

➢ Foods high in **complex carbohydrates** are not only satisfying, they are an extraordinary fat-burning tool.

➢ The amount of **fat** you eat, not total calories, will determine whether or not you gain weight.

➢ Simple, moderate **exercise** on a regular basis will keep your metabolism high enough to ensure maximum fat-burning.

➢ Slow and steady wins the weight-loss race. When you continue to lose at a rate of two pounds a week, **you'll keep those pounds off.**

➢ Losing weight is **good** for your health! This program will cut your risk of contracting such life-threatening diseases as cancer, heart disease, and high blood pressure.

Best of all, this program is incredibly easy to follow. It involves no calorie-counting, no complicated calculations, and no specialized foods or food combinations. It also promises you no more hunger pangs and no more growly stomach. In fact, **you will not be hungry during this program!**

Your 30 Miracle Foods

This amazing program is based on 30 "miracle" foods high in complex carbohydrates. Foods such as rice, potatoes, and pastas, as well as fruits and vegetables, are not only nutritious, satisfying, and inexpensive. They're also high in fiber and may well reduce your exposure to diseases such as cancer. You'll learn how these foods, when combined with simple exercise, will actually "teach" your body to burn fat and lose weight.

Here's a list of 30 fat-burning foods you can eat until you're fully satisfied.

Apples
Bananas
Beans (all varieties)
Bread (plain)
Broccoflower
Broccoli
Cabbage
Cauliflower
Celery
Citrus fruit
Corn, including air-popped popcorn
Cranberries
Frozen low-fat waffles and pancakes
Grains and grain products
Grapes
Jam (sugar-free, low-cal only)
Leeks
Lettuce
Melon
Mushrooms
Pasta (low-fat, preferably whole grain)
Pears
Peas
Peppers
Pineapple
Potatoes
Root vegetables
Spinach
Tomatoes
Zucchini

In the pages ahead, you'll learn about studies that prove your body handles complex carbohydrates differently than it does other types of food. Complex carbohydrates seem to lose many of their calories as they're being digested. That means you can eat until you're completely satisfied–and still lose weight!

But, of course, one cannot live by bread alone. This program also includes moderate amounts of protein (eggs, low-fat cheese, fish, and chicken) and very low amounts of fat, especially saturated fats (the kind found in red meat and butter).

Another key step towards a successful slimdown is cutting down on fats. Scientists have discovered that fat actually hangs on to its calories while moving through your body. Again, you'll learn more details in the pages ahead. For now, just remember that calories from fat in foods are more likely to "stick to your waistline" than calories from carbohydrates and protein.

Finally, you'll learn that food alone won't do the trick. Regular activity brings your metabolism high enough to keep the fat-burning action going. This book will provide you with practical tips on exercise that you can easily incorporate into your life. They're an essential component of this program.

Why Diets Don't Work

Americans are just plain diet crazy. And yet, most diets don't work. Believe it or not, over one-third of American women and a quarter of a million American men are dieting each day. Yet, more than 90 percent of these diets will be unsuccessful.

By now, you've probably tried a grapefruit diet, a food-combining diet, a Scarsdale diet, a liquid diet . . . the list goes on and on. You've weighed every morsel of food that went into your mouth for weeks at a time, or you've counted calories until your calculator went on the fritz. You may have tried "diet pills," which suppressed your appetite and kept you awake all night. Or diuretics, which made you lose water and salt, not fat. Or laxatives, which may have damaged your digestive system and seriously risked your health. Or hormones, which may have created a wide range of physical problems.

What did you achieve? Chances are, you ended up with a thicker waistline and wider hips than you had before!

The fact is, "fad-of-the-month" diets cause you more harm than good, mostly because they suddenly deprive your body of food. When your body thinks it's starving, your survival instinct kicks in and tries to preserve your fat stores to maintain the status quo.

As your hunger continues, your body reacts to "starvation" by decreasing its *basal metabolic rate* (the rate at which your body burns calories) in order to conserve energy. Your body becomes super-efficient at storing whatever calories it doesn't use as body fat. The less you eat, the harder your body tries to retain fat.

Then, when you go off one of the diets—and eventually you'll want to eat "normally" again—not only will you gain all the weight back, but you'll likely end up heavier than before.

It's a vicious cycle—one that puts you back at square one every time. The only permanent loss you might experience is in your bank account. Have you ever noticed that fad diets or pills are not cheap?

The fat-burning foods approach is completely different. One of the most important keys to success in this exciting new program is that you're not going to be hungry. Whenever you feel the urge to munch, you can grab one of the 30 fat-burning foods and eat until you're satisfied. Your body never "starves," so your basal metabolic rate stays high and you keep burning off extra fat slowly and steadily.

Best of all, this simple program will fill you up with satisfying foods and delicious tastes. You'll learn how your body reacts to fat-burning foods and why they are perfect for easy weight loss. You'll also learn about "diet foes"—foods and other factors that make you gain weight. Best of all, you'll find that making a commitment to good health is easy. Read on to discover . . .

The secret of permanent weight loss: The basic ideas behind this amazingly simple weight-loss and weight-maintenance plan.

The step-by-step plan to a slim new you: A detailed plan for getting started, including essential hints for success, shopping tips, food preparation tips, and an easy-to-begin activity program.

Sure-fire ways to keep excess pounds off: Suggestions for fast meals, eating out, and coping with social situations.

Delicious recipes and tantalizing menus: A seven-day menu and easy-to-prepare recipes feature delicious fat-burning foods to help you enjoy taking off those pounds.

A Word of Caution

Following this program will improve your health. But before making changes to your diet or activity level, it's always wise to discuss your decision with your physician. This book is designed to *supplement* your physician's prescribed treatment, not replace it.

CHAPTER 1

THE SECRET OF PERMANENT WEIGHT LOSS

Why You Need to Lose Weight—Starting Right Now!

IF YOU'RE READING THIS BOOK, you're probably tired of carrying extra weight. It's discouraging to find your clothes getting tight, and to feel like shunning your image in the mirror.

Carrying extra weight is also a major health risk. If you're overweight, you probably have excess fats in your blood. This builds up in the arteries of your heart, leading to angina and heart attacks. Obesity also strains your heart, which is forced to pump blood through all the extra arteries your body grows to feed your fat deposits.

Furthermore, if you are suffering from diabetes, high triglycerides, or high blood pressure, you can't afford to be even moderately overweight. A portly frame can result in hypertension, cardiovascular disease, gallbladder disease, diabetes, and some types of cancers. **Obesity can kill you. But losing weight can reduce and ultimately eliminate that potential!**

Test your weight-loss savvy

True or false?

1. Foods labeled "cholesterol-free" or "no cholesterol" are better for weight loss than other products.
2. Foods that have one of the new labels stating they're "light" or "lite" are ideal for weight-loss programs.
3. Vegetable oils or margarine are better for weight loss than butter.
4. Lasagna and other pasta products are too fattening for any weight-loss diet.
5. Half a croissant is less fattening than a large plate of rice.
6. Dairy products are always fattening.
7. If you really want to lose weight, eliminate red meat.
8. Chicken is a good source of dietary fiber.
9. A lean cut of beef is always bright red.
10. If you really want to lose weight, eat a lot of cheese.

All false. Here's why:

1. *False.* All vegetable oils, for instance, are "cholesterol-free." They're still all fat, and should be avoided.
2. *False.* "Light" could refer to less sugar or salt, or less of a particular nutrient than that contained in the regular version. The words "lite" or "light" may even describe its color, taste, or texture. Current FDA regulations stipulate, however, that if the label "lite" or "light" describes fat content, the food must have one-third fewer calories, or 50 percent less fat, than the standard version.
3. *False.* Vegetable oils and margarine are equally fattening.

4. *False*. Pasta is an excellent diet food. It's when you load it up with high-fat cheeses and ground beef that you add pounds and inches.

5. *False*. Croissants are approximately 45 percent fat. Rice is more filling and satisfying, and has only trace amounts of fat.

6. *False*. Although you can't eat unlimited amounts of milk and cheese, you can get your calcium and protein from skim milk, low-fat yogurt, and low-fat cheeses. These should be eaten in limited quantities.

7. *False*. Red meat is a good source of protein. You can eat small amounts of beef, pork, and chicken, and still lose weight.

8. *False*. There's no dietary fiber in meat or in dairy products. Dietary fiber derives from plants.

9. *False*. Lean beef has very little marbling and white fatty bits; the color of the beef itself does not indicate leanness.

10. *False*. Most hard cheeses are high in fat.

Risky business

Now that you've evaluated your weight-loss savvy, the next step is to determine whether your excess pounds are putting you at risk for serious health problems. Here's how:

A. Enter your current weight: ______ pounds

B. Find your ideal weight, according to Metropolitan Life Insurance Company's chart on page 15: ______ pounds

C. Subtract your ideal weight (B) from your current weight (A): ______ – ______ = ______
A B C

If C is greater than 25, those extra pounds you're carrying may be affecting your health.

Another method to determine whether your excess pounds are putting your health at risk is to calculate your Body Mass Index (BMI) and your Waist-Hip Ratio.

The BMI, the ratio of your weight to your height, is most useful for people ages twenty to sixty-five. It is not appropriate for very muscular people, endurance athletes, or pregnant or nursing women. Here's how to figure your BMI using the chart on page 17.

1. On line A, mark an X at your height.
2. On line B, mark an X at your weight.
3. With a ruler, join the two Xs.
4. Extend the line with the ruler to line C. This is your BMI.

If you have a BMI higher than 27, you are probably overweight. You are more likely to develop problems such as heart disease or high blood pressure than someone whose BMI falls below that range.

A high BMI alone does not necessarily mean you need to lose weight. The amount of fat you have and where it is distributed on your body is the other critical factor. If your body resembles an "apple" rather than a "pear," you may be at increased risk of health problems.

STANDARD METROPOLITAN LIFE INSURANCE HEIGHT/WEIGHT TABLES

Women

Height Feet	Inches	Small Frame*	Medium Frame	Large Frame
4	10	102–111	109–121	118–131
4	11	103–113	111–123	120–134
5	0	104–115	113–126	122–137
5	1	106–118	115–129	125–140
5	2	108–121	118–132	128–143
5	3	111–124	121–135	131–147
5	4	114–127	124–138	134–151
5	5	117–130	127–141	137–155
5	6	120–133	130–144	140–159
5	7	123–136	133–147	143–163
5	8	126–139	136–150	146–167
5	9	129–142	139–153	149–170
5	10	132–145	142–156	152–173
5	11	135–148	145–159	155–176
6	0	138–151	148–162	158–179

Men

Height Feet	Inches	Small Frame	Medium Frame	Large Frame
5	2	128–134	131–141	138–150
5	3	130–136	133–143	140–153
5	4	132–138	135–145	142–156
5	5	134–140	137–148	144–160
5	6	136–142	139–151	146–164
5	7	138–145	142–154	149–168
5	8	140–148	145–157	152–172
5	9	142–151	148–160	155–176
5	10	144–154	151–163	158–180
5	11	146–157	154–166	161–184
6	0	149–160	157–170	164–188
6	1	152–164	160–174	168–192
6	2	155–168	164–178	172–197
6	3	158–172	167–182	176–202
6	4	162–176	171–187	181–207

See page 16 to determine frame size.

STANDARD METROPOLITAN LIFE INSURANCE ELBOW MEASUREMENTS FOR MEDIUM FRAME

* To determine your frame size, bend your forearm upward at a 90 degree angle. Keep fingers straight and turn the inside of your wrist toward your body. Place thumb and index finger of other hand on the two prominent bones on either side of the elbow. Measure space between your fingers on a ruler. Compare with the tables below listing medium-framed men and women. Measurements lower than those listed indicate small frame. Higher measurements indicate large frame.

Height in 1" Heels	Elbow Breadth
Women	
4'10"–5'3"	2 1/4"–2 1/2"
5'0"–5'3"	2 1/4"–2 1/2"
5'4"–5'7"	2 3/8"–2 5/8"
5'8"–5'11"	2 3/8"–2 5/8"
6'0"	2 1/2"–2 3/4"
Men	
5'2"–5'3"	2 1/2"–2 7/8"
5'4"–5'7"	2 5/8"–2 7/8"
5'8"–5'11"	2 3/4"–3"
6'0"–6'3"	2 3/4"–3 1/8"
6'4"	2 7/8"–3 1/4"

Source: 1979 Build Study, Society of Actuaries and Association of Life Insurance Medical Directors of America, 1980. Copyright 1983, 1993 Metropolitan Life Insurance Company.

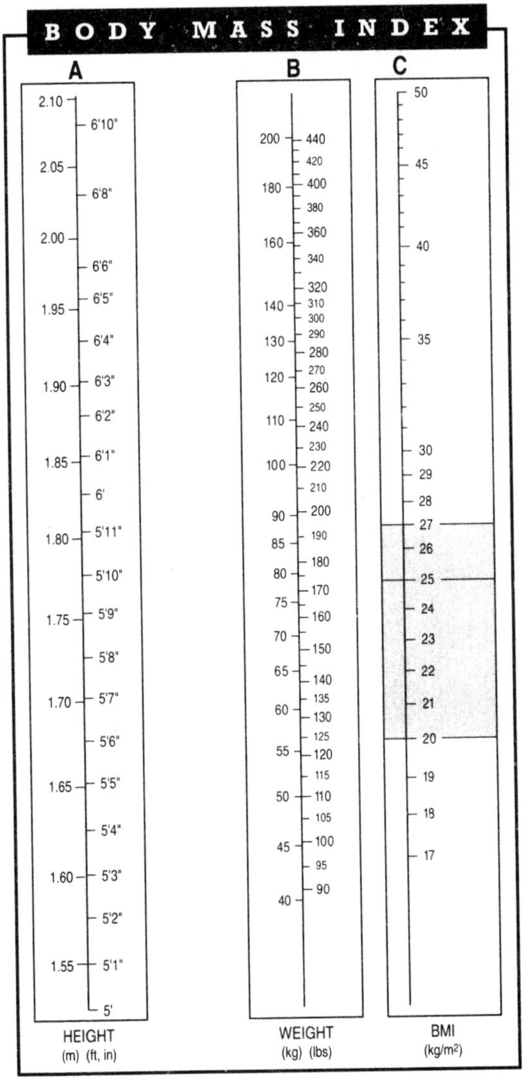

BODY MASS INDEX

A

2.10 — 6'10" — 2.05 — 6'8" — 2.00 — 6'6" — 6'5" — 1.95 — 6'4" — 1.90 — 6'3" — 6'2" — 1.85 — 6'1" — 6' — 1.80 — 5'11" — 5'10" — 1.75 — 5'9" — 5'8" — 1.70 — 5'7" — 5'6" — 1.65 — 5'5" — 5'4" — 1.60 — 5'3" — 5'2" — 1.55 — 5'1" — 5'

HEIGHT
(m) (ft, in)

B

200 — 440 — 420 — 180 — 400 — 380 — 360 — 160 — 340 — 320 — 140 — 310 — 300 — 290 — 130 — 280 — 270 — 120 — 260 — 250 — 110 — 240 — 230 — 100 — 220 — 210 — 90 — 200 — 190 — 85 — 180 — 80 — 170 — 75 — 160 — 70 — 150 — 65 — 140 — 135 — 60 — 130 — 125 — 55 — 120 — 115 — 50 — 110 — 105 — 45 — 100 — 95 — 90 — 40

WEIGHT
(kg) (lbs)

C

50 — 45 — 40 — 35 — 30 — 29 — 28 — 27 — 26 — 25 — 24 — 23 — 22 — 21 — 20 — 19 — 18 — 17

BMI
(kg/m2)

generally acceptable range

Source: Health Canada, 1991. Reproduced with permission of the Minister of Supply and Services Canada 1995.

To determine whether you're an "apple" or a "pear," calculate your Waist-Hip Ratio. Here's how:

A. Measure the circumference of the smallest part of your waist: ______ inches
B. Measure the circumference of the widest part of your hip: ______ inches
C. Divide your waist measurement (A) by your hip measurement (B) to get your Waist-Hip Ratio (C):

______	÷	______	=	______
A		B		C

Your health is at increased risk due to excess weight if C, your Waist-Hip Ratio, is 1.0 or greater (for men), or 0.8 or greater (for women).

The Calorie-Counting Game

Starvation diets don't work because you need nourishment just to stay alive. The energy from food—calories—provides your body with the energy it needs to breathe, to keep your blood pumping, and to carry on other important life functions.

On other diets, you probably spent hours calculating the calories in your food. According to the theory, calories are the basic unit of energy that food can provide. The higher the calories in a particular food, the more energy it contains. This energy can fuel your body's basic functions. But, if calories are not burned off, they can accumulate as unwanted fat.

According to the Food and Nutrition Board, the average American adult male of 154 pounds requires between 1,440 to

1,728 calories a day—just to lie around! The average inactive female of 128 pounds uses up 1,296 to 1,584 calories a day. So most conventional diets tell you to consume fewer calories than you need, and supposedly, you'll lose weight.

Wrong! If calories alone made you overweight, Americans would all be thin. Believe it or not, we actually consume fewer calories now than we did 100 years ago. The difference between then and now, however, is more than just calorie consumption. A century ago, people were far more physically active. They also ate no processed foods, which tend to be high in sugar and fat.

In theory, the fewer calories you eat, the more weight you lose. But that theory won't work if you have a relatively low basal metabolic rate. As you've already learned, when you starve yourself your system copes by dropping your basal metabolic rate. Starvation dieting makes your body hang on to every bit of body fat it can. **That's why starvation diets are the worst possible solution for an overweight person.**

Ideally, your diet should contain at least 10 calories per pound of your ideal body weight. In other words, if you want to weigh 120 pounds, you should be eating at least 1,200 calories every day. But nobody wants to count calories, and that leads us to the beauty of this program.

By eating fat-burning foods and keeping up your physical activity, your body will use up your calories **before** they turn to fat. So put away your calorie counter and read on.

Pyramids and the Power of Three

The U.S. Department of Agriculture's (USDA) new Food Guide Pyramid provides a practical set of eating guidelines for

FOOD GUIDE PYRAMID

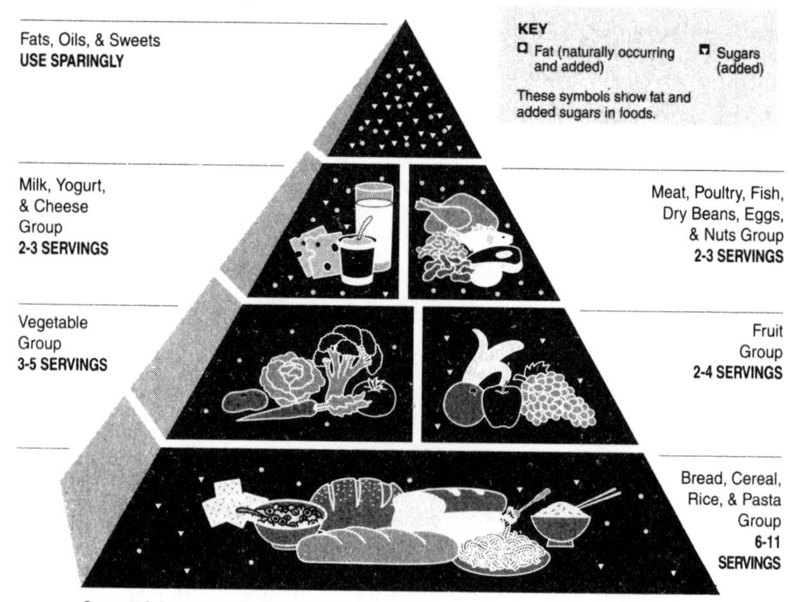

Source: U.S. Department of Agriculture/U.S. Department of Health and Human Services

all Americans. At the base of the pyramid—the foundation of every good diet—the USDA recommends 6 to 11 daily servings of grain-based foods (bread, cereal, rice, and pasta). The second most important food groups, one tier up, are vegetables (3 to 5 servings) and fruit (2 to 4 servings). The next level is shared by milk, yogurt, and cheese (2 to 3 servings) as well as meat, poultry, fish, dry beans, eggs, and nu (2 to 3 servings). At the top point of the pyramid are fats, oi and sweets that are to be used sparingly.

The truth is, only three kinds of foods provide your body with the calories it needs to sustain life: carbohydrates, fats, and proteins. We will discuss each of these.

Complex Carbohydrates: Nature's Fat-Burners

Next to water, your body needs more carbohydrates than any other nutrient. Doctors and nutritionists say carbohydrates are invaluable sources of these nutrients:

Iron	Vitamin A	Magnesium
Phosphorous	Vitamin B_6	Iodine
Thiamine	Vitamin C	Folacin
Niacin	Copper	Protein

There are two kinds of carbohydrates: *simple* and *complex. Simple carbohydrates* include jelly beans and sugary soft drinks. They're generally low in nutritional value. Complex carbohydrates, on the other hand, include pasta, potatoes, broccoli, bran, and rice. These provide more even-burning fuel than simple carbohydrates. They're also packed with more nutrients and fiber. They're key players in a successful fat-burning program.

FAT-BURNING FOOD TIP #1

At least 65 percent of the calories in your diet should come from carbohydrates, preferably complex carbohydrates.

In general, *complex carbohydrates* are a happy union of natural sugars, starches, and fiber. They include:

- *Sugars,* primarily sucrose, glucose, and fructose, found in fruits, sugar, honey, most syrups, and molasses.

- *Starches,* found in bread, pasta, rice, potatoes, and cereals.

- *Dietary fiber,* found in whole grains, whole grain products, fruits, vegetables, nuts, seeds, and legumes (seeds of plants such as lentil, pea, and bean).

Ounce for ounce, these foods provide the same amount of energy as protein, yet have fewer than **half** the calories of fat. For every gram of carbohydrate or protein you eat, you get about 4 calories of energy, a considerable savings over the 9 calories you get from fats.

ENERGY FROM FOOD

1 gram of carbohydrate = approximately 4.5 calories of energy
1 gram of protein = approximately 4 calories of energy
1 gram of fat = approximately 9 calories of energy

The bulk of your diet should come from complex carbohydrates. These are the ideal fat-burning foods. Because complex carbohydrates break down easily into glucose (blood sugar)—a main source of energy—they are like high-octane, clean-burning fuel for your body.

In addition, although you don't need to count calories on this program, fruits, vegetables, grains, breads, and cereals don't have a lot of calories. You can eat as much as you want of these foods to satisfy your appetite. In fact, your appetite is "cued" to

Carol Kaufman: Crazy for Protein

AT FORTY-THREE, Carol had been on every diet that came along, and she was *still* 30 pounds overweight. Although she loved bread, rice, and potatoes, she was afraid to eat them because she thought these foods were fattening.

Of course, she paid no attention to the fact that she enjoyed her favorite foods with a generous dollop of fat. She always applied a thick layer of butter or mayonnaise to sandwiches. Likewise, she buried baked potatoes under a mound of sour cream.

In fact, she enjoyed rich foods so much that she decided a high-protein approach was the way to lose weight. So her breakfast consisted of eggs and bacon. Lunch was cold cuts, more eggs, and cheese slices. Dinner was meat, meat, and more meat, accompanied by a salad topped with dressing.

She did lose weight at first. But her doctor was not happy when Carol's cholesterol level shot through the roof. Eventually, Carol wasn't happy, either. A month into her high-protein regimen, Carol was constantly fatigued and frequently constipated.

Fortunately, Carol decided to give carbohydrates another chance. But this time, she decided to use good old common sense. For breakfast, she ate bread, jam, fruit, and cereal. For lunch, she filled up with a huge bowl of noodle soup. At dinner, she splurged on two baked potatoes (topped with low-fat sour cream), a small portion of broiled chicken, microwaved vegetables, and a salad splashed with low-fat dressing. Fruit and air-popped popcorn saw her through snack times.

Much to her amazement, Carol lost three pounds the first week. She felt so good that she started looking forward to a half-hour morning walk. The second week, another two pounds disappeared, and she maintained a steady loss of one to two pounds a week for the next few months.

Today Carol is slim, active, and very proud of herself. She hasn't lost her craving for bread, rice, and potatoes; now, she knows they're good for her!

tell your body to stop eating while your body converts energy from carbohydrates into glucose for energy.

A menu loaded with carbohydrates is chock-full of wonderful fat-burning foods. As far back as 1975, Dr. Olaf Michelsen, professor of nutrition at Michigan State University, made a surprising discovery. He found that bread—and lots of it—can be the ideal diet food. A published study demonstrated that overweight young men lost weight easily on a menu that included 12 slices of bread a day! Within eight weeks, the eight men who were given high-fiber bread lost almost 20 pounds, on average. The eight who ate low-fiber bread lost less—13.7 pounds. But they all lost weight, even though they were filling up on bread.

More recently, in 1981, University of Virginia scientists fed adult laboratory rats food identical in calorie and fat content. Some, however, had diets rich in carbohydrates, while others had diets rich in protein. The animals on the carbohydrate-rich diets gained much less weight and put on considerably less body fat than those on diets rich in protein. One of the researchers' explanations was that on a high-carbohydrate, low-protein diet, more calories may be "burned up" as body heat while fewer are stored as energy reserves, or fat.

How can this be? The most likely explanation is that **meals high in complex carbohydrates raise the metabolic rate of overweight people more than meals containing the same number of calories, but composed mostly of fats or proteins.**

Scientists have many theories about why complex carbohydrates have such a magical effect on our weight. One theory is that fat consumption changes your body chemistry to slow down your metabolism. Another theory is that fatty foods somehow interfere with your body's ability to use its fat stores for energy.

Still another theory is that when you eat foods high in complex carbohydrates, you tend to eat enough calories to provide the energy you need. When you eat fatty foods, on the other hand, you are eating for pleasure, rather than for energy. Eating chocolate cake for no other reason than because it tastes good has nothing to do with hunger or your energy requirements.

Other research by Dr. Michael Levitt at Minneapolis Veterans Administration Hospital has shown that up to one-third of the calories in starchy foods are not absorbed by the human body. He suggests that bacteria in the gut "digest" them and eliminate them as gas.

The most compelling theory is that your body seems to "prefer" complex carbohydrates to fats, for energy. One research team, for instance, learned that the body had to use 28 percent of its high-carbohydrate calories to convert them into fat. But the body only had to use 7 percent of its dietary fat calories to convert *them* into fat. Doctors from Stanford University School of Medicine found that complex carbohydrates appear to lose up to one quarter of their calories while being digested. Fat, on the other hand, loses only 3 percent of its calories as it moves through your body (and settles on your waist).

Obviously, it's "easier" for the body to convert carbohydrates into energy and dietary fat into body fat for future use. Perhaps dietary fat is so similar in chemical composition to our body fat that it just takes less energy to convert it into flab.

Whatever theory you choose, two important facts are clear:

➢ **Calories from starch, sugar, and other carbohydrates are not stored in your body as easily as calories from fat.**

➢ **Your body prefers to fuel itself with carbohydrate calories.**

Fill up on fiber!

Complex carbohydrates are essential for another very important reason. These foods are a good source of dietary fiber—the part of the plant which is not digested or is only partially digested by our enzymes.

There are two main types of dietary fiber: *water-soluble* and *insoluble.* Both are excellent for weight control and are superb for your health.

Water-soluble fiber can dissolve in water. It's found in foods such as oat bran, white beans, and many legumes, fruits, and vegetables. In general, these foods help regulate blood sugar levels and may also lower cholesterol in your blood. The soluble fiber in apples and oats has also been linked to reduced risk of heart disease.

How do water-soluble fibers do this? Oat bran appears to form a gel-like substance in the intestines that binds with bile acids. These acids are manufactured by your body's cholesterol stores for use in digesting cholesterol. When you eat a food like oat bran that contains water-soluble fibers, the indigestible fiber attaches itself to the bile acids that carry cholesterol. The whole mass then passes right through your body.

Insoluble fiber is found in foods like wheat bran, lima beans, peanuts, and many legumes, fruits, and vegetables. It provides the roughage your digestive system needs to stay healthy, acting like a toothbrush on the interior of your digestive tract. This action reduces your risk of developing constipation, hemorrhoids, diverticular disease, and possibly some cancers. Eating insoluble fiber in wheat bran has been linked to reduced risk of colon cancer and possibly breast cancer.

Like other complex carbohydrate foods, fiber helps satisfy

SOLUBLE FIBER CONTENT OF COMMON FOODS

Food	Grams of soluble fiber
Oat bran, 1/3 cup	2.01
Whole-wheat bread, 1 slice	0.34
White rice, raw, 1/6 cup	0.25
Garbanzo beans, canned, 1/7 cup	0.16
Kidney beans, canned, 1/2 cup	1.45
Lentils, dried, cooked, 1/2 cup	0.56
Navy beans, dried, cooked, 1/2 cup	2.29
Pinto beans, canned, 1/2 cup	1.10
Broccoli, frozen, 1/2 cup	0.98
Potato, white, raw, 1/2 cup	0.77
Apple, raw, 1 small	0.97
Orange, California seedless navel, 1 small	1.13

hunger, and thus helps you resist the temptation to overload on fat. Fiber in your diet adds necessary bulk and is satisfying. It also takes a long time to chew most fibrous foods, which allows time for the "I'm full" signal to reach your brain.

Furthermore, the fiber in complex carbohydrates absorbs water and slows down the speed at which your stomach can empty itself of food, staving off hunger pangs. The longer the food stays in your stomach, the longer you will feel full.

High-fiber foods also help keep your blood sugar level stable, which makes you feel full and less inclined to keep on eating. The American Physicians' Association has found that fibers in whole grains, some fruits, and vegetables keep sugars in the intestinal tract for longer periods. This makes your blood glucose level go up more slowly than if you ate a simple sugar. Your blood glucose level also takes longer to drop down to the lower level again.

Also, high-fiber foods keep your insulin levels stable. Your body releases insulin after you eat. The more food you consume at one sitting, the more insulin your body releases. Insulin is a hormone that encourages your body to burn carbohydrates for energy. It also prevents your body's fat cells from breaking down their fat; indeed, it encourages these cells to "plump up" with the fat you've eaten. So it's a good idea to eat small, high-fiber meals during the day to keep insulin levels low and stable. By doing this, you will burn more carbohydrates and store less fat.

BEST SOURCES OF FIBER

Fruits (fresh, not canned)
Vegetables (fresh, not canned)
Legumes (lentils, beans, and peas)
Nuts or seeds
Whole grains
Whole-grain products

Meet your new best friend—fiber!

What this means, in short, is that you should plan to eat considerably more fiber than you consume now. Thirty to forty grams of fiber is more than double the amount most Americans eat at present.

It's easy to accomplish this if you eat the recommended fat-burning foods. Former diet no-nos like bread, pasta, and cereal will become your new friends. As long as you don't load them up with fat-ridden sauces, fillings, and spreads, or purchase brands that are high in fat, you may fill up on them and still lose weight.

FAT-BURNING FOOD TIP #2

Plan to eat 30 to 40 grams of fiber every day.

To make sure that the breads and cereals you choose are a good source of fiber, read the label and choose those with at least 2, but preferably 4, grams of fiber per serving. Always choose bread made from whole-wheat flour, which has three times as much fiber (1.4 grams per slice) as plain white bread. There's actually very little fiber in white flour or baked goods made with white flour.

You should also start switching your priorities at mealtimes. Instead of protein as dinner's central focus, put the spotlight on carbohydrates, such as pasta or rice dishes. Add at least two vegetables, and enjoy fruit for dessert. You can still eat protein, but consider it an accent, rather than the centerpiece.

If you're adding high-fiber foods to your diet for the first time, be sure to use a variety of sources, and to go slowly until your system adjusts. Try adding one new high-fiber food per meal for a few days, and then build up your fiber intake from there. Some of these foods can stimulate the formation of intestinal gases, which can make you feel bloated and flatulent until your system adjusts.

It's also essential to drink plenty of fluids. If you consume too much insoluble fiber without drinking enough water to carry it along, the fiber will become dry and constipating.

Satisfying Your Sugar Tooth

SUGAR, BELIEVE IT OR NOT, will not make you gain weight. As a matter of fact, studies indicate that overweight people eat less sugar than lean people do. Although obesity has increased some five-fold in the past forty years, sugar consumption has remained constant.

This doesn't mean you should stuff yourself with jujubes or sugary candies, which are made of refined and/or processed sugars and have no nutritional value (they're also terrible for your teeth). Sugar alone makes your blood glucose level go up very fast and drop just as fast, leaving you as hungry as you were before.

Instead, enjoy the natural simple sugars in apples, grapes, pineapple, and other fruit, which provide vitamins and minerals along with fiber, to satisfy your hunger. Eat as much of them as you like. But the odd sugary treat won't hurt your weight loss, as long as the sugars are not accompanied by fat. Cake, cookies, brownies, and chocolate bars, all of which are high in fat, will make you gain weight. The occasional vanilla wafer or sugar in your tea will not slow down your weight loss on this program.

Your 30 Fat-Burning Foods

Now that you understand why fat-burning foods are key to losing weight, look over this expanded list of your 30 miracle foods. These fat-burning foods are all high in complex carbohydrates and low in fat, and they keep stomachs full.

- Apples
- Bananas
- Beans (all varieties, fresh, sprouted, and dried)
- Bread (plain, preferably whole grain)
- Broccoflower
- Broccoli
- Cabbage
- Cauliflower
- Celery
- Citrus fruit (includes lemons, oranges, grapefruit)
- Corn, including air-popped popcorn
- Cranberries
- Grains and grain products (barley, bran, bulgur, couscous, quinoa, rice, rolled oats, corn tortillas, wheat, high-fiber, low-fat cereals)
- Grapes
- Jam (sugar-free, low-cal only)
- Leeks
- Lettuce
- Melons
- Mushrooms
- Pasta (low-fat, preferably whole grain)
- Pears
- Peas (all types)
- Peppers
- Pineapple
- Potatoes
- Root vegetables (beets, carrots, onions, parsley, pumpkins, squash, turnips)
- Spinach
- Tomatoes (includes salt-free, sugar-free tomato sauce and salsa)
- Waffles and pancakes (frozen, low-fat)
- Zucchini

Fats: First in Your Mouth, Then on Your Hips

Fats, found in most meats, dairy products, nuts, and grain products, are necessary for your health. They help transport some of the vitamins you need, and are an essential part of your cell membranes, some hormones, and digestive acids. They insulate and cushion your major organs, and regulate your temperature. Fat also makes food taste better and keeps you from getting hungry between meals.

FAT-BURNING FOOD TIP #3

Remember that the more fat you eat, the more likely you are to be overweight—and stay overweight.

Many foods that contain fat also contain other valuable nutrients. Red meat is rich in iron and zinc, for example. Dairy products are your most concentrated source of calcium, necessary for strong bones and teeth as well as nerve and muscle health. So it's foolish to cut fat out of your diet altogether.

Trim your fat intake

The trouble is, you don't need nearly as much fat as you're eating. All you really need to satisfy your body's minimum requirements for fat is the equivalent of a daily teaspoon of canola oil, which is pure, unadulterated polyunsaturated fat. You'll get at least that if you eat the minimum protein recommendations of this program.

Researchers have found that the main difference between overweight and slender people is the amount of fat they eat. The average North American diet is about 35 to 40 percent fat, thanks to our fondness for red meat, fried foods, dairy products, and desserts. Overweight people tend to get 40 percent or more of their calories from such fatty foods. Slim people tend to eat more vegetables, fruits, and grains, which are all low-fat foods.

One recent major study has found that there is no relationship between how many calories people eat (relative to body size) and how likely they are to be fat. Another study, from Stanford University School of Medicine, even found that the fewer calories people eat per pound of body weight, the more likely they are to be fat. But both studies came to a common conclusion: **the more fat that people ate, the more likely they were to be overweight.**

FAT-BURNING FOOD TIP #4

Consume no more than 20 to 30 percent of calories from fat per day.

FAT CONSUMPTION IS THE CRITICAL FACTOR IN OBESITY. You must reduce your fat intake to 20 to 30 percent of your daily calories, preferably less.

One important reason why fats make you fat is that they are a very "expensive" form of energy for your body: they provide 9 calories per gram, as opposed to the 4 calories per gram you get from proteins and carbohydrates. Ounce for ounce, you take in more than twice as many calories when you eat fats as when you eat carbohydrates.

Furthermore, as you have already learned, your body tends to use up the calories from carbohydrates, and store the fats. Fat calories are harder to burn off than carbohydrates and protein. They're also more readily converted to body fat, since your body prefers to use carbohydrate calories for fuel.

To calculate how much fat you're allowed, remember that each gram of fat contains 9 calories. Now perform the following calculation:

A. Number of calories you usually consume daily: _____

B. To determine the allowable daily amount of calories as fat, multiply the number of daily calories (A) by 30 percent: ______ x 0.3 = ______
   A B

C. To find out how many grams of fat you're allowed daily, divide the total allowable daily calories from fat (B) by 9 calories: ______ ÷ 9 = ______
   B C

What this means is that a woman consuming 1,200 calories a day should aim to eat no more than 40 grams of fat daily (preferably less), while a man consuming 1,800 calories may eat 60 grams (preferably less).

Antonia Barnes: After-the-Baby Fat

ANTONIA NEVER had a weight problem until her son, Ryan, was born. She and her husband, Bill, nicknamed him "the boy who doesn't sleep." Antonia's days and nights were a whirl of feeding and changing.

Leisurely mealtimes with Bill became a thing of the past. At dinnertime, they relied on take-out meals of fried chicken, hamburgers, hot dogs, and burritos. When Bill was at work, breakfast and lunch consisted of whatever Antonia could grab on the fly from the fridge, which was usually leftovers from the previous night's dinner.

By Ryan's first birthday, Antonia was finally starting to get a little rest. Then, she got pregnant with Laurie. Little Laurie was born prematurely. Antonia spent two months after her daughter's birth at the hospital, waiting for opportunities to hold the child. Whenever her baby fell asleep, she'd nip down to the hospital cafeteria and load up on lasagna, noodles Alfredo, and meat loaf soaked in gravy. Between meals, vending machines were a rich source of nuts, chocolate bars, and chips.

By the time Laurie left the hospital, Antonia was 50 pounds heavier than she'd ever been. Discouraged by her weight gain, Antonia decided that she had to make time for herself. Bill agreed to watch the children on Saturday afternoons while Antonia visited friends and gossiped over a huge salad. For quick fixes, Antonia had a bowl of whole-grain cereal topped with fruit. She discovered low-fat lasagna and took up stir-frying with a vengeance.

It took a year, but soon she was back to her original (pre-baby) weight. Best of all, the program was terrific for her marriage. She rejoined Bill and their volleyball cronies on Wednesday nights. Last time we checked in, Bill and Antonia were just about to enjoy a regular evening's half-hour bicycle ride together.

Where fat lurks

Animal fat is the most obvious source of fat in your diet. You must cut down your intake of red meat to a maximum of 5 ounces per serving, no more than twice a week. In fact, the upper limit of .your red meat consumption should be one or two dinners of red meat per week. The rest of your meat intake should consist of chicken and fish.

The fat in dairy products is another enemy. You must switch to skim milk and low-fat cheese products, and limit your consumption of them to a maximum of 2 cups of milk, or the equivalent, daily.

Oils, margarine, butter, and other "pure" fats, such as those found in most commercial salad dressings, have no place in this program, either. You'll learn so many healthy alternatives that you'll lose your taste for them in no time.

Although vegetables are one of the mainstays of this program, some vegetables, such as avocados and olives, are loaded with fat and should also be avoided.

For the purposes of this program, you should eat as little fat as possible, from all sources. All fats are bad for your waistline.

"Good" fats versus "bad" fats

First, a quick biology lesson. When you eat foods that contain any kind of fat, that fat is digested and transported through your blood to every cell in your body. Unfortunately, fat doesn't dissolve in blood. Some fat is transported in your blood in the form called "triglycerides." The rest is conveyed via one of three different types of fat-carrying molecules called "lipoproteins"—fats in the form of blood cholesterol. Lipoproteins are

FAT CONTENT OF COMMON FOODS

Food	Grams of fat	Percentage of calories from fat
Apple	—	—
Banana	less than 1	5%
Navy beans, 1/2 cup, boiled	less than 1	4%
Red beans, 1/2 cup, canned	—	—
Light bran bread, 1 slice	less than 1	11%
Pumpernickel bagel, 3" diameter	0.5	3%
Broccoli	—	—
Cabbage	—	—
Cauliflower	—	—
Celery	—	—
Orange	—	—
Grapefruit	—	—
Corn, 1 ear, cooked	1.0	10%
Frozen low-fat waffle	1.0	13%
Rice, brown, long-grain, 1 cup cooked	0.9	5%
Spaghetti, 2 oz.	1.0	4%
Lasagna noodles, 2 oz.	1.0	4%
Couscous, 1/2 cup	—	—
Tortilla, 1 small corn	—	—
1 small wheat	2.0	21%
Seedless Thompson grapes, 1/2 cup	—	—
Jam (sugar-free, low-cal)	—	—
Romaine lettuce, 1/2 cup	—	—
Leeks, 1/2 cup	—	—
Cantaloupe, 1 cup	less than 1	8%
Mushrooms, fresh	—	—
Bartlett pear	1.0	9%

Food	Grams of fat	Percentage of calories from fat
Green peas, 1/2 cup	—	—
Pepper, raw	—	—
Pineapple, fresh, 1 cup	0.66	8%
Baked potato, 1 medium	—	—
Beets, fresh	—	—
Pumpkin, fresh, 1 cup	—	—
Spinach, fresh, 1 cup	—	—
Tomatoes	—	—
Squash, summer or winter	—	—
Approach With Caution!		
Top round beef, 3 oz., broiled, lean only	5.0	29%
Eye of round steak, 3 oz., lean only, roasted	5.0	30%
Round tip of beef, 3 oz., lean only, roasted	6.0	35%
Sirloin steak, 3 oz., lean only, broiled	7.0	36%
Tenderloin, 3 oz., broiled, lean only	7.0	38%
Parmesan cheese, 1 tbsp., grated	1.5	59%
Mozzarella cheese, 1 oz.	5.0	64%
Chicken breast, 3 oz.,		
no skin, roasted	3.0	19%
skin on, roasted	7.6	35%
Sole, 3 oz., cooked	1.0	11%
baked with butter	0.6	45%

composed of fat (lipid) encased in protein and other fats.

Three main types of lipoproteins are found in your blood:

- *High-density lipoproteins (HDLs):* HDLs are the so-called "good" cholesterol. They benefit your heart because they clean up excess cholesterol from body tissues and take it to the liver for processing and elimination.

- *Low-density lipoproteins (LDLs):* LDLs are the so-called "bad" cholesterol. If you have too many of them in your blood, they start depositing cholesterol on the walls of your coronary arteries, which enlarges fatty deposits that are already there.

- *Very-low-density lipoproteins (VLDLs):* VLDLs are also not good for you, because they are lipoproteins that eventually turn into "bad" LDLs. When you consume more carbohydrates, alcohol, or protein than you need for energy, your body stores the excess calories as fat, or adipose tissue. VLDL molecules carry excess calories from the liver to the fatty tissue, in the form of fats called triglycerides. Once triglycerides are delivered, what remains of the VLDL molecule is an LDL molecule—the "bad" cholesterol.

Dietary Fats in Food

There's a difference between the types of fat in your food and the lipoprotein molecules that ultimately carry fat through your blood. What's important to understand is that the type of fat in your food has an effect on which type of lipoprotein your blood carries. Which types of fat are less harmful to eat than others? Read on to find out.

FAT-BURNING FOOD TIP #5

Avoid fat in your diet whenever possible.

Saturated fats, also known as hydrogenated fats, raise your "bad" cholesterol level in your blood more than unsaturated fats.

Saturated fats are the solid kind found in meats and dairy products such as butter and cheese. They're also found in hydrogenated or partially hydrogenated margarines, shortenings, peanut butter, and certain tropical vegetable oils, including palm, palm kernel, coconut oil, and coconut butter. The process of hydrogenation is used to turn liquid oils into solid margarine. Margarine, shortening, and many cookies, crackers, chips, and other processed foods are made with hydrogenated or partially hydrogenated vegetable oil.

Furthermore, a report out of Harvard University shows that another fat lurking in margarine and other processed foods could be responsible for 30,000 heart disease deaths annually in the United States. The hydrogenation process apparently creates a new type of fat not found in nature: "trans fat." In the American Journal of Public Health, researchers pointed out that trans fatty acids not only raised the "bad" LDL cholesterol level just like saturated fat, but also lowered the "good" HDL cholesterol.

Dorothy Sobel: Nighttime Pastry Fiend

DOROTHY HAD A TROUBLED ADOLESCENCE. Her family moved frequently, so she had to develop new friendships, from scratch, at a dozen different schools. Her mother didn't enjoy the frequent moves any more than she did. There were frequent fights, and her dad moved out a few times.

Dorothy spent many a sad evening in her bedroom, listening to her parents quarrel and feeling sorry for herself. During those lonely nights, her favorite companions were cookies, cakes, and doughnuts. She would lie in bed, sadly contemplating her solitude, while she stuffed her face.

By the time she hit her twenties, Dorothy was 20 pounds overweight—a huge amount for her petite frame—and lonelier than ever. One New Year's, alone as usual, she made her usual New Year's resolution—to lose weight. This time, however, she read up on fat-burning foods.

Fortunately, Dorothy's daytime eating habits were already healthy. She loved salads, pasta, vegetables, grilled fish, and chicken. The problem was that late-night lonely hour. There was no way she could make it to morning without a few munchies between dinnertime and bedtime.

Her main solution was to eat plenty of air-popped popcorn, sprinkled with a butter substitute. She satisfied her hunger for sweets with fruit and the occasional sugar-free jam sandwich on whole-wheat bread. She also joined a bowling club, getting her out of the house at least once a week. And she made it a priority to take a long walk after dinner.

Within a few months, Dorothy's nights were no longer lonely! She had made a few friends at the bowling club, and some of them were available to keep her company on other evenings, too.

The excess weight slid off in plenty of time for summer swimming. By July, Dorothy was in the water, in a bikini!

FAT-BURNING FOOD TIP #6

Keep your intake of saturated fats at or below 10 percent of your daily calorie intake, and your total fat consumption at or below 20 to 30 percent of your daily calorie intake.

You don't need a drop of saturated fat in your diet for good health, so try to keep these types of fat to an absolute minimum.

Foods High in Saturated Fats

- Beef (fattier cuts)
- Bologna
- Butter
- Cakes (most)
- Cheese
- Chicken (dark meat, skin)
- Chips (most)
- Chocolate
- Coconut butter
- Coconut oil
- Cookies (most)
- Corned beef
- Crackers (most)
- Cream
- Fried foods
- Granola
- Gravy
- Hot dogs
- Ice cream
- Lamb
- Lard
- Margarine (hydrogenated)
- Milk (whole, 2%, 1%)
- Non-dairy creamers
- Non-dairy whipped cream
- Palm kernel oil
- Palm oil
- Peanut butter (hydrogenated)
- Pizza
- Popcorn (microwave type, buttered)

Pork
Processed meats
Pudding
Quiche
Shortening (hydrogenated)
Soybean oil
Turkey (dark meat)
Veal (fattier cuts)
Vegetable oils (hydrogenated)
Whipped cream

Unsaturated fats are the liquid type of fat. In general, they're not as harmful to your health as saturated fats. There are four types, mostly found in vegetable products.

1. *Monounsaturated fats,* found in certain vegetable oils such as olive oil and canola oils, not only don't raise blood cholesterol levels, but lower them when they replace saturated fats in your diet. They don't lower the "good" cholesterol, HDL, and therefore are not as bad for your health. But you won't lose weight unless you cut them way back in your diet.

Foods High in Monounsaturated Fats

Beef (leaner cuts)
Canola oil
Chicken
Croissants
Eggs
Nuts (almonds, cashews, chestnuts, hazelnuts, macadamias, peanuts, pecans, pistachios)
Olive oil
Olives
Peanut butter (nonhydrogenated)
Peanut oil
Pies (most)
Popcorn (popped in vegetable oil)
Pork
Rapeseed oil
Shortening (vegetable)
Veal (leaner cuts)

2. *Polyunsaturated fats,* found in other liquid vegetable oils, such as liquid safflower, canola, corn, soybean, nut, or cottonseed oil, have the same good effect on overall blood cholesterol levels as monounsaturated oils. Again, too much of them is not good for your health. In fact, some studies have shown a link between polyunsaturates and breast cancer.

Foods High in Polyunsaturated Fats

Canola oil
Corn chips
Corn oil
Cottonseed oil
Mayonnaise
Nut oil
Potato chips
Safflower oil
Salad dressings (most types)
Seeds (pumpkin, sesame, squash, sunflower)
Soybean oil
Soybeans
Tofu

3. *Omega-3 fatty acid,* which is another type of polyunsaturated fat, is the type found in fish oil. It received a lot of attention a few years ago as a cure-all for heart disease. Fish oil may reduce your triglyceride levels, but there's no convincing evidence that it reduces cholesterol levels in your blood. Large doses of fish oil supplements may even increase "bad" cholesterol in people who have high triglyceride levels. Fish, however, contains less fat than many other forms of protein, and it may even help prevent blood clots from forming.

Foods High in Omega-3 Fatty Acid

Bluefish
Cod
Haddock
Herring

Mackerel
Mussels
Oysters
Salmon
Sardines
Scallops
Trout
Whitefish

4. *Dietary cholesterol* in food (which is not the same as the lipoproteins in your blood) is a source of fat that actually has no calories, so it doesn't make you gain weight. Dietary cholesterol, however, still isn't good for you in excess quantities. It is absorbed, circulates in your body, and is then deposited in your blood vessels. Dietary cholesterol is found in foods of animal origin. Egg yolks, butter, lard, whole milk, meat, shellfish, and poultry are particularly high in it. Dietary cholesterol is also found in pastries and cakes made with butter or lard and milk products made with whole milk.

Foods High in Dietary Cholesterol

Butter
Chicken
Eggs
Lard
Lobster
Milk (whole)
Scallops
Shrimp
Turkey

Protein—Too Much, Too Often

You need some protein in your daily diet. This important nutrient is a major component of muscles, bone, cartilage, skin, brain tissue, blood, lymph, enzymes, and many hormones. In fact, the only body substances that normally lack protein are bile and urine.

Proteins are composed of building blocks called "amino acids." There are twenty amino acids, some of which the body cannot make by itself. You need a new supply of protein every day to repair and build almost all body tissues, and to produce virtually every chemical in your body.

Animal products contain all the essential amino acids, so sources such as meats, poultry, cheese, and eggs provide your body with what is called "complete protein." A complete protein can supply all twenty amino acids in a single serving.

Other sources of protein, including legumes (beans, lentils, and peas), whole grains, and milk and milk products, can be an incomplete source. That doesn't mean animal products are your best source of protein. It does mean, however, that if you cut back on animal sources of protein, you must eat a variety of other proteins every day to ensure you're getting your quota. This is especially important for vegetarians, who do not use meat sources for protein.

FAT-BURNING FOOD TIP #7

A maximum of 10 to 15 percent of your daily calories should come from animal sources of protein.

If your daily intake is 2,000 calories, you need only 200 to 400 calories of protein from animals a day, which you can get from 6 ounces of broiled fish and an ounce or two of cottage cheese. Alternatively, you only need about 1 ounce of protein

Johnny Burston: Greasy Kid Stuff

JOHNNY ACQUIRED HIS TASTE for fatty foods in college. Before he had graduated, he had a Ph.D. in grease! That included expertise in the merits of many a double-cheese-with-everything-on-it pizza, as well as a diet of french fries, hamburgers, fried chicken, chicken-fried steak, potato chips, and, for roughage, cole slaw drowning in mayonnaise or salads drenched in oil and vinegar.

Fortunately for Johnny's waistline (not to mention his long-term health), he married Jocelyn, a woman who had discovered a few fat-burning secrets on her own.

On their wedding day, Johnny was 40 pounds overweight. Although she loved him as he was, Jocelyn was concerned about the long-term health risks of his excess weight. She was especially concerned once she learned that heart disease ran in Johnny's family. But she realized that Johnny was never going to give up all his old habits completely. She decided that she would come up with fat-burning versions of his usual diet.

To begin with, she began turning out "no-cheese" pizzas, topped with tomato sauce and a wide selection of interesting vegetables. French fries were an interesting challenge: she prepared the potatoes, lightly sprayed them with a small amount of vegetable oil, and broiled them in the oven. Johnny never realized that the "hamburgers" she prepared so lovingly were in fact chicken burgers, broiled in the oven. Fried chicken was easily replaced with spicy grilled chicken. Jocelyn made sure that plenty of celery and carrots were always around to replace the potato chips, and she stocked up on fat-free salad dressing to top Johnny's greens.

Her ingenuity became a standing joke between them. And it still gets plenty of laughs among their friends, now that Johnny can boast about his successful weight loss.

for every 18 pounds of ideal body weight. In other words, a 126-pound woman only needs about 7 ounces of protein a day, while a 162-pound man needs about 9 ounces of protein.

Your diet is unlikely to be deficient in proteins. Most Americans eat a diet that contains too much protein, and certainly too much animal protein. In fact, in America, most of us eat at least twice as much animal protein as we need. And too much protein is almost as hazardous as not enough. Your body cannot store protein, so excess quantities put a strain on your liver and kidneys, the organs that process and eliminate what your body doesn't need. Excess protein also promotes the loss of calcium from bones (which can eventually lead to bone loss, fractures, and osteoporosis).

FAT CONTENT IN COMMON SOURCES OF PROTEIN

Food	Percentage of calories from fat
T-bone steak	80%
Hard cheese	75%
Whole milk	48%
Tuna packed in oil	64%
Fillet of sole	10%
Chicken (white and dark), skinless	31%
Peanut butter	66%
Bacon	75% or more
Cream cheese	75% or more
"Extra lean" ground beef	54%

FAT CONTENT IN COMMON SOURCES OF VEGETABLE PROTEIN

Food	Percentage of calories from fat
Rice	1%
Dried beans	3 to 4%
Rice, brown, long-grain, cooked, 1 cup	5%
Italian pasta salad	7%
Whole-wheat spaghetti with tomato sauce	5%

Too much protein from animal sources will make you gain weight because meats and cheeses—the most common sources—are also high in fat and calories. Remember, animal protein seldom travels "solo." Usually, it takes plenty of fat along for the ride.

You don't have to eliminate steak and roast chicken from your menu. But you can reduce your protein intake relatively painlessly by filling up instead on those healthy, fat-burning complex carbohydrates. Consider replacing high-fat protein with low-fat sources. Dried peas, beans, and many whole grains, for instance, not only are excellent sources of vegetable protein, they are practically fat-free and terrific sources of complex carbohydrates.

Change your protein habits

One mistake many people make is to eat most of their day's protein at dinner. You'll feel better if you eat protein earlier, because it will stabilize your blood sugar throughout the day.

In other words, instead of eating meat, chicken, or fish only at dinnertime, consider starting the day with a small portion of leftovers from last night's supper. Be sure to include another small helping of additional protein at lunch and dinner.

For maximum nutrition, eat a variety of protein sources. If you're a vegetarian, have as much variety as possible—eggs and dairy products, grains, legumes, and nuts—every day, to make sure you're getting complete protein.

One of the best sources of protein is red meat. This includes beef, pork, veal, lamb, and mutton. They are important sources of iron and zinc, two nutrients Americans have trouble getting in sufficient amounts. But because red meat is high in fat, you'll have to limit your servings to 5 ounces, once or twice a week.

FAT-BURNING FOOD TIP #8

Plan to eat one or two dinners of lean red meat weekly, another one or two dinners featuring chicken, another one or two of fish, and at least one vegetarian dinner a week, preferably two.

Meat today is much leaner, especially if you trim off excess fat and cook it in lower-fat ways (you'll learn more about food preparation in the next chapter). Many lean cuts of beef and pork have less fat per serving than fatty fish like trout and salmon.

One meat you might consider substituting for beef is pork, which can be almost as low in fat as chicken in terms of its content of total and saturated fat.

FAT-BURNING FOOD TIP #9

Never eat more than 5 ounces of animal protein in a day.

Dairy Dilemma: Getting Calcium Without the Fat

Dairy foods provide many vital nutrients, including protein, vitamin A, riboflavin, niacin, vitamin B-12, and folacin. Their most significant nutrient, however, is calcium and, in fortified milk, vitamin D.

You need calcium, which is stored in your bones, for muscles, nerves, blood, and cell membrane functioning. If you don't eat enough of it, your body will take calcium from your bones, eventually making them so porous that you could develop osteoporosis. Women especially must ensure there is sufficient calcium in their diets. After menopause, they must have a good source of calcium for prevention of osteoporosis.

FAT-BURNING FOOD TIP #10

Avoid whole milk and hard cheese.

PERCENTAGE OF CALORIES FROM FAT IN COMMON DAIRY FOODS

Dairy food	Calories	Percentage of calories from fat
Whole milk, 1 cup	150	49%
2% milk, 1 cup	121	35%
1% milk, 1 cup	102	22%
Skim (nonfat) milk, 1 cup	86	5%
Light cheddar cheese, 1 oz. (a slice)	90	56%
Mozzarella cheese, 1 oz. (a slice)	70	64%
Parmesan cheese, 1 oz.	129	59%
Fat-free cheddar cheese, 1 oz.	40	—
Fat-free mozzarella cheese, 1 oz.	40	—
1% cottage cheese, 4 oz. (1/2 cup)	90	10%
Fat-free process cheese spread, 1 oz.	30	—

The trouble is, the most common sources of calcium—whole milk and hard cheese—are very high in fat.

Skim milk is just as nutritious as whole milk, and has a fraction of the fat. If you switch from drinking two glasses of whole milk a day to two glasses of skim milk, you'll save yourself 18 grams of fat. You can drink up to two glasses of skim milk a day, or the equivalent amount of low-fat yogurt or cottage cheese. Eat low-fat cheese products in moderation.

It's advisable to eat as little hard cheese as possible on this program, and only low-fat varieties.

Many people, particularly African-Americans and those

Christine Timmons: Too Busy to Diet

CHRISTINE IS A SUCCESSFUL BUSINESSWOMAN. Her work takes her into the highest social circles, not only in her native New York, but all over the world. Unfortunately, it also takes her into the world's best restaurants, and keeps her so busy that exercise during the day is out of the question. Nonetheless, once she noticed that she was 20 pounds overweight, she began to fear that the "price" of those excess pounds could be her next big promotion.

Her "diet" of choice was 600-calorie-a-day starvation, even though constant hunger cravings made her late-night business dealings a real challenge. Usually she'd lose five pounds the first week and two pounds the second week, but after that, the pounds would start creeping back again.

She'd wait a month or two, then try again. Each time a new diet came out, she was the first on the bandwagon, all to no avail.

Then she decided to do one thing and one thing only: cut out fat, whenever possible. She started by eliminating the butter on her toast in the morning and on her sandwiches at lunch, as well as cake for desserts. That one change alone enabled Christine to lose four pounds within a month.

Then she got even more serious. Instead of steak dinners, she started ordering broiled fish. She began to enjoy the taste of foods without sauces over them, and made it a point of ordering salad, with diet dressing, for at least one meal daily.

Another six pounds dropped off within a month, and Christine realized that most days she could probably add in a morning walk, if she set her alarm to ring a half-hour earlier.

Two months later, Christine fits into her best dress-for-success wardrobe. And she hasn't been hungry since!

from Mediterranean areas, are not able to drink milk at all because they are "lactose-intolerant." Their systems cannot handle the natural sugar in milk. Lactose-intolerant people can get the calcium they need by using an over-the-counter product that neutralizes the lactose in milk.

Fortunately, dairy products require no preparation: for a thirst-quenching, energizing snack, just grab a glass and pour out milk, spoon yogurt into a bowl, or nibble on a slice of low-fat cheese.

Here are a few tips to help you incorporate low-fat dairy products into your diet:

➢ Make drinks or soups using skim milk.

➢ Add a dollop of low-fat yogurt to cold soups.

➢ Replace oil or mayonnaise with low-fat yogurt in a dip for fruits and vegetables, or as a base for salad dressings.

➢ Combine low-fat grated cheeses with wheat germ or whole-wheat bread crumbs as toppings for casseroles.

➢ Spread your morning toast with fat-free cream cheese instead of butter.

Understanding Food Labels

When you buy packaged food, read the label to look for fat and fiber content. The new nutrition labels that began appearing in 1994 (see sample label) show the number of calories per serving. You'll also learn how much fat, cholesterol, sodium, carbohydrates, and protein the food contains, by weight and percentage.

The new labels not only indicate the total calories in food, but the amount of calories from fat. They also list the grams of fat per serving and provide a Daily Value (% Daily Value) for that fat. This is the percentage of daily fat intake each serving contains. Always choose the product that has the lowest possible % Daily Value (DV) of fat.

But don't let a low DV figure fool you; it's only the amount considered "healthy" if you're on a 2,000-calorie-a-day diet and eating 65 grams of fat per day. As the label itself indicates, your daily values may be higher or lower, depending on your calorie needs. Sixty-five grams of fat per day on a 2,000-calorie diet means you'll eat 30 percent fat from calories, the very upper limit we recommend for weight loss.

Remember too, that if you eat twice as much as the suggested serving size, you're also eating twice of everything in that food, including the fat.

On this program, the food should be no more than 20 to 30 percent fat, preferably closer to 20 percent. To ensure this is the case, perform the following calculation based on label information:

A. Calories from fat: ______
B. Total calories: ______
C. To determine the percentage of food composed of fat, divide the total calories from fat (A) by the total calories (B), then multiply by 100: ______

THE NEW FOOD LABEL AT A GLANCE

Nutrition Facts

Serving Size 1 cup (228g)
Servings Per Container 2

Amount Per Serving

Calories 260 Calories from Fat 120

	% Daily Value*
Total Fat 13g	**20%**
Saturated Fat 5g	**25%**
Cholesterol 30mg	**10%**
Sodium 660mg	**28%**
Total Carbohydrate 31g	**10%**
Dietary Fiber 0g	**0%**
Sugars 5g	
Protein 5g	

Vitamin A 4%	•	Vitamin C 2%
Calcium 15%	•	Iron 4%

* Percent Daily Values are based on a 2,000 calorie diet. Your daily values may be higher or lower depending on your calorie needs:

	Calories:	2,000	2,500
Total Fat	Less than	65g	80g
Sat Fat	Less than	20g	25g
Cholesterol	Less than	300mg	300mg
Sodium	Less than	2,400mg	2,400mg
Total Carbohydrate		300g	375g
Dietary Fiber		25g	30g

Calories per gram:
Fat 9 • Carbohydrate 4 • Protein 4

Source: Food and Drug Administration, 1994

Here's an example, based on information from the food label on page 52.

A. Calories from fat: 120
B. Total calories: 260
C. Percentage of food composed of fat:
(120 ÷ 260) x 100 = 46%

The label also shows the ingredients in the food, listed in order of their proportion by weight. A product that lists apples before sugar contains more apples by weight than sugar.

Look for the total fat content on the label. It will tell you how many grams there are of polyunsaturates, monounsaturates, saturates, cholesterol, and trans fatty acids. Because you want to restrict your purchases to products with little or no fats in them, look for—and avoid—foods that contain items such as oil, shortening, butter, chocolate or milk chocolate, cocoa butter, cream, egg and egg-yolk solids, glycerolesters, lard, mono- or diglycerides, suet, or whole milk solids.

To avoid unnecessary sugars in your diet, look for—and avoid—foods that contain the following, especially if one appears first, or if several are listed:

Corn syrup	Gluco-fructose	Maple syrup
Dextrose	Glucose	Molasses
Fructose	Honey	Sucrose
Fruit juice concentrate	Lactose	Sugar
	Maltose	Syrup

The art of label reading

New USDA food label regulations have standardized the application of certain terms used by food manufacturers on products. Here's what those terms mean to you:

If it says **fat-free, without fat, no fat,** or **zero fat,** the food has fewer than 0.5 grams of fat per serving.

If it says **calorie-free, without calories, no calories,** or **zero calories,** the food has fewer than 5 calories per serving.

In general, **low** means the same as **little, few,** and **low source of. Low-fat** means 3 grams of fat (or less) per serving. **Low calorie** means 40 calories or less per serving. **Low cholesterol** means 20 milligrams or less, and 2 grams or less of saturated fat per serving. **Low saturated fat** means 1 gram or less per serving.

Lean means fewer than 10 grams of fat, 4 grams of saturated fat, and 95 milligrams of cholesterol per serving and per 100 grams. If the serving size is relatively small, these foods may still contain a relatively high percentage of fat calories per serving.

Extra-lean means fewer than 10 grams of fat, 2 grams of saturated fat, and 95 milligrams of cholesterol per serving and per 100 grams.

Less or **fewer** means the food contains 25 percent less of a nutrient or of calories than a comparative product. The label may say, for example, that pretzels have 25 percent less fat than potato chips.

Reduced means the product contains at least 25 percent less of a nutrient or of calories than the regular product. This claim can't be made if the regular food already meets the requirement for being **low** in fat, calories, or cholesterol.

Percent fat-free should provide an accurate description of the amount of fat present in a low-fat or fat-free product. If a food contains 5 grams of fat per 100 grams, for instance, the label would say 95 percent fat-free.

Don't be fooled by labels such as **light** or **lite.** These words may refer to color, texture, flavor, alcohol content, sodium content, or fat content. **Light** soy sauce, for instance, could be low in sodium. **Light** olive oil could be light in color; it's still 100 percent fat. If the label **light** or **lite** does refer to fat content, this means the food has one-third fewer calories, or no more than half the fat, of the higher-calorie, higher-fat version.

Likewise, the label **cholesterol-free** can be deceptive. It means the food has no more than 2 milligrams of dietary cholesterol and 2 grams (or less) of saturated fat per serving. The product could still contain unsaturated or some saturated fats. Vegetable oils, for instance, are cholesterol-free, but they are almost entirely unsaturated fat.

Even a label like **95% fat-free** could be deceptive, because it may refer to the percentage fat-free by weight, not the percentage fat-free by calories. Turkey ham, for instance, which is advertised as "95% fat-free," still provides more than half its calories from fat.

Dairy products must contain between 0.5 and 2 percent milk fat to be labelled **low-fat. Low-fat** meat can be no more than 10 percent fat by weight.

The truth about health claims

New food labels can carry claims about the relationship between nutrients and diseases. However, they can only suggest the relationship by using words such as "may" or "might." They also imply that other factors can play a role in causing disease.

Here's a guide to health claims you may find on labels:

Osteoporosis prevention and calcium intake. The label can point out that people who need calcium most for prevention of osteoporosis include teens and young adult white and Asian women. Calcium-rich foods that claim to prevent or delay the onset of osteoporosis must contain 20 percent or more of the Daily Value for calcium, have a calcium content equal to or greater than its phosphorous content, and contain a form of calcium our bodies can easily absorb and use. If the food has 40 percent or more of the Daily Value for calcium, the label must further state that a total dietary intake greater than 200 percent of the Daily Value has no further known benefit.

Cancer prevention and fat intake. Only **low-fat** foods or **extra-lean** fish and game meats may make this claim.

Cancer prevention and eating fiber-containing grain products, fruits, and vegetables. Food must be or must contain a grain product, fruit, or vegetable, be a good source of dietary fiber (without fortification), and be **low-fat.**

Cancer prevention and eating fruits and vegetables. The fruits must be **low-fat** and a **good source** (without fortification) of dietary fiber and/or vitamins A or C.

Coronary heart disease prevention and eating foods low in saturated fat and cholesterol intake. These foods also meet the criteria for **low saturated fat, low cholesterol, low fat,** or, if fish and game meats, **extra lean.**

Jeffrey Binley: Milk Shake Man

IN HIS YOUNGER DAYS, when Jeff was into weightlifting, football, and other energetic pursuits, he quaffed a quart of milk a day. He thought he needed that much milk to keep his bones strong.

By the time he entered his forties, Jeff's athletic career was long behind him, but not his fondness for dairy products. He still downed that same quart of milk daily, but also enjoyed milk shakes, sour cream, and lots of cheese. He was 30 pounds overweight when he had his first heart attack.

His doctor prescribed a daily walk and a low-fat diet as part of his recovery process. He explained to Jeff that all the dairy products he was consuming were high in saturated fat—the worst possible kind of fat for people with heart conditions. Jeff learned that a low-fat diet can make fatty deposits in coronary arteries start to shrink, especially if the sufferer also quits smoking, exercises sensibly, and keeps stress under control.

His doctor also pointed out that being overweight was exactly the kind of strain Jeff's body didn't need: his heart had to pump blood through all the extra arteries his body had grown to feed his fat deposits.

Jeff decided to replace the whole milk he'd been drinking with skim milk. He started whirling low-fat yogurt and fruit in the blender to replace the milk shakes of old. He discovered that thickened low-fat yogurt was practically indistinguishable from sour cream on top of baked potatoes and in chicken stroganoff dishes. And he learned to love beans, instead of cheese, on toast.

Because his work was so high-stress, Jeff also decided to take up yoga on his lunch hours. The stretching and relaxing poses helped keep him calm and collected, and away from double martinis.

Today he's trim, energetic, and—best of all—healthy.

Coronary heart disease prevention and eating fiber-containing grain products, fruits, and vegetables. Aside from containing grain products, fruits, and vegetables, the food has to meet the criteria for **low saturated fat, low cholesterol,** and **low fat,** and contain (without fortification) at least 0.6 grams of soluble fiber per serving.

Hypertension (high blood pressure) control and eating a low-sodium diet. The food must be **low sodium.**

Active Benefits: Get a Move On!

There's one simple fact that you need to know about exercise. **Regular activity keeps your basal metabolic rate high enough to burn off body fat.** Even hours after activity, your basal metabolic rate remains raised.

As you have learned, the diets you might have followed in the past encouraged your body to call on its "hunger troops" to maintain the *status quo,* thinking it is "fighting for survival." As the hunger continued and your body thought it was starving, it decreased its metabolic rate in order to conserve energy. That's where exercise comes in: it increases your metabolic rate to keep those pounds rolling off.

Exercise also encourages your body to burn fat stores instead of carbohydrate stores or muscle. Studies have shown that weight loss from dieting alone leads to a loss of about 75 percent fat and 25 percent muscle. When physical activity is added, muscle loss can be reduced to 5 percent.

And, of course, exercise burns off calories. If you perform 500 calories of exercise a week, you'll lose 4 to 5 pounds within a year even on your present diet—weight you wouldn't have lost without that activity. The more active you are, the more calories you can consume and still lose or maintain your weight.

Furthermore, physical activity changes your body composition by building muscle and reducing fat. It's in your interest to keep your muscle mass up and the amount of fat in your body down. Muscle requires more energy to sustain itself than fat stores. So the more muscle you have in your body, the easier it is to stay slim. An increase in your musculature increases your daily caloric burn-off, even when you're not exercising, because muscle requires more energy to maintain than fat.

As you get older, some of your muscle will be replaced by fat, a natural part of the aging process. This means it's even more important to keep active in order to prevent or slow down the replacement of muscle by fat. Muscle weighs more than fat and occupies less space.

Furthermore, exercise keeps food moving along quickly through your digestive tract, which means foods that might otherwise add calories to your body may not be fully absorbed.

Not insignificantly, exercise also makes you feel more energetic and good about yourself and your eating program. You'll sleep better, cope with stress better, deal with the ups and downs of life more calmly. This vitality can only help you in the long run.

What type of exercise is best for weight loss? Believe it or not, you don't have to "go for the burn" to maximize fat-burning potential. In fact, if you work too hard at your workout, your body could stop drawing on your fat stores for food and start depending on your carbohydrate supplies.

That's why an activity like walking is the absolutely best

form of exercise. The idea is to decrease the intensity of a workout and increase the amount of time you spend at moderate activity. In the next chapter, you'll learn about specific activities that can keep weight rolling off.

What About My "Bad Genes"?

Most overweight people blame their problem on bad genes or bad eating habits when they were growing up. They've got a point.

If one of your parents is overweight, the likelihood of your being overweight is 40 to 50 percent. If both your parents are overweight, the likelihood jumps to 70 to 80 percent. It's hard to determine whether this happens because of heredity or the family environment. The chances of being overweight when you come from a family that had a weekend ritual of going for walks is certainly lower than in one whose favored activity is eating out.

Dr. Albert Sunkard, obesity specialist at the University of Pennsylvania, studied hundreds of adopted people in Denmark. He discovered there was no relationship between how overweight adoptees were, compared to their adoptive parents. But there was considerable correlation between overweight and natural parents. In other words, children of heavy parents who were adopted by thin folks still tended to end up overweight. Here is more confirmation that heredity strongly influences your adult body shape.

Nonetheless, **no matter what your gene pool, no matter how you were brought up, you can still lose weight!**

Although your genes—or your childhood home environ-

EXERCISE AND CALORIE EXPENDITURE

Activity	Calories expended per hour[1]	
	Man[2]	Woman[2]
Sitting quietly	100	80
Standing quietly	120	95
Light activity:	300	240
Cleaning house		
Office work		
Playing baseball		
Playing golf		
Moderate activity:	460	370
Walking briskly (3.5 mph)		
Gardening		
Cycling (5.5 mph)		
Dancing		
Playing basketball		
Strenuous activity:	730	580
Jogging (9 min./mile)		
Playing football		
Swimming		
Very strenuous activity:	920	740
Running (7 min./mile)		
Racquetball		
Skiing		

[1]May vary depending on environmental conditions. [2]Healthy man, 175 lbs; healthy woman, 140 lbs. Source: McArdle, et al., Exercise Physiology, 1986.

ment—may determine your basal metabolic rate and how much fat you carry and where, this program will help you develop a healthy attitude towards food and will certainly help you lose weight if you have a genetic predisposition to amass body fat. This program is an effective combatant to heredity. It will work for anyone.

Furthermore, if you believe a hormonal problem accounts for your figure size, or that your metabolism is the problem, you should have a doctor examine you. But almost certainly, you'll find out this program will take off those pounds.

Once you get used to the taste of fresh foods prepared without fatty sauces—and once you start making food selections from our list of 30 fat-burning foods—you'll quickly get rid of your taste for grease.

Best of all, if you raise your children in an environment where they eat lots of vegetables and little meat, and drink 1 percent milk instead of whole milk, there's a good chance they can remain slender when they get older, despite their genetic heritage.

That's My Cue!

There are two different kinds of "cues," or appetite stimulators, that eaters respond to: internal or external.

Internally cued eaters are people who eat when their bodies need food. They eat in response to "hunger" signals the body sends, such as a grumbling tummy.

Unfortunately, many overweight people are *externally cued eaters,* or ECEs (pronounced "Eeks," as in "Eeks! I want to eat!"). ECEs tend to eat in response to cues from the world around them. Their situation, rather than their body's needs, frequently "tells" ECEs to consume food, whether or not they're hungry. Externally cued eaters will have lunch at the stroke of noon, for example, instead of waiting until they're hungry. They'll eat "because it's there," or in response to a hundred other distractions, such as depression, social anxiety at a party, even the presence of other people.

A study at Georgia State University, for instance, found that when six or more people ate together in a group, their food intake soared by 76 percent! Even when two people ate together, their food intake was 28 percent greater than when they ate alone. (Not surprisingly, this effect is particularly noticeable at dessert time.)

If you're an externally cued eater, you can try alternative activities to overeating. Many of these are provided for you in the next chapter.

There's no point in starting a diet if you don't feel good about yourself. Although you'll probably like yourself better once you've lost weight, you need self-esteem to help you stick to any self-improvement program. At first, you may need lots of support from friends, or even professional help, in order to stick to this program. If you're a compulsive eater, Overeaters Anonymous has helped thousands of participants break their food addictions. There's probably a chapter near you!

The fact is, psychological disturbances are more likely to be caused by being overweight than by compulsive overeating. You'll find yourself more emotionally healthy after you've lost weight.

Fat-Burning Basics

You've now learned the ten basic rules of this amazing new weight-loss program:

- Eat as much as you want of the 30 amazing fat-burning foods.
- Enjoy just about as much complex carbohydrate foods as you need in order to feel full. These foods must provide at least 65 percent of your daily calories.
- Aim to eat at least 30 to 40 grams of fiber every day. To keep your fiber level up, read the label of packaged foods, and always buy the higher-fiber product (it's also usually the lower-fat item).
- Consume 20 to 30 percent of your total daily calories as fat. To keep life simple, avoid fat whenever possible. For health reasons, you should keep your intake of saturated fats (the "solid" type found in animal fat, butters, cheeses, "hydrogenated" margarine, and tropical vegetable oils) at or below 10 percent of your daily calorie intake.
- Eat a maximum of 10 to 15 percent of your daily calories in animal protein.
- Stick to fewer than 5 ounces of animal protein daily, and no more than two dinners of lean red meat weekly.

- Eat at least one vegetarian dinner a week, preferably two.

- Eat as little hard cheese as possible, and low-fat varieties in moderation.

- Drink up to two glasses of skim milk a day, or the equivalent amount of low-fat yogurt or cottage cheese.

- Enjoy regular activity, which will keep your metabolism high enough to burn off body fat.

CHAPTER 2

STEP-BY-STEP TO A SLIMMER YOU

YOU'VE NOW LEARNED EVERYTHING you need to successfully lose weight. On a day-to-day basis, however, temptation in the form of your old habits is your biggest obstacle to permanent weight loss.

Here are some suggestions that will *guarantee* diet success!

1. Slow and steady wins the diet race. As you've already learned, losing too much weight too quickly is a sign that you're starving yourself. Such dieting makes your body hang on to every bit of body fat it can. A 1- or 2-pounds-a-week loss will ensure that you lose weight, keep it off, and stay healthy.

2. Weigh yourself once a week—or less. Your weight will fluctuate on a daily basis, and this may discourage you when, in fact, you're losing weight on a weekly or monthly basis.

3. Take the program one day at a time, but make a long-term commitment to successfully lose your excess weight. You'll enjoy this program and feel proud of your decision to become a new, healthy you. **You can do it!**

4. Do it for yourself—not to make your husband or wife happy, get a new job, or impress your former classmates at your high school reunion.

5. Variety is important. Remember the grapefruit-only diet? No one can live like that for long—and you deserve better. The fat-burning foods on this plan will provide you with hundreds of exciting meal combinations.

6. If the support of others trying to lose weight will help you, join a group like Overeaters Anonymous, or form your own group.

7. Be kind to yourself. The night you go on a chocolate cake binge is not the end of the world. It's also not the end of this program. The very next day, pick yourself up again and renew your commitment.

8. Experiment to discover the meal pattern that works for you. If you're sure of your pattern, eat a good breakfast. Then, eat just enough to satisfy your appetite for the other two meals of the day, keeping track of your food intake. Monitor your resulting hunger. If you find dinner is your hungry time, plan to eat a little extra at lunch and an afternoon snack. You may discover that you're hungry in the morning, but satisfied with a snack for dinner. Alternatively, you may find that you wake up with no appetite at all, but crave food before bedtime.

Replace Old Habits With Fat-Burning Activities

Because new habits extend well beyond the dinner table, it's often helpful to observe which situations trigger your bad overeating ways, and then substitute other behaviors.

Consider keeping a food diary for a week or two. Record every bit of food you eat, the amount, the time of day, the place, who you were with at the time, what you were doing, how you were feeling, and what might have made you eat (aside from hunger).

You'll learn a lot about your own special "triggers" for overeating. You may discover that cookie binges almost always follow a fight with your children. Or that you never eat when you're alone. Or that you tend to gulp down leftovers, rather than toss them into the garbage.

Make a point of discovering one of your "triggers" and working on *only* that problem. After a month, see if you can discover another trigger, and tackle that one. (If you try to change everything at once, you may get discouraged and give up.) By taking on one trigger a month, you'll have changed your eating habits for the better within a year!

To get you started, here are just a few "alternative behavior" suggestions for overeating:

- Force yourself to eat regular meals and then, when the urge to snack hits, go for a walk, play tennis, or write an angry entry in your diary. Do anything but eat to handle your stress (as long as it's legal and doesn't hurt anyone). "Train" yourself to eat from hunger, not from other factors.

- Instead of snacking while you watch TV, start crocheting, basketweaving, sketching, doodling, or embroidering—any activity that'll keep your hands busy.

- Walk the dog after dinner, instead of reading that novel accompanied by a bag of potato chips.

- ➢ Put leftovers away immediately after mealtime. You don't need them tempting you when you're not hungry. Forget about "clean plate" clubs and starving children in other countries.

- ➢ Alternatively, feed leftovers to the dog or actually throw them out. That makes a lot more sense than using yourself as a human garbage can, doesn't it?

- ➢ If you can't resist eating leftovers "just to get rid of them," talk your spouse or children into clearing the table.

- ➢ Treat yourself to flowers, a novel, a new dress, or tickets to a baseball game instead of a box of cookies.

- ➢ Figure out ways that do not involve food to show your children and spouse that you love them. Your children would probably enjoy a game of Frisbee with you more than your home-baked cookies.

- ➢ Prepare your low-fat snacks ahead of time, so you don't find yourself getting hungry with no fat-burning foods to eat in the house.

- ➢ Ask your kids to make their own snacks, or make them yourself at mealtime and package them for later snacking.

- ➢ Stay clear of the cafeteria or junk machines at work if they offer nothing healthy to eat. Bring your own lunch to work, or find a restaurant that serves fat-burning foods.

- If your kids like to eat high-fat cookies, make sure you buy them varieties you don't like.

- Change the route of your daily walk if it takes you past an inviting bakery or restaurant.

Healthy Mealtime Tricks to Stave Off Temptation

You've spent a long time developing the poor eating habits that made you overweight. Be patient with yourself as you develop healthy new eating habits at mealtime; soon you'll lose your taste for unhealthy foods. But in the meantime . . .

DO

- Eat enough to satisfy yourself, and then stop.

- Put less food than you're used to on your fork or spoon, chew it thoroughly, and put your fork down between bites. It takes at least 20 minutes for your brain to tell your stomach it's full, so eat slowly.

- Serve your food on a smaller plate than you're accustomed to. You may find the smaller portions will fill you up.

- Set your table properly, and eat only at the kitchen table. Don't watch TV or read, even if you eat alone. This will reduce the number of locations you associate with eating.

- Concentrate on your meal. Inhale it (with your nose!), enjoy the look of it, feel its texture in your mouth, eat it slowly.

- Serve from the stove or countertop, not from a serving platter loaded with food you don't need.

- Take only one helping, and leave the table as soon as your hunger is satisfied.

DON'T

- Skip meals. Overweight people typically skip breakfast, eat a modest lunch and a generous dinner, and then snack all night long. Always start your day with breakfast, and eat according to your body's natural hunger patterns throughout the day.

- Eat when you're not hungry.

- Eat foods you really don't want to eat out of politeness or obligation.

- Eat because you're bored, upset, depressed, anxious, or otherwise emotional.

- Eat because you're afraid you might be hungry later.

- Put more on your plate than you want to eat at that meal.

Diet-Proofing Your Home

One way to ensure you will not return to your unhealthy eating habits is to get rid of those "fat-making" foods. Toss out food that's not good for you! Then, replace the food that's bad for your waistline with substitutes.

➢ Toss out your stash of chocolates, hard candies, packaged fruit snacks, cookies, cakes, danishes, even granola bars. Ditto for regular mayonnaise, sour cream, regular salad dressings, and guacamole.

➢ Although you can enjoy limited quantities of dairy products, discard your whole milk, dairy creamer, whipped cream, regular cheese, and regular yogurt.

➢ Processed meats are a no-no. That includes bacon, bologna, corned beef, hot dogs, liverwurst, pastrami, pepperoni, salami, and sausage.

➢ Say goodbye forever to regular ground beef, chicken wings and backs, high-fat cuts of beef or pork, creamy soups, gravies made with drippings, pastry, cake or ice cream, chips, and cheese puffs.

➢ Say hello to all the fat-burning alternatives that are just as tasty, just as filling, and are guaranteed to make you lose weight.

If other people in your life (like your slender spouse or your teenager) must keep food in the house that's not good for you, rearrange your fridge and cupboard to keep them out of sight. You can also store tempting foods in containers you can't see through.

Shopping for Success

The main thing you'll want to do, of course, is to stock up on the 30 fabulous fat-burning foods that will enable you to lose weight. You'll want lots of these foods around the house so you can grab a snack or create a filling meal without having to fight temptation.

Buy a variety of fruits and vegetables and eat them raw as often as possible. If you're short on time, buy cleaned and chopped vegetables from your supermarket's salad bar. You'll spend a little more, but you'll cut down on time-consuming food preparation.

As for meeting protein requirements, try these tips:

- Buy enough fish or white meat of poultry to make them your protein source. After all, aside from one or two meals a week, you will be replacing red meat with the white meat of chicken or turkey, fish, or vegetable proteins.

- Buy more modest portions of meat than you used to. You don't need more than 5 ounces of animal protein a day.

- Buy the leanest cuts of meat available. Cuts from a young animal, such as veal, or from the parts of an animal that are more muscular, such as round or foreshank, are leaner than cuts from the loin area and breast.

➢ Ask your butcher to grind sirloin, or buy ground turkey or chicken breast instead.

➢ Choose ground chicken or turkey over higher-fat ground beef, veal, or pork, but only if the meat has been ground without the skin. The label should specifically say "breast meat."

➢ Choose chicken over pork. A cut of trimmed pork has one-third more fat than skinless chicken and twice as much fat as skinless turkey.

➢ Plan to replace animal proteins with vegetable proteins for at least one meal a week—preferably two. Foods such as tofu, soybeans, lentils, chickpeas, and beans are low in fat, less expensive than meat, yet just as tasty, and rich in fiber and nutrients.

Poultry picks

In general, choose turkey over chicken, and white meat over dark meat. Remove the skin, which is all fat, before you indulge.

What's the matter with chicken? It has one-and-a-half times more fat than turkey! Similarly, breast meat is considerably lower in fat than dark meat. Chicken breast (without skin) has approximately 23 percent of its calories from fat, while dark meat (without skin) has about 43 percent of its calories from fat. Chicken thigh, in contrast, is as high in fat as many red meats. In fact, 47 percent of its calories come from fat, which makes it fattier than grade round steak, sirloin, or chuck arm pot roast. It also has nearly as much fat content as pork tenderloin, top loin, or the rump of a ham leg—assuming you trim every bit of fat off the red meats. As for chicken wings, they're 36 percent fat, even when roasted; the figure jumps to 39 percent fat when fried.

FATS AND CHOLESTEROL IN COOKED POULTRY

Type	Percent of fat by weight	Percent of calories from fat
Turkey, light meat (roasted)		
without skin	3	19
with skin	8	38
Turkey, dark meat (roasted)		
without skin	7	35
with skin	12	47
Chicken, light meat (roasted)		
without skin	5	23
with skin	11	44
Chicken, dark meat (roasted)		
without skin	10	43
with skin	16	56

Source: U.S. Department of Agriculture Handbook No. 8-5

Not all turkeys, however, are created equal. Avoid self-basting or deep-basted turkey. As you'll see from the label, it has been injected with butter, oil, or turkey broth. Likewise, prestuffed birds are a no-no; the stuffing is generally high-fat.

The best of beef

Even after you trim all visible fat, beef is still relatively high in fat compared to your fat-burning foods. You may eat up to 5 ounces (6 ounces raw) of the following cuts once or twice a week. (That's a piece of meat about the size of your hand.)

Choose From the Leanest Cuts of Beef (Choice Grade)

Top round (29% fat)
Eye of round steak (30% fat)
Round tip (sirloin tip, tip steak, or tip roast) (36% fat)
Top sirloin steak (36% fat)
Top loin (New York steak, strip steak) (40% fat)
Tenderloin (filet mignon, chateaubriand) (38% fat)

Avoid the Fattiest Cuts of Beef

Chuck blade roast (72% fat)
Flank steak (51% fat if lean; up to 58% if lean and fat)
Ribs (75% fat)
Brisket (48% if whole and lean; 75% if lean and fat-braised)
Porterhouse steak (44 to 64% fat)
T-bone (68% fat)
Tongue (66% if simmered; 98% if medium-fat and braised)

At the supermarket, choose meat with the least amount of "marbling." The higher the concentration of marbling, the more fat it contains.

Be careful when purchasing ground meat. Regular ground beef can be 30 percent calories from fat. Switch to lean ground meat and the percentage drops to 17 percent calories from fat.

Pork possibilities

Pork has received bad press at times, but it can be as low in fat as chicken if you select carefully, trim visible fat, and avoid frying it.

Choose From the Leanest Cuts of Pork

Center loin pork chops (26% fat)
Center loin pork roast (26% fat)
Tenderloin (26% fat)

Avoid the Fattiest Cuts of Pork

Loin blade steaks (50% fat)
Ribs (54% fat)
Top loin (36% fat)
Shoulder blade steaks (51% fat)
Bacon (40 to 90% fat)

Lean on lamb

When selecting and preparing lamb, look out for marbling, trim the fat, and avoid frying. Ribs and chops are especially

Shopping Tips

TRY THESE GROCERY SHOPPING suggestions to help you lose weight and win.

- Make a rough menu for the week and shop from that list, checking for the foods you need that are not already on hand.
- Divide your shopping list into the same areas as the grocery store departments.
- Shop alone so you can get in and out of the store quickly.
- Do your grocery shopping after mealtime, not before. Never shop on an empty stomach.
- Shop strictly from your shopping list, and never buy anything that is not on your list.
- Read all labels on the foods you buy to determine if they have any hidden sugars. Sugars include corn syrup, dextrose, fructose, gluco-fructose, glucose, honey, maple syrup, molasses, maltose, and sucrose.
- Also read all labels to ensure that you are avoiding hidden fats. Fat information on the label will include grams of total fat per serving, as well as the amount that is saturated fat and cholesterol. The list of fats in the ingredients include any oil or shortening, butter, chocolate or milk chocolate, cocoa butter, cream, egg and egg-yolk solids, glycerolesters, lard, mono- or diglycerides, suet, and whole milk solids.
- Whenever possible (for example, with foods such as cereal and bread), buy the higher-fiber product; it's listed on the label as "dietary fiber."

high in fat. You should also avoid lamb breast. Your best bets are shanks (44 percent fat) and the sirloin portion of the leg (39 percent fat).

Focus on fish

In general, fish is a good low-fat alternative to red meat and even poultry. Shellfish, however, are high in dietary cholesterol, which may be bad for your heart. Avoid marinated fish or those canned in oil.

Healthy Hardware

Aside from the new foods you'll be eating, it's wise to stock up on the basic equipment you'll need in order to prepare these foods. You'll need nonstick frying pans, cookie sheets, loaf pans, casserole dishes, and baking dishes. Plastic utensils and a plastic scrubber are necessary in order to prevent scratching.

A good blender, food processor, or food-chopper is a time-saver when making delicious dressings and chopping up vegetables and fruit.

If your budget permits, a microwave oven is not only a time-saver, but will enable you to create low-fat meals in minutes.

Substitute, Don't Sacrifice

If you really crave the taste of fat in your food, there's no reason why you can't use one of the FDA-approved fat substitutes now available on the market. They have no nutritional value, of

SHOPPING ALTERNATIVES

Instead of	Buy
Whole milk, dairy creamer	Skim milk
Regular cheese	Low-fat cheese
Regular yogurt	Low-fat yogurt
Pork, beef, ham, or cold cuts	Turkey, chicken, fish
Processed meats (such as bacon, bologna, corned beef, hot dogs, salami, sausage)	Sliced chicken, turkey, low-fat meat substitute
Ground beef	Ground trimmed cuts of beef
Your usual cuts of beef and pork	Top round steak, sirloin steak, eye of round, pork tenderloin
Your usual cuts of pork, bacon	Pork tenderloin
Creamy soups, gravies made with drippings	Clear soups and broths
Pastry, cake, or ice cream	Fruit
Eggs	Egg whites or low-fat egg substitutes
Chips, cheese puffs	Air-popped popcorn, low-fat pretzels
Chicken wings and backs	Turkey breast, chicken breast

course, but they're not bad for you.

Olestra, an experimental fat substitute, tastes, feels, and acts like fat. Your body doesn't have enzymes to break it down, so you can eat as much of this substitute as you want and it will be eliminated. According to one study, replacing fat with Olestra not only makes people's fat intake go down, but also makes their carbohydrate intake go up. *Simplesse* is also harmless, but you can't cook with it and it's only available in a few products.

As you learned in the last chapter, you can enjoy the occasional treat like sugary candy, which is made of refined and/or processed sugars, and not worry about gaining weight. The trouble is, such treats not only damage your teeth, they have no nutritional value. Sugar alone makes your blood glucose level go up very fast and drop just as quickly, leaving you as hungry as before. Furthermore, dietary sugar is usually accompanied by plenty of fat. You must avoid high-fat sugary treats, such as cakes, pies, and chocolate bars.

Substitute diet soft drinks for sugary ones, and use NutraSweet or other sugar substitutes when possible. Artificial sweeteners, such as NutraSweet and saccharine, won't harm you unless you suffer from phenylketonuria, a relatively rare disease.

Kill Those Caffeine Cravings!

Strictly speaking, caffeine is not a food, but a chemical found in coffee, tea, chocolate, soda, and many drugs. It acts as a stimulant, increasing alertness and raising blood pressure. In excess amounts, caffeine may cause heartburn or indigestion, increase the rate of calcium loss from bone (a serious side effect if you're suffering from osteoporosis), and put you at risk for cardiovascular disease. Caffeine can also cause premature or irregular heartbeats. You should avoid caffeine if you have any heart problems, especially heart rhythm irregularities.

If you have no such health problems, there's no reason to avoid coffee, tea, and other drinks that have moderate amounts of caffeine in them. Caffeine has no calories. It may even start a complex hormonal reaction that accelerates your body's release of fat from its fat stores. But caffeine would be unlikely to help you lose weight because the fat would still be in your body.

Thirst-Quenching News

Drinking water can be good for your waistline! Drinking up to eight 8-ounce glasses daily helps to flush out your system and keeps tummy-rumbling at bay.

Also consider fruit juice, vegetable juice, plain mineral water, or mineral water or soda pop made with artificial sweeteners. You're also allowed up to two cups of skim milk on this program. Exercise restraint with soda pop or alcohol, which have no nutritional value. Soda pop is loaded with sugar, and alcohol is a relatively high-calorie, nutrition-free snack. It has 7 calories per gram, fewer than in fat but more than in carbohydrates and protein.

In fact, drinking alcohol works against losing weight, because spirits tend to enhance your appetite. Alcohol also dehydrates your body, which means that it's unwise to use it as a thirst-quencher during hot weather. Instead, replenish your body fluid with water, fruit or vegetable juice, or milk.

The USDA recommends that women limit themselves to a

maximum of one drink per day of alcohol (pregnant women should avoid alcohol). Men may have two drinks per day. This assumes "one drink" is a 12-ounce bottle of beer, 5 ounces of wine, or $1^1/_2$ ounces of hard liquor. Beer labeled "light" contains fewer calories than the same brand of regular beer.

Organic Food: Is it Really Safer?

Organic fruits and vegetables, which are considerably more expensive than non-organic produce, have been grown from soil that has not been treated with pesticides or chemicals for at least three years. But there's nothing to stop the farmer in the field next door to an organic farm from using pesticides on his or her crops. In fact, there's no official regulatory process to protect consumers of organic products and no standard definition of "organic."

There are no additives, preservatives, or coloring in fresh American meat. Low levels of antibiotics are sometimes given to livestock to control or prevent disease, but the antibiotics are stopped for a period before slaughter.

There's no such thing as hormone-free meat. Like humans, animals naturally produce hormones, and they're given to some livestock in order to promote growth and to reduce the fat content of the meat.

Additives, preservatives, and coloring found in packaged or canned foods have been stringently tested for safety by the FDA. Though you should use fresh food as often as possible, don't hesitate to use packaged foods to add convenience to your nutritional intake. After all, if the only way you're going to eat a salad is with salad dressing and you don't have time to make your own, it's time to consider using bottled low-cal dressing. It'll make the salad taste better and you'll get the nutritional benefits of the fresh vegetables.

Save on Supplements

Can vitamin and mineral supplements help you to lose weight? There's a simple answer: no. If you follow our guidelines for weight loss, you're going to get all the vitamins and minerals you need from fat-burning foods and other sources. You don't need vitamin pills unless your doctor prescribes them to treat a specific condition.

There are two types of vitamins: fat-soluble (vitamins A, D, E, and K) and water-soluble (all others). Almost all foods contain some of the vitamins and minerals your body needs, so if you enjoy a variety of foods on this program, you should be getting all the nutrients you need. In fact, since your body can use vitamins and minerals only in small amounts, you excrete all the extra water-soluble ones in your urine. Excess fat-soluble vitamins are stored in your fat, may never be needed, and can become toxic if you take too many.

If you must take multivitamin supplements, take ones that contain iron and as broad a range of vitamins as possible, including all the B vitamins, in amounts not exceeding federally suggested limits.

Don't think that because a little is good, a lot would be better. When you get vitamins from your food, you get them in the minute amounts you need. Once you start taking megadoses from supplements, you're no longer taking a vitamin. You're taking a drug.

I've Got My Supplies: Now What Do I Do?

The shopping's done and now it's time to put it all together and create fabulous fat-burning meals. Preparation is the key to keeping food low in fat and rich in nutrients. Here are some tips.

Preparation Tips for Meats

- Trim fat from meat before and after cooking.
- Remove skin from poultry.
- Replace stuffings and breaded toppings or coatings with herbs and spices.
- Refrigerate overnight stews, soups, boiled meat, and chili. Then, skim the fat off the top and enjoy.
- Broil, poach, stew, or roast, rather than fry or sauté. If you must sauté, use no more than half a teaspoon oil, in a non-stick pan.
- When a recipe tells you to sauté the meat in butter and/or oil, cook it in wine instead. Try red wine with onions for red meats, white wine with tarragon for chicken or fish. Or, cook the meat in broth or tomato juice.
- To keep red meat as moist as possible, braise or stew. To keep natural juices in, avoid pricking or searing steaks.

➢ Marinades that include wine, vinegar, or lemon juice make meat more tender.

Preparation Tips for Vegetables, Pastas, and Grains

➢ Fill up on raw vegetables. They're better for you—and more filling—than cooked vegetables. They also take very little time to prepare and leftovers make great snacks.

➢ If you prefer vegetables with a cooked taste and texture, steam, stir-fry, broil, microwave, poach, or roast until they're barely tender. Avoid frying, basting, and sautéing.

➢ If you must boil vegetables, use the cooking liquid, which is where most of the nutrients end up, to make soup.

➢ Replace rich cream sauces with herbs, tomato sauce, or low-fat dressing.

➢ Make lasagna with low-fat cheese and/or cottage cheese, and lots of vegetables.

➢ Avoid rice mixes and fried rice. Season with herbs.

➢ Flavor baked potatoes with low-fat salad dressing or low-fat yogurt and herbs, not butter, margarine, mayonnaise, or sour cream.

➢ If a recipe tells you to sauté vegetables in butter or oil, cook them in wine. Mushrooms and onions are particularly delicious simmered in white wine.

Preparation Tips for Sandwiches

- ➢ Add flavor to low-fat cheese sandwiches by using a low-fat whole-grain bun, mustard, tomatoes, sprouts, and lettuce.
- ➢ Use lettuce and tomato, salsa, mustard, light mayonnaise, onion slices, or horseradish instead of butter or margarine.
- ➢ To moisten toast, use a little sugar-free jam or low-fat cream cheese instead of butter or margarine.

Fat-Burning Flavor Boosters

You can still enjoy many condiments and sauces to spice up your mealtimes. You can also use unlimited amounts of the following condiments and sauces to zip up your food. Buy low-sodium products whenever available, to prevent fluid retention. Try these flavor boosters:

Bouillon cubes
Chili sauce
Clear broth
Cocktail sauce
Cranberry sauce
Herbs
Horseradish
Ketchup
Lemon juice
Lime juice
Low-fat mayonnaise
Mint sauce
Mustards
Pickles
Relishes
Salsa
Soy sauce
Spices
Steak sauce
Sweet and sour sauces
Vinegars
Worcestershire sauce

The old days of creamy or oil-based dressings are now behind you. So are the days of butter, mayonnaise, sour cream, cheese, and cream sauces. Welcome to the world of herbs, mustards, lemon juice, vinegar-based dressings, diet salad dressing, nonfat yogurt, light sour cream, and whipped cottage cheese.

Here are a few tips on boosting flavor with condiments, sauces, and dressings:

- Fruit juices, vinegars, and herbs add zip to the flavor of dressings.
- Buttermilk, low-fat yogurt, and reduced-calorie mayonnaise can create creamy dressings.
- For cold salads, try reduced-calorie dressings or a specialty vinegar, such as balsamic or tarragon.
- Beer, wine, and tomato purée or broth, jazzed up with spices, make terrific marinades.
- Fruit juices or puréed fruits can replace sugar.
- Mustard and salsa can replace cream sauces and dips.

Enjoying Mealtimes

Breakfast—your most important meal

Study after study has shown that you run on empty when you wake up in the morning. You wouldn't jump in your car and go on a big trip without filling your gas tank. There's even evidence that the nutrients you miss at breakfast are never compensated for during the day. So why would you even consider starting your day without a good breakfast?

A good breakfast is also essential for safe and effective weight loss. One study in the Midwest showed that overweight people who received their entire allotment of calories at breakfast lost weight, while those who took in all their calories at dinnertime gained weight.

Break away from the expected, and eat leftovers from last night's dinner. Vegetables, lentil soup, or chickpea salad are just as nutritious in the morning as the night before. Or, try throwing a banana, low-fat yogurt, and orange juice in the blender, accompanied by sugar-free jam on toast for a quick-fix breakfast. A bowl of low-fat enriched cereal loaded with fruit and a bit of skim milk is not only convenient but rich in minerals and fiber.

Microwaveable oatmeal plus low-fat milk is a terrifically filling start to your day. Oatmeal has lots of high-quality protein compared to other grains, but is relatively low in fiber. To add fiber, throw in oat bran, wheat germ, or soy grits while the oatmeal is cooking.

Add fruit to cereal for flavor instead of butter, with low-fat milk. Add egg whites to eggs when making omelettes, beat in nonfat milk and flour to thicken the mix. Fill it with lots of vegetables.

Other alternatives include homemade waffles and pancakes, low-fat yogurt with cereal, low-fat cottage cheese combined with fresh fruit, a bagel or English muffin topped with Neufchatel or light cream cheese, homemade low-fat muffins, or fruit.

Lunch options

Some of the same people who skip breakfast also believe a quick lunch on the go will help them lose weight. They're wrong. Lunches on the go tend to be long on fat and short on satisfaction. Plan a fat-burning meal that you can enjoy, if only for 20 minutes.

Consider fresh fruit, grains, a sandwich of low-fat cheese, turkey or chicken breast, a fillet of fish with lettuce and tomato, sliced vegetables, or leftovers warmed up from dinner.

Our recipe section has a variety of low-fat sandwich fillings. No matter what sandwich filling you use, spice it up with low-fat mayonnaise, ketchup, salsa, or mustard rather than butter or margarine. If you're in a rush, consider beans on toast or cold rice salad.

If you're a soup fan, how about a huge bowl of noodle soup? A big bowl of chicken noodle soup (heavy on the noodles) will fill you up and keep you going. Dry soup to which you add water is also a good low-fat meal. Whatever soup you choose, stick to clear broths rather than cream soups.

Dinner à la thin

For most people, the temptation to overeat is strongest when the sun goes down. You're relaxed and perhaps a little tired after the challenges of your day, and stuffing yourself into oblivion looks appealing. Stop! There's nothing wrong with relaxing over a good dinner, but you're going to have to redefine your definition of "good dinner" to include plenty of fat-burning foods.

The section of this book on preparing protein is loaded with important tips on preparing and cooking poultry, fish, or red meat. In general, stop frying and start broiling, poaching, and roasting. And don't allow protein to be the star of the meal. Instead, splurge on relatively large portions of baked potatoes, whole grains, vegetables, salads splashed with low-fat dressing, and fruits. Eat dinner no later than 6 p.m., in order to give your body time to digest the meal before bedtime.

Get your snack attack on track

Try to stop snacking by 8:30 p.m. in order to give your body 11 or 12 hours to burn off all food before breakfast. The following foods are all fat-burning, low-fat treats. Exercise reasonable restraint, but enjoy them when you crave a treat.

- Air-popped popcorn
- Animal crackers
- Bagels
- Breadsticks
- Canned or frozen fruit
- Fat-free baked goods
- Fig bars
- Frozen fruit bars
- Gelatin (regular or sugar-free)
- Ginger snaps
- Graham crackers
- Hard candy
- Hot cocoa mix (regular or sugar-free)
- Ice milk
- Melba toast
- Nonfat yogurt
- Nonfat frozen yogurt (plain or sugar-free)
- Popsicles
- Pretzels
- Raw vegetables
- Rice cakes
- Saltine crackers
- Sorbet
- Tomato juice
- Vanilla wafers
- Vegetable juice

Seven-day Sample Menu

The sample menu on pages 94-95 provides a whole week's worth of ideas for fat-burning success. (See Chapter 4 for complete recipes.) These menus will get you started on the program. You can also develop your own recipes using what you have learned to keep them low in fat and high in complex carbohydrates.

Exercise: Fat-Burning in Action

As you have learned by now, what you put into your mouth is the most important component of this plan. But exercise is an amazing fat-burner as well. As you learned in the last chapter, **regular exercise keeps your metabolism high enough to burn off body fat. Exercise also encourages your body to burn fat instead of carbohydrate stores or muscle.**

Aside from helping you lose weight and keep it off, regular activity can:

- reduce stress and improve circulation and digestion,
- cut your risk of developing heart disease and diabetes,
- keep your bad blood cholesterol levels low, and
- just plain make you feel better.

There are many different types of exercise, but to maximize weight loss, choose aerobic activities. They provide a workout

SEVEN-DAY SAMPLE MENU

	Monday	Tuesday	Wednesday
Breakfast	orange	apple juice	grapefruit
	frozen waffle	Cornmeal Muffin	Fruit Cocktail Muffin
	hot cereal	oatmeal	farina
Lunch	Pasta Fagioli	Quick Jamaican Chicken	Special Turkey Salad
	Steamed Asparagus	Marinated Vegetable Salad	Danish Salad
	Spicy Rutabaga Bread	Herbed Biscuit	Speckled Brown Bread
		banana	pear
Dinner	Mixed Chinese Vegetables	Vegetable Lasagna	Shrimp and Asparagus
	Carrot-Poppy Seed Bread	Basic Green Salad	brown rice
	Cool Cucumber Pasta Salad		Cucumber and Onion Salad
	Apple-Grape Salad	Three Fruit Sherbet	Crocked Acorn Squash

Thursday	Friday	Saturday	Sunday
apple	melon	grapefruit	melon
Carrot-Oat Muffin	frozen pancake	Mini-Bran Fruitcake Muffin	Wheat Bran Bread
prepared cereal	hot cereal	oatmeal	prepared cereal
Mexican Stuffed Pepper	Lunch Box Minestrone	Hot Chinese Noodles	Chunky Chicken Salad
Famous Bean Salad	Basic Green Salad	Bean Sprout Salad	Sprout Soup
Wheat Bran Bread	Whole-Wheat French Bread	Carrot-Poppy Seed Bread	Carrot Salad
orange	apple	peach	Cranberry Applesauce
Chicken with Tomatoes and Chickpeas	Stuffed Zucchini	Monkfish Kebabs	Burrito Bundle with frijoles
Potato Bread	Rice Salad	Rice Pilaf with Onion	Green Rice
Eggplant Salad	Gourmet Peas	Molasses Oat Muffin	
Lemon Sherbet	Cranberry Applesauce	Apple-Grape Salad	Pineapple-Grape Parfait

for your heart, lungs, and large muscle groups. Brisk walks, swimming, cycling, and fitness classes (if you're really ambitious) burn off fat, and are important preventives for heart disease—the largest killer in North America. Water exercises, such as aqua-aerobics, are also great fat-burners, providing people who have painful joints with a terrific cardiovascular workout.

You don't need to become a jock. **Regular, low-key, aerobic exercise will help you lose weight far more efficiently than high-powered workouts.** If you're older than forty-five, you must avoid high-impact aerobic activities, such as jogging and jumping. These force too much weight suddenly onto joints and the lower back. Also, take competitive sports with a grain of salt. They're hard on your system and are not necessary in order to lose weight. Your victory will be a slim new body, not first prize at the Boston Marathon.

It's not even necessary to get to the gym for a 30- to 45-minute cardiovascular workout three to five times a week. Find a half-hour once a week, mark it in your calendar, and set aside the time in your schedule for the next few months. Even if you can only commit yourself to a 30-minute walk, your waistline will reap the benefits.

The key word is balance. Just 90 minutes of walking or gardening per week for a 156-pound person can boost metabolism enough to roll off pounds and keep them off. If you're heavier, you need to spend even less time at these activities because you will spend more energy in burning off fat.

When you consider that the following modest activities are enough to keep your weight loss going, how hard would it be to incorporate some of them into your weekly routine?

- $1^1/_2$ hours walking at a normal pace
- $1^1/_2$ hours gardening, hedging
- 45 minutes of swimming, fast crawl
- 1 hour 50 minutes leisure bicycling, at 5.5 miles per hour
- 2 hours 20 minutes ballroom dancing
- 1 hour 20 minutes golf
- 1 hour cross-country skiing
- 1 hour tennis
- 2 hours 20 minutes volleyball

Better yet, make a point of doing something physical every day or at least every other day. And always choose activities you enjoy. Variety will make these activities fun and exhilarating!

Walking—fat-burning in motion

A brisk daily walk is the ideal exercise for most people. Injuries are unlikely, the only equipment you need is a good pair of shoes, and you can stay active anywhere, alone or with company.

The latest research shows that walking, at a moderate pace, is just as good a weight-loss strategy as a tough workout—maybe better. According to a study published by the *Journal of the American Medical Association,* a brisk 20-minute walk at least three times a week can help people live longer than any other form of exercise. As well, you'll be slim and fit during the years you add to your life.

Regular walking raises your metabolic rate just as effectively as attending an exercise class, which is what you need to continue your weight loss. What's critical is the amount of time you spend at it. You're far more likely to lose weight if you walk at a moderate pace for, say, 30 minutes a day, three times a week, than if you take an hour-long jog once a week. Walking for more than an hour a day doesn't seem to add to the benefits, either. Overdoing it isn't going to help you.

All you need is a good pair of walking shoes and comfortable clothing. Make sure your shoes have good arch support and adequate room for your toes. If you're walking in cold weather, cover the lower part of your face with a scarf, to avoid inhaling cold air into your lungs.

At first, you may want to walk slowly and just enjoy the scenery. Eventually, your pace should be brisk enough to carry on a conversation without having to catch your breath. For better back health, maintain good posture: hold your head up proudly, tuck in your pelvis, and straighten your back.

Exercise tips

Here are some easy ways to include regular exercise in your routine:

- Park the car a few blocks away from the office and walk the rest of the distance.

➢ Get off the bus one stop before the office and walk to work from there.

➢ Walk or run up the stairs to your office instead of taking the elevator.

➢ Take the kids to the park to play Frisbee.

➢ Use your feet instead of the car. When you need to pick up some milk at the last minute, walk to the grocery store instead of driving.

➢ Use your bicycle instead of the bus.

➢ Start a garden or build a deck onto your house instead of having someone else do the work.

➢ Play hockey with your kids instead of sending them to Little League games.

➢ Use a regular broom instead of an electric broom to sweep floors.

➢ Help your neighbor bring in the hay this fall.

➢ Walk your children to school in the morning.

Eventually, you may become ambitious enough to set up an exercise program. Here's how to make it appealing:

➢ If you want to exercise at home, select a room or part of a room that you don't visit often. Decorate it with bright colors, which are stimulating. It will be invigorating just to walk in the room.

➢ To help time pass more pleasurably while you're exercising, listen to your favorite music or even watch television.

➢ Exercise with a partner or a group. Take a regular bike ride after dinner with a friend, or join a walking group.

➢ Motivate yourself with realistic short-term goals ("I'm going to bicycle to the grocery store for milk on Saturday mornings") as well as an achievable long-term goal ("by August, I'll be bicycling to work three times a week").

You're Off to a Great Start

You are now prepared to start slimming down. Focus on eating fat-burning foods, cutting fat and protein intake, and exercising regularly, and get ready to start taking in your clothing. Now that you've got the knowledge—and the tools to use that knowledge—nothing can hold you back!

CHAPTER 3

KEEPING IT OFF— YOU CAN DO IT!

WITHIN A WEEK OR TWO ON THIS PROGRAM, you're going to feel so much better about yourself—and your waistline—that you won't believe the change! You'll have succeeded in replacing the irritability you felt in the old days, during one of your many starvation diets, with pride in your appearance.

Because fat-burning foods tend to be less expensive than fatty, processed, high-protein foods, the only weight-gainer around your place should be your wallet.

Although this program is easy and satisfying, it can be difficult to resist backsliding, especially once you've lost all the weight you need to lose. Social occasions, stress, the rush of modern life, and the difficulty in finding the "right foods" in restaurants are all challenges you will have to face on an ongoing basis.

Read on to learn valuable tips on coping with the challenge of keeping that weight off for a lifetime. You're worth it!

Satisfy the Party Animal in You

The party is in full swing and the canapé tray is loaded with tiny mouthfuls of temptation. Most people at parties stuff themselves with so much food they can't even estimate their intake! Studies have shown that many people will consume more than 2,000 calories of unnecessary food over the course of an evening! The trick is to prepare yourself beforehand.

Keep these suggestions in mind at the next party or social outing you attend:

- Don't skip lunch because you know you're going to be eating dinner out. You'll arrive starving and probably overeat.

- Before you leave for the party, eat some fruit or a jam sandwich so you don't arrive hungry.

- If you don't think there will be anything you can eat at the party, offer to bring fresh vegetables, along with a low-fat dip. Then, at the party, eat only your contribution.

- Try to eat slowly and enjoy your food.

- Drink lots of soda water, diet drinks, or fruit juice. (Note: If you choose a diet drink that has caffeine in it, such as Coke, expect to react as if you've drunk coffee.)

- Avoid the bar. Alcoholic beverages have no food value, and may impair your judgement about what to eat.

De-stress for Success!

Although you're going to feel and look better than ever, change is not easy. You're going to need the support of your family, friends, and co-workers, and you will have to work together to keep your motivation up. You're allowed to make mistakes! You're human. Don't be ashamed to ask for help.

Compulsive overeaters, however, may need more help than any one friend can offer. If it's within your budget, a few sessions with a therapist might help you understand why you overeat. Or, you may consider joining a support group, such as Overeaters Anonymous, which uses a twelve-step program in helping overeaters break their habits. Overeaters Anonymous is listed in your local phone book, or you can write P.O. Box 92870, Los Angeles, California, 90009, for information on the meeting place nearest you.

If you tend to overeat to cope with stress, depression, loneliness, or just plain boredom, turn to one of the alternative activities you learned about in the previous chapter. Take a walk, call a friend, or take up a hobby. It's far healthier to do something about your problems than it is to bury them under a mound of unhealthy food.

You may need to look more closely at managing your stress before you can stick to this amazing program. Stress can be a positive force, providing the extra spurt of energy you need to finish a job, the drive that keeps you going on an important project, or the enthusiasm to provide moral support to your family and friends.

The problem with stress is not so much the actual source—your mortgage, the traffic jam on the way home, your teenager's attitude—as how you deal with it. Everyone gets upset over major calamities. But if you are regularly using the small irritations of everyday life as an excuse to overeat, then you're giving stress too much power over your life—and your waistline.

Time management, career planning, or assertiveness training may help you feel calmer. Time management, for instance, offers practical techniques for scheduling activities so you don't feel rushed and out of control of your time and life.

Career planning could help you explore your skills, aptitudes, and interests, and to identify occupational choices that will satisfy your personal and professional ambitions. This will make you feel more in control of your own destiny.

Assertiveness training will teach you how to clearly communicate your opinions, ideas, and feelings, without backing down, in an effective, non-threatening way.

Progressive relaxation is another effective, easy technique for total body relaxation. It's a method of systematically tensing and relaxing your body, one part at a time.

Visualization is a method of creating a positive mental environment by imagining you have already achieved a specific, identifiable goal. The effectiveness of this technique for coping with serious illness has been widely promoted in books such as Dr. Bernie Siegel's best-seller *Love, Medicine, and Miracles.*

If you still can't relax, try breath control, self-hypnosis, yoga, meditation, tai chi, even listening to music or doing color-by-number paintings.

Check your local library or bookstore for self-help guides on these and similar topics, or ask about personal development courses or seminars at community centers, night schools, or other learning institutions.

Another way of reducing stress—and sticking to this program—is to plan ahead.

Help! Half an Hour Until Dinnertime!

What to do when you arrive home, kids in tow, with nothing in sight for dinner? Don't despair. A great weight-loss meal could be 30 minutes away, and the entire family will enjoy it. Here are a few tips to help you along the way:

- Store meal-sized portions of cooked rice, beans, peas, low-fat corn tortillas, broths, tomato sauce, and soups in your freezer. Stock up on frozen vegetables, cooked leftover chicken, turkey, pork, beef, veal, and fish. You can easily combine two or more portions into one satisfying meal, with a little help from your microwave.

- Take frozen chicken or meat out of the freezer in the morning to use as a satisfying touch of protein in a quick stir-fry. Cook up garlic, onions, ginger, soy sauce, and a little oil in a wok, throw in frozen vegetables and chopped up meat or tofu, and serve over rice or another grain.

- Likewise, fish poached in water and lemon juice, spiked with celery, carrots, and onions, cooks quickly. If it's not a strongly flavored fish, you can drain the broth through a cheesecloth and freeze it. Fish broth is a great foundation for fish chowder, which is a fast fat-burning meal. Just add cooked carrots, onions, celery, potatoes, other vegetables of your choice, skim milk, and fish bits to the stock.

- Pastas are so fast and nutritious they should become a regular part of your "fast food" diet. While you're boiling the noodles, cook up garlic and onion in a little oil, and, in another pan, warm a can of plum tomatoes, frozen vegetables, and some oregano, basil, and pepper. Toss it all together, top with low-fat Parmesan, and you have a meal in 15 minutes. Add a small quantity of ground meat, chopped meat, or canned fish if you want.

➢ Pasta primavera is an even faster meal. A few minutes before your dried pasta is cooked, throw in a bag of frozen mixed vegetables and cook until the vegetables have just thawed. Drain well, then toss with diet dressing and dust lightly with low-fat Parmesan.

➢ Microwave-baked potatoes are fast, healthy vehicles for tasty fillings. Stuff with low-fat cottage cheese, low-fat yogurt, and broccoli, or cooked vegetables, a small amount of water-packed canned salmon, and a sprinkle of low-fat Parmesan.

➢ Stock up on dehydrated refried beans and low-fat tortillas for another easy meal. Defrost the tortilla in the microwave, add water to the beans, and cook up some onions, pepper, and tomatoes in water. Stuff the tortilla with beans and vegetables, top with grated low-fat cheese, and you have burritos in five minutes.

➢ "Under-10-minute" alternatives to plain brown rice include quick-cooking barley, quick-cooking brown rice, bulgur, and couscous.

➢ Combine a can of beans with half a can of tuna, chopped peppers, onions, minced parsley, other fresh herbs, and a splash of low-fat salad dressing for a delicious, satisfying dinner on the go.

- Combine bite-sized pieces of chicken breasts, canned chicken broth, ginger, frozen vegetables, and egg noodles for a nourishing dinner soup.

- Marinate tofu in the refrigerator all day to jazz up its flavor, then put it under the broiler. Here's a marinade that's simplicity itself: a combination of 1 tablespoon fresh rosemary, 1 tablespoon olive oil, 1 tablespoon raspberry vinegar, and 1 teaspoon Dijon mustard.

- If you only have time to make complicated dishes on the weekend, make twice as much as you need and freeze one meal, to be enjoyed during the week.

- During barbecue season, replace skewered beef with tofu chunks that have been marinated all day in 1/4 cup soy sauce, 1/4 cup red wine, 3 tablespoons rice vinegar, 1 tablespoon sesame oil, a dash of hot pepper sauce, and 2 cloves of minced garlic.

Quick, Low-Fat Fixings From (Gasp!) the Convenience Store

If it's 30 minutes to dinnertime and you have no dinner fixings, don't despair. Just stop in at the corner store for some, or all, of these quick fixings:

- Low-fat canned soup, doctored with canned or frozen vegetables, rice, and beans, is a terrific meal-in-a-bowl.

- Pasta, prepared tomato sauce, and canned or frozen vegetables, topped with grated low-fat Parmesan, can be your main course, followed by canned fruit (make sure it's packed in fruit juice or water, not syrup) for dessert.

- Liquid eggs, low-fat cheese, and lots of frozen vegetables make a tasty omelette.

- A rice casserole made with beans, tomato sauce, and water-packed tuna will satisfy any growling tummy.

- Skim milk can be the basis for low-fat custards, quiches, puddings, and blender drinks.

Fat-Burning Lunches—in the Bag!

A nutritious and filling lunch will keep you on track. Consider these suggestions:

- Stave off sandwich blahs by using your freezer to store a variety of ready-to-use breads and fillings: cut low-fat rolls or bagels in half and put them in the freezer. Freeze low-fat corn tortillas, pita bread, and sliced bread.

- Dinnertime leftovers can provide plenty of interesting sandwich fillings. Slice and freeze uneaten cooked chicken, fish, turkey, or tofu, along with cooked vegetables. The next morning, just grab them on your way out the door. Heat them in the office microwave, and spice them up with a fat-burning flavor booster.

- Stuffed pita bread can be more interesting than a plain old sandwich. To fill it, bring along containers of vegetables, water-packed tuna, broiled chicken, and diet dressing. That way, the pita won't be soggy by lunchtime.

- Whenever you prepare food, make extra and recycle it into lunches. Make extra dinner vegetables, which can be combined with diet dressing into appetizing lunchtime salads. Or cook extra noodles at dinnertime, and add canned water-packed tuna, broiled chicken, chickpeas, beans, tofu, vegetables, and dressing.

- If your office has a microwave oven, take along a thermos of soup prepared the night before, along with crackers or bread, and a fruit.

- Keep cut-up raw vegetables, such as celery, carrots, and cucumber, in a closed container in the fridge ready to be tossed into your lunch bag.

- Make low-fat muffins and cookies on the weekend to satisfy your lunchtime sweet tooth. Alternatively, take along fresh fruit, low-fat puddings, yogurt, or fruit salad.

- A box of crackers at your desk, combined with low-fat cheese, vegetables, fruit, and popcorn, is good for snacking.

Renovate Your Recipes for Easy Weight Loss

Chapter 4 contains meal suggestions and recipes that will stoke your flavor furnace and guarantee steady weight loss. But there's no need to toss out the rest of your cookbooks. Often, you can replace protein with carbohydrates, or at least a lower-fat protein. You can get most of the fat out of a recipe—or at least minimize it—without affecting the flavor that much. For example:

- Experiment with butter-flavored sprinkles such as Butter Buds. You probably won't taste the difference on popcorn or artichokes. In fact, air-popped popcorn, sprinkled with butter-flavored sprinkles and low-fat Parmesan (plus a touch of garlic salt if you're feeling adventurous), is a terrifically satisfying late-night snack.

- A puréed boiled potato added to soup broth is a wonderful thickener.

- When baking cookies or cakes, experiment with fewer eggs, sugar, or fat than the recipe calls for.

The Recipe Renovation Guide offers a few other suggestions, just to get you started. Soon you'll be renovating all your recipes with ease and confidence.

RECIPE RENOVATION GUIDE

Replace	With
Ice cream	Sherbet or ice milk
Creamy soups	Clear soups
Creamy or oil-based salad dressings	Lemon juice, vinegar-based, or diet salad dressings
Butter, margarine, or oil	Broth, low-fat yogurt, light mayonnaise, fruit juice, or wine
Bacon, bologna, corned beef, hot dogs, liverwurst, pastrami, sausages, pepperoni, and salami	Sliced chicken or turkey and meat substitutes found in health food stores
Gravies made from meat drippings	Herbs, spices, and clear broths
Mozzarella, cheddar, and other hard cheeses	Cheeses made of non-fat or skim milk, including cottage cheese

continued →

Replace	With
Cream cheese	Neufchatel cream cheese, light cream cheese
Whole milk ricotta cheese	Skim ricotta
Whole milk	Buttermilk, low-fat, and non-fat milk
Dairy creamers	Low-fat milk or non-dairy creamers made without coconut oil
Sour cream	Low-fat yogurt
Chocolate	Cocoa powder mixed with non-fat milk
Hot chocolate mix	Non-fat dry milk powder, unsweetened cocoa powder, and sugar
Regular potato chips	Polyunsaturated potato chips
Eggs	Egg whites, liquid eggs
Mayonnaise	Low-fat yogurt, low-fat (light) mayonnaise

Avoid the Pitfalls of Dining Out

Eating out can pose a special challenge now that your eating habits have changed. You can't expect a restaurant to improvise a dish not on the menu, but you can politely request that your food be prepared and served the way you need it. After all, you're paying for food as well as service. These hints should help:

- Contact the restaurant in advance to ask about the food and if special requests are honored.
- Don't be embarrassed to order an appetizer or a half-portion instead of a full meal (or share a full portion with a friend).
- Don't be embarrassed to send food back to the kitchen if it's not prepared according to your specifications. You're the one paying for it.
- Indulge in the bread basket. Believe it or not, you'll lose weight if you fill up on breadsticks, rolls, French bread, pita bread, or toast that show up on your table before the meal—*as long as you pass on butter or any other high-fat spread.*
- Ditto to vegetable sticks. Stuff yourself with carrots, celery, and so on. Enjoy.
- Select small amounts of margarine made from corn, safflower, sunflower, soybean, cottonseed, or sesame oils. Better yet, use condiments like mustard or salsa.

➢ If you wish to order meat, fish, or poultry, make sure it's steamed, prepared in its own juice, broiled, roasted, or poached. Once it arrives, trim visible fat off the meat or skin off the poultry.

➢ A fresh green or fruit salad, accompanied by several side dishes of vegetables, beans, pilafs, and other grains is a terrific fat-burning meal. If the restaurant has no fat-free salad dressing or sauce, ask for salad dressings and sauces to be served on the side, and use only small amounts, if any at all.

➢ Ask for low-fat yogurt to top your baked potato, instead of butter or sour cream.

➢ Choose clear broth soups, such as noodle, bean, or minestrone, instead of cream-based soups.

➢ Choose fresh fruit or sherbet for dessert.

➢ Ask for skim milk for your coffee instead of whole milk, cream, or non-dairy creamer, which are high in saturated fat.

➢ Avoid deluxe anything. It usually means extra fat.

➢ Avoid creamy, breaded, batter-dipped, or fried foods.

➢ Avoid casseroles and foods with heavy sauces.

➢ Ask for a doggie bag for food you can't eat.

➢ If the meal comes with several courses, some of which you

can't eat, order à la carte even if you have to pay extra for it.

- If your business requires you to take people to lunch, take your clients to restaurants that serve foods you can eat. Salad bars, buffets, and smorgasbords are a safe bet; you can make your own selection.

In a **fast food restaurant,** order:

- fruit or regular salad, with dressing on the side
- plain baked or mashed potatoes, topped with a small container of low-fat yogurt you bring yourself
- broiled chicken on an unbuttered roll, accompanied by lettuce and tomato
- noodle soup
- corn on the cob
- fruit juice

Sorry, but you're going to have to pass on the hot dogs, hamburgers, cheeseburgers, milk shakes, and french fries.

In an **Italian restaurant,** order:

- pasta with tomato or marinara sauce

- vegetables
- salad
- broiled fish or chicken
- mushroom spaghetti
- vegetable pizza with half the normal amount of cheese and extra herbs

In a **Mexican restaurant**, order:

- corn (not flour) tortillas
- rice
- beans (even refried beans aren't bad in moderation)
- broiled chicken
- salads
- chicken taco or tostada, made with a baked or steamed tortilla
- vegetarian burrito (a steamed tortilla filled with beans, rice, salsa, and a little cheese)

In a **Chinese restaurant**, order:

➢ stir-fried dishes

➢ lots of steamed rice

Most Chinese food is very high in fat. Choose another type of restaurant if possible.

In a **steakhouse**, order:

➢ plain baked potato

➢ vegetables

➢ salads

In a **French restaurant**, order:

➢ chicken breast or fish fillet, poached in wine

➢ steamed mussels

In a **Japanese restaurant**, order:

➢ yakimono (broiled seafood)

➢ soba soup (noodle soup in broth, accompanied by spinach,

bean sprouts, other vegetables, and a little chicken, beef, or tofu)

- sushi (vinegared rice rolled up with raw fish and vegetables inside a thin sheet of seaweed)

- rice

In a **Greek restaurant,** order:

- chicken shish kebab

- salad without feta cheese, anchovies, or olives, with dressing on the side

- plaki (fish cooked with tomatoes, onions, and garlic)

- pilaf or other rice dish

At the local **breakfast diner,** order:

- toast or English muffins and jam

- cereal with fruit and skim milk

- three or fewer pancakes, with syrup only

- fruit salad and cottage cheese

Keep on Moving!

Once you've become the slender person you always knew you were, you'll still want to continue your activity program. That's the only way your metabolism can stay high enough to keep weight off.

Studies of extremely overweight people show that pound for pound, they need one-third to one-half fewer calories to maintain their weight than people who are not overweight. The reason is, body fat needs fewer calories to maintain itself than lean muscle tissue.

Now that you have more muscle tissue than fat, you'll need regular activity to keep burning off excess calories before your body converts them into fat. As long as you stay active, you'll be able to eat as much as you want of the fat-burning foods on this program.

Final Words: Nip Temptation in the Bud

If you stick to the program outlined in this book, the pounds will melt away. Be patient, and watch the needle on the scale plunge downward gradually. If, however, several weeks go by and you're not losing weight, ask yourself these questions:

1. Have any excess fats "sneaked" onto your plate? If fried foods and buttered rolls have found their way back into your diet, or if you've stopped reading labels to track down hidden fats, the pounds will stop dropping off. Whether it's whole milk instead of skim milk or butter on your toast, get rid of it!

2. Are you stuffing yourself out of boredom? You should not be hungry on this diet, but you do have to stop eating when your stomach is full.

3. Have you kept your activity level up? Your daily walk or other routine is an essential component of your fat-burning program. If your life has suddenly become too busy for a regular walk, remember some of the other tricks suggested in Chapter 2. Park the car a couple of blocks away from the office, for instance, or use the stairs instead of the elevator at the office.

4. Have you kept your protein consumption down? If that weekly 3-ounce steak has become a fat-marbled 6-ouncer several times a week, the extra fat in your diet will keep you from losing weight. Instead, start filling up on carbohydrates.

5. What about your serving sizes? If you're basing your fat intake on the new labels but eating twice as much as the label serving size, you're deluding yourself.

Happy eating!

CHAPTER 4

MENUS AND RECIPES FOR FAT-BURNING SUCCESS

Seven-Day Menu

Day 1

Breakfast	1 sliced orange 1 low-fat frozen waffle 1/2 cup hot cereal
Lunch	1 serving Pasta Fagioli (page 167) 1 cup Steamed Asparagus (page 160) 1 slice Spicy Rutabaga Bread (page 142)
Dinner	1 serving Mixed Chinese Vegetables (page 165) 1 slice Carrot-Poppy Seed Bread (page 134) 1 cup Cool Cucumber Pasta Salad (page 149) 1 serving Apple-Grape Salad (page 175)
Snack	1 medium-sized pear

Day 2

Breakfast	3/4 cup apple juice
	1/2 cup cooked oatmeal with cinnamon and raisins
	1 Cornmeal Muffin (page 135)
Lunch	1 serving Quick Jamaican Chicken (page 168)
	1/2 cup Marinated Vegetable Salad (page 153)
	1 Herbed Biscuit (page 136)
	1 banana
Dinner	1 serving Vegetable Lasagna (page 172)
	1 cup Basic Green Salad (page 145)
	1/2 cup Three Fruit Sherbet (page 178)
Snack	1/2 cup grapes

Day 3

Breakfast	1/2 grapefruit 1 Fruit Cocktail Muffin (page 135) 1/2 cup farina
Lunch	1 serving Special Turkey Salad (page 170) 1 slice Speckled Brown Bread (page 141) 1/2 cup Danish Salad (page 150) 1 medium-sized pear
Dinner	1 serving Shrimp and Asparagus (page 169) with 3/4 cup short-grain brown rice 1 cup Cucumber and Onion Salad (page 149) 1 quarter Crocked Acorn Squash (page 177)
Snack	1 cup air-popped popcorn

Day 4

Breakfast	1 medium-sized apple 1 Carrot-Oat Muffin (page 133) 1 ounce prepared cereal with 1/4 cup non-fat milk
Lunch	1 Mexican Stuffed Pepper (page 164) 1/2 cup Famous Bean Salad (page 152) 1 slice Wheat Bran Bread (page 143) 1 medium-sized orange
Dinner	1 serving Chicken with Tomatoes and Chickpeas (page 163) 1 slice Potato Bread with Caraway Seeds (page 139) 1/2 cup Eggplant Salad (page 151) 1 serving Lemon Sherbet (page 177)
Snack	1 cup carrot sticks

Day 5

Breakfast	1 slice honeydew melon 1 low-fat frozen pancake 1/2 cup hot cereal
Lunch	1 cup Lunch Box Minestrone (page 155) 1 cup Basic Green Salad (page 145) 1 slice Whole-Wheat French Bread (page 144) 1 medium-sized apple
Dinner	1 serving Stuffed Zucchini (page 171) 1/2 cup Gourmet Peas (page 157) 1/2 cup Rice Salad (page 160) 1 cup Cranberry Applesauce (page 176)
Snack	1 slice cantaloupe

Day 6

Breakfast	1/2 grapefruit 1 Mini-Bran Fruitcake Muffin (page 137) 1/2 cup cooked oatmeal with cinnamon and raisins
Lunch	1 cup Hot Chinese Noodles (page 158) 1 serving Bean Sprout Salad (page 146) 1 slice Carrot-Poppy Seed Bread (page 134) 1 medium-sized peach
Dinner	1 serving Monkfish Kebabs (page 166) 3/4 cup Rice Pilaf with Onion (page 159) 1 Molasses Oat Muffin (page 138) 1 serving Apple-Grape Salad (page 175)
Snack	6 vanilla wafers

Day 7

Breakfast	1 slice melon 1 slice Wheat Bran Bread (page 143) 1 ounce prepared cereal with 1/4 cup non-fat milk
Lunch	1 serving Chunky Chicken Salad (page 148) 1 cup Sprout Soup (page 156) 1/2 cup Carrot Salad (page 147) 1/2 cup Cranberry Applesauce (page 176)
Dinner	1 Burrito Bundle with Frijoles (pages 161 and 162) 1 cup Green Rice (page 158) 1 Pineapple-Grape Parfait (page 178)
Snack	1 slice Pumpkin Bread (page 140)

Bountiful Breads

Carrot-Oat Muffins

- 3/4 cup quick-cooking oats
- 1 cup low-fat buttermilk
- 1 1/4 cups unbleached flour
- 3 teaspoons baking powder
- 1/2 teaspoon salt
- 1 egg
- 3 tablespoons honey
- 1/2 cup carrot, finely shredded
- 1 teaspoon orange rind, grated

Combine oats and buttermilk in a mixing bowl and let stand for 15 minutes. Beat egg with honey. Meanwhile, combine flour, baking powder, and salt. Stir with egg into the oat mixture. Fold in carrots and orange rind, stirring only enough to moisten all ingredients. Spoon into muffin cups sprayed with low-fat cooking spray. Bake at 400°F for 20 to 25 minutes. Serves 12.

Carrot-Poppy Seed Bread

- 2 packages active dry yeast
- 1/4 cup lukewarm water
- 2 cups hot water
- 1/4 cup molasses
- 2 teaspoons salt
- 1/4 cup oil
- 2 cups carrot pulp
- 3 teaspoons poppy seeds
- 5 1/2 cups whole-wheat flour

In a small bowl, soften yeast in lukewarm water. Separately, combine hot water, molasses, oil, salt, carrot pulp, and poppy seeds in a large mixing bowl. Stir until well mixed, then stir in yeast mixture and blend thoroughly. Add flour, 1 cup at a time (retain 1/2 cup for kneading). When dough is well mixed, turn out on a floured board and knead for 6 to 8 minutes. (Dough will be slightly sticky.) Transfer to an oiled bowl, cover, and let rise until doubled in bulk, about 90 minutes.

Punch dough down and divide into two oblong or round loaves. Place in bread pans or on cookie sheet sprayed with low-fat cooking spray; cover and let rise for 30 minutes. Bake in a pre-heated oven at 425°F for 10 minutes. Then, reduce heat to 350°F and bake for 35 to 40 minutes, or until bread is nicely browned. Makes two loaves. Serves 16.

Cornmeal Muffins

1 package corn meal mix
1 cup cream-style corn
1 egg, beaten
low-fat sharp cheese, grated, to taste
pepper, to taste

Mix ingredients together, place in muffin tins sprayed with low-fat cooking spray. Bake at 425°F for 12 to 15 minutes. Serves 8.

Fruit Cocktail Muffins

1 8-ounce can fruit cocktail, well-drained
1 3/4 cups flour, sifted
2 tablespoons sugar
2 teaspoons baking powder
3/4 teaspoon salt
1 egg, well-beaten
3/4 cup milk
1/3 cup vegetable oil

Sift dry ingredients into mixing bowl. Make a well in the center. Mix milk, egg, and oil, and add to dry ingredients. Stir quickly, just enough to moisten. Add the drained fruit cocktail. Fill nonstick or paper-lined muffin tins two-thirds full. Bake at 400°F for 25 to 30 minutes. Serves 12.

Herbed Biscuits

- 2 cups flour
- 3 teaspoons baking powder
- pinch of salt
- 1 teaspoon brown sugar
- 2 tablespoons dried parsley flakes
- 1 teaspoon dill weed
- 1/2 cup and 3 tablespoons margarine, softened
- water

Mix together dry ingredients. Cut in margarine until mixture has a coarse consistency. Add enough water to make a workable dough. Shape and place on a nonstick baking sheet. Bake at 400°F until tops are browned. Serves 8.

Mini-Bran Fruitcake Muffins

1/2 cup unsweetened applesauce
1/2 cup bran cereal buds
1/2 cup wheat cereal flakes
1/3 cup nonfat dry milk powder
1 teaspoon baking soda
1/2 teaspoon baking powder
1 tablespoon all-purpose flour
2 tablespoons dried currants or raisins, or chopped mixed dried fruit
1 teaspoon rum or brandy flavoring, or vanilla extract
1 teaspoon pumpkin pie spice, optional
pinch of grated orange peel, optional

Combine all ingredients in a bowl and mix thoroughly. Spoon into six paper-lined muffin tins, three-quarters full. Bake in a preheated oven at 350°F for 25 minutes. Serves 6.

Molasses Oat Muffins

1 1/2 cup quick-cooking oats, toasted*
1 cup all-purpose flour
3 teaspoons baking powder
3/4 teaspoon salt
3/4 teaspoon cinnamon
1/3 cup dark brown sugar, firmly packed
1 large egg
2/3 cup milk
1/3 cup molasses
1/3 cup oil

Toast oats.* In a medium bowl stir together the flour, baking powder, salt, and cinnamon; then stir in the sugar and toasted oats. In a small bowl, beat the egg until yolk and white are blended. Add milk and molasses, and beat to blend. Add these and the oil to the flour mixture, and stir until dry ingredients are moistened. Fill muffin tins (each 1/3 cup capacity) sprayed with low-fat cooking spray about two-thirds full. Bake in a preheated oven at 400°F until a cake tester inserted in center of muffin comes out clean, or about 15 to 18 minutes. Serves 12.

*To toast oats, spread 1 1/2 cups quick-cooking oats in an ungreased rectangular cake pan. Bake in a preheated oven at 350°F until golden brown, or about 14 to 18 minutes. Cool. Makes 1 1/2 cups.

Potato Bread with Caraway Seeds

1 medium potato, peeled and diced
1 1/2 cups water
1 package active dry yeast
2 tablespoons sugar
2 tablespoons margarine, softened
1/2 cup liquid eggs
1 1/2 teaspoons salt
2 teaspoons caraway seeds
4 1/2 cups all-purpose flour

Place potato in small saucepan with water, cover and bring to boil, then reduce heat to low. Cook 10 to 12 minutes or until tender. Drain, reserving 1 cup of boiled potato water. Steam diced potato a few minutes in saucepan until dry; mash alone.

When potato water has cooled to lukewarm, pour into mixing bowl. Add yeast and stir until dissolved. Add mashed potato, sugar, margarine, eggs, salt, caraway, and 2 cups flour. Beat with electric mixer on low speed for 1 minute, scraping bowl frequently. Increase speed to medium; beat 2 minutes. Mix in enough remaining flour to form dough that can be easily handled. Turn out onto floured board; knead until smooth and elastic. Place in greased bowl and cover. Let rise in warm place until doubled in bulk, 60 to 90 minutes.

Punch down dough. Turn out onto floured board; form into round loaf. Lightly spray 2-quart round casserole with low-fat cooking spray. Place loaf in casserole and cover. Let rise until doubled in bulk.

Bake at 375°F for 30 to 35 minutes or until golden. Remove from casserole; cool on wire rack. Makes one large loaf. Serves 12.

Pumpkin Bread

1 cup honey
1 cup date sugar
1 cup oil
3 cups pumpkin purée
1 cup dates, chopped
1 cup walnuts, chopped
1 teaspoon salt
1 teaspoon cinnamon
1 teaspoon ground cloves
4 teaspoons baking soda
2 cups unbleached white flour
2 1/2 cups whole-wheat flour
1/2 cup wheat germ

Mix together honey, date sugar (available at health food stores), oil, pumpkin purée, chopped dates, chopped walnuts, salt, cinnamon, cloves, and baking soda. Add flour and wheat germ. Put into three loaf pans sprayed with low-fat cooking spray and bake for one hour at 350°F. Serve warm. Makes three loaves. Serves 20.

Speckled Brown Bread

- 1 1/2 cups flour
- 1 1/2 teaspoons salt
- 1 1/2 teaspoons soda
- 1 teaspoon baking powder
- 2 cups Zante currants, seedless grapes, or raisins
- 1 cup wheat germ
- 3/4 cup yellow corn meal
- 3/4 cup regular oatmeal
- 1 cup low-fat buttermilk
- 1 egg
- 3/4 cup molasses
- 1/4 cup maple syrup
- 2 tablespoons vegetable oil

Sift flour, salt, soda, and baking powder in a large bowl. Add Zante currants, wheat germ, corn meal, and oatmeal. Beat one egg lightly and add buttermilk, molasses, maple syrup, and vegetable oil. Add to dry mixture and stir until flour is moistened. Pour into a 9- by 5-inch loaf pan sprayed with low-fat cooking spray and floured. Bake at 350°F for one hour. Cool in pan 10 minutes before turning out. Makes one loaf. Serves 12.

Spicy Rutabaga Bread

- 1 cup all-purpose flour
- 2/3 cup sugar
- 1/2 teaspoon baking soda
- 1/4 teaspoon allspice, ground
- 1/4 teaspoon cinnamon
- 1/4 teaspoon nutmeg
- 1/4 teaspoon salt or to taste
- 1/4 teaspoon baking powder
- 1 egg
- 1/2 cup rutabaga, cooked and puréed
- 1/4 cup vegetable oil

Spray an 8- by 4-inch baking pan with low-fat cooking spray, and line with wax paper. Combine flour, sugar, baking soda, allspice, cinnamon, nutmeg, salt, and baking powder, and mix well. In separate bowl, beat egg and add rutabaga and vegetable oil. Add moist ingredients all at once to dry ingredients. Stir just enough to blend. Pour into prepared pan and bake in oven preheated to 350°F for one hour, or until toothpick inserted in center comes out clean. Makes one loaf. Serves 10.

Wheat Bran Bread

- 1/4 cup warm water
- 1 package active dry yeast
- 2 tablespoons margarine
- 2 tablespoons brown sugar
- 1 teaspoon salt
- 1 cup skim milk, scalded
- 1/2 cup unprocessed wheat bran
- 3 cups whole-wheat flour

Place warm water in large bowl, sprinkle yeast over, and stir to dissolve. Let stand 5 to 10 minutes or until foamy. Add margarine, brown sugar, and salt to hot milk. Stir until margarine is melted, then let cool to room temperature.

Stir milk mixture into yeast until blended. Stir in bran and enough whole-wheat flour to make soft dough. Place dough on a lightly floured surface and knead in enough whole-wheat flour to make smooth dough. Knead until smooth and elastic. Place in bowl lightly sprayed with low-fat cooking spray, and turn to coat. Cover and let rise in a warm, draft-free place until doubled in bulk, about 90 minutes.

Spray an 8- by 4-inch loaf pan with cooking spray. Punch dough down. Shape dough into a loaf and place in prepared pan. Cover and let rise until dough reaches rim of pan.

Preheat oven to 375°F. Brush top of loaf with water and bake in preheated oven 30 to 35 minutes or until bread sounds hollow when tapped on bottom. Remove from pan and cool on wire rack. Makes one loaf. Serves 12.

Whole-Wheat French Bread

- 2 cups whole-wheat flour
- $1\frac{1}{2}$ cups all-purpose flour
- 2 teaspoons salt
- 1 package active dry yeast
- $1\frac{2}{3}$ cups warm water (105 to 115°F)
- additional all-purpose flour for kneading

Combine whole-wheat flour, all-purpose flour, and salt in large bowl. Dissolve yeast in warm water. Add yeast to flour mixture; mix well with wooden spoon until dough no longer clings to sides of bowl. Turn onto lightly floured board; knead until smooth and elastic, about 10 minutes. Place in greased bowl; cover and let rise until doubled in bulk, about 90 minutes. Punch dough down; cut dough in half.

Turn each half onto lightly floured board; sprinkle with flour. Roll each half into a 15- by 3-inch rectangle; dust off flour. Knead each half approximately 10 minutes. Then bring edges up and pinch together tightly. Carefully place loaves, pinched side down, on lightly floured baking sheet. Cover with cloth towel; let rise 45 minutes.

Cut three diagonal slashes, about one-fourth inch deep, in each loaf. Preheat oven to 450°F, and spray with water from a plant mister to create steam. Put loaves in oven; spray oven again to create steam. Bake until loaves sound hollow when tapped, about 25 to 30 minutes. Remove loaves from oven and spray lightly with water. Cool on racks. Makes two loaves. Serves 12.

Fresh Salads

Basic Green Salad

1 head lettuce or other greens
1 teaspoon salt
1 clove garlic, peeled
1 tablespoons olive oil
freshly grated black pepper
2 tablespoons wine vinegar

Wash lettuce in cold water. Shake well; pat dry with paper towel. Put salt in bottom of large wooden salad bowl. Grind garlic into salt until half the clove is gone; discard the remainder. Tear lettuce into bite-sized pieces and drop into salad bowl. Pour olive oil over lettuce; toss gently until all the leaves are coated. Sprinkle pepper over lettuce, add vinegar, and toss.

Greens. Experiment with different greens: Bibb lettuce, leafy romaine or escarole, curly chicory, tart endive, rich spinach, pungent watercress. For the crispiest salad greens, wash leaves gently, then pat dry with paper towels and refrigerate in plastic bags until ready to use.

Extras. The basic green salad is often perfect. But when "something extra" suits the meal, try these "extras": tomato wedges; chopped green onion; slices of sweet onion, green pepper, cucumber, or fresh mushrooms; artichoke hearts, broccoli, or cauliflower.

Bean Sprout Salad

- 1 pound fresh bean sprouts
- 1/2 pound fresh mushrooms, sliced
- 1/4 cup vegetable oil
- 2 tablespoons vinegar
- juice of one lemon
- 2 tablespoons soy sauce
- 1 teaspoon prepared mustard
- 1/2 teaspoon paprika
- 2 tablespoons pimentos, chopped
- 1 teaspoon salt
- 1/2 teaspoon pepper
- 1/2 green pepper, chopped

Rinse sprouts under cold water and let drain. Rinse mushrooms and let dry.

Put oil, vinegar, lemon juice, soy sauce, mustard, paprika, pimentos, salt, and pepper in a jar with a lid. Shake well.

Combine sprouts and mushrooms. Before serving, pour dressing over salad and toss. Garnish with chopped green pepper. Serves 6.

Carrot Salad

3 cups carrots, grated (7 medium carrots)
1/2 cup raisins
1 cup non-fat yogurt
1/4 cup orange juice
1 teaspoon lemon juice

Combine carrots and raisins. Take 1/2 cup of carrot-raisin mixture and blend with yogurt, orange juice, and lemon juice. Combine yogurt mixture with remaining carrot-raisin mixture and mix well. Chill, serve cold. Serves 6.

Chunky Chicken Salad

2 cups cooked white rice
1 16-ounce can of chicken broth
2 teaspoons lemon juice
1/2 teaspoon rosemary, crumbled
1 bay leaf
1 1/2 cups chicken, cooked and cut into chunks
1 6-ounce jar marinated artichoke hearts, undrained
1/3 cup green pepper strips
1/3 cup carrot, shredded
1/4 cup green onion, chopped
lettuce
1 tomato or several cherry tomatoes

Prepare rice, substituting the canned chicken broth for the water called for in package directions. Add lemon juice, rosemary, and bay leaf. Cook for 45 minutes. Remove bay leaf. Combine chicken with artichoke hearts, green peppers, carrots, and onion. Toss chicken and vegetables in rice. Serve on leafy lettuce and garnish with tomato wedges or cherry tomatoes. Serves 4.

Cool Cucumber Pasta Salad

1 8-ounce box pasta
1 cucumber, diced
1 tomato, diced
3 stalks scallions, diced
salt
pepper
1/2 cup light mayonnaise

Boil pasta until soft. Rinse under cold water and drain. Add mayonnaise, diced vegetables, salt and pepper to taste. Refrigerate until 30 minutes before serving. Serves 4.

Cucumber and Onion Salad

4 medium cucumbers, thinly sliced
2 red onions, thinly sliced
salt
1 cup water
1 cup vinegar
4 tablespoons sugar

In a 2-quart casserole, layer cucumbers, then onions. Sprinkle with salt. Repeat layers and salt. Cover tightly and drain off liquid every hour for three hours. Combine water, vinegar, and sugar. Cover vegetables and refrigerate overnight. Serves 6.

Danish Salad

Salad:

1 16-ounce can French-style green beans
1 16-ounce can small tender peas
6 stalks celery, chopped
1 large onion, chopped
1 small can pimentos, chopped

Dressing:

2 cups vinegar
1 tablespoon water
3/4 cup sugar
1 teaspoon salt
3/4 teaspoon pepper

Combine beans, peas, celery, onion, and pimentos in large salad bowl. Mix vinegar, water, sugar, salt, and pepper, and pour over salad. Marinate 24 to 48 hours before serving. Serves 8.

Eggplant Salad

1 medium eggplant
1 tomato, chopped
1/4 green pepper, chopped
1/4 onion, chopped
pepper, to taste
vinegar, to taste

Bake eggplant at 350°F for 45 minutes or until soft. Cool. Cut lengthwise, scoop out insides, and chop. In a large bowl, mix eggplant with tomato, green pepper, onion, pepper, and vinegar. Chill. Serve on crackers or bed of lettuce. Serves 4.

Famous Bean Salad

1 8-ounce can green beans
1 8-ounce can wax beans
1 8-ounce can kidney beans
1 8-ounce can chickpeas
1 2-ounce jar pimentos
1 cup onion, finely sliced
1 cup celery, sliced
1 cup vinegar
1 teaspoon salt
1 cup sugar, or substitute

Heat vinegar, salt, and sugar in a small saucepan. Cool. Set aside. Drain beans, chickpeas, and pimentos. Combine with onion and celery. Add vinegar mixture. Cover and refrigerate before serving. Serves 8.

Marinated Vegetable Salad

Salad:

4 small zucchini
2 small yellow squash
1/2 head broccoli
1/2 head cauliflower
2 small carrots
1 red onion
1/2 pound fresh mushrooms

Dressing:

1 cup white vinegar
1/2 cup wine vinegar
1/4 cup lemon juice
salt, to taste
1/2 teaspoon oregano leaves
1/2 teaspoon dry mustard
1/2 teaspoon garlic powder
1/4 teaspoon anise seed

Slice salad vegetables and place in a large bowl. Combine all dressing ingredients in large jar. Shake well and pour over vegetables several hours before serving. Refrigerate. Stir once every hour. Serves 8.

Nutritious Soups

Lunch Box Minestrone

- 2 tablespoons olive oil
- 1/4 cup celery
- 1/4 cup onion
- 1/4 cup zucchini
- 1/4 cup carrot
- 1 small clove garlic, minced
- 3/4 cup cabbage, shredded
- 1 cup tomatoes, peeled, seeded, and chopped
- 2 teaspoons fresh basil, chopped (or 1/2 teaspoon dried)
- 2 teaspoons fresh oregano, chopped (or 1/2 teaspoon dried)
- 1/4 cup small pasta
- 3 cups beef broth
- 3/4 cup chickpeas
- grated Parmesan cheese, to taste

Dice celery, onion, zucchini, and carrot. Sauté vegetables in oil with garlic and cabbage until tender, but not brown. Add remaining ingredients except chickpeas and cheese and simmer 15 minutes. Add chickpeas and simmer another 5 minutes. Stir in a dash of grated Parmesan cheese. Serves 6.

Sprout Soup

1 medium potato, cut into chunks
1 medium carrot, cut into chunks
1 small onion, diced
1 stalk celery, chopped
1 cup vegetable or chicken stock
1/4 teaspoon salt
dash of pepper
2 cups sprouts, coarsely chopped
2 tablespoons soy sauce
2 tablespoons parsley, chopped

Cook potato, carrot, onion, and celery in stock for about 10 minutes. Add salt and pepper. Process in blender until thick and smooth. Return to saucepan; add sprouts and soy sauce and simmer for 3 minutes. Garnish with parsley and serve immediately. Serves 3.

Savory Side Dishes

Gourmet Peas

- 2 cups peas, fresh or frozen
- 1 teaspoon onion, finely chopped
- 1/2 teaspoon mint leaves, dried and crushed
- watercress
- fresh mushrooms, to taste
- 2 tablespoons white wine

Combine peas, onion, and mint leaves in a saucepan. Cook in lightly salted water until just tender. Sauté fresh mushrooms in white wine. Add mushrooms and a handful of snipped watercress to drained, cooked peas just before serving. Serves 4.

Green Rice

- 3/4 cup green onions with tops, thinly sliced
- 1/2 cup green pepper, finely chopped
- 1 cup rice, uncooked
- 1/4 cup parsley, snipped
- 1 teaspoon salt
- 1/4 teaspoon pepper
- 2 cups chicken broth, boiling

Steam onions and green pepper over boiling water until soft but not brown. Place rice in a 2-quart baking dish. Add steamed vegetables, parsley, seasoning, and broth. Stir. Cover with tight-fitting lid or heavy-duty foil. Bake at 350°F for 25 minutes or until rice is tender and liquid is absorbed. Toss lightly with a fork before serving. Serves 6.

Hot Chinese Noodles

- 1 pound medium spaghetti or linguini, cooked and cooled

Garlic Ginger Mix:

- 12 garlic cloves
- 3 inches ginger roots
- 3/4 teaspoon salt
- 4 to 5 tablespoons water

Chop garlic and ginger, and mash with water and salt. Stir Garlic Ginger Mix into linguini. Serves 4 to 6.

Rice Pilaf with Onion

2 tablespoons olive oil
1 cup long-grain or converted rice, uncooked
2 cups chicken broth, or 2 cups hot water and 2 teaspoons chicken-broth granules
2 tablespoons green onion tops, thinly sliced
1/8 teaspoon garlic powder

Heat oil in a medium-sized saucepan over medium-low heat. Add rice and cook until golden in color, stirring occasionally. Meanwhile, heat chicken broth to boiling, and add to rice. Add green onion tops and garlic powder. Cover and simmer for 25 minutes or until all liquid is absorbed. Fluff rice with a fork, and serve. Serves 4.

Rice Salad

4 cups cooked rice
1 chicken bouillon cube
1/2 cup onion
2 tablespoons vinegar
2 teaspoons salt
3/4 cup green pepper
2 cups celery
1 cup green peas, cooked
1 small jar pimentos, chopped

Cook rice according to package directions, adding chicken bouillon cube to water. Mince onion in food processor. Mix together rice, onion, vinegar, and salt. Refrigerate for three hours or overnight. Mince green pepper and celery in food processor. Add to rice mixture along with peas and pimentos. Serves 6.

Steamed Asparagus

1 pound fresh asparagus

Place raw asparagus standing up in a tall steamer. Pack enough asparagus to nearly fill the diameter of the steamer basket. Add water to boiler and drop basket in boiler. Bring water to a boil and cook until the lower part of the asparagus stems are just tender. Serves 4.

Exciting Entrees

Burrito Bundles with Frijoles

- 1/2 cup frijoles (see recipe on page 162)
- 1/2 cup onion, chopped
- 1 8 3/4-ounce can whole kernel corn, drained
- 4 10-inch corn tortillas
- 1 cup green pepper, diced
- 1 1/2 cups lettuce, shredded
- 1 1/2 cups low-fat sharp Cheddar cheese, shredded

Brown onion. Add corn and heat through. Place tortillas between two damp tea towels and warm in oven at 300°F for 3 to 5 minutes or until soft. Divide frijoles, corn, pepper, lettuce, and cheese among tortillas; fold envelope-style to eat. Serves 4.

Frijoles

- 2 1/2 cups pinto, black, or red kidney beans
- 2 onions, finely chopped
- 2 cloves garlic, chopped
- 1 bay leaf
- 2 or more serrano chiles, chopped, or 1 teaspoon dried pequin chiles, crumbled
- 1 tablespoon vegetable oil
- 1 medium tomato, peeled, seeded, and chopped

Wash beans, but do not soak. Put in cold water to cover. Add bay leaf, chiles, and half of the chopped onions and garlic. Cover and simmer gently, adding more water as needed. When beans begin to wrinkle, add oil. When beans are soft and almost done, add seasonings. Cook another 30 minutes without adding more water; there should be little liquid remaining when beans are cooked.

Steam remaining onion and garlic until limp. Add tomato and cook for 1 to 2 minutes; add a tablespoon of beans and mash into the mixture. Add a second tablespoon of beans without draining so that some of the bean liquid evaporates in this cooking process. Add a third tablespoon of beans without draining and continue to cook until the mixture becomes a smooth, fairly heavy paste. Return mixture to the bean pot and stir into beans over low heat, thickening the remaining liquid. Serves 6 to 8.

Chicken with Tomatoes and Chickpeas

1 pound boneless chicken breasts
2 tablespoons olive oil
1/2 pound mushrooms, sliced
1 8-ounce can chickpeas
1 tomato, chopped
1 green pepper, chopped
2 cloves fresh garlic, minced
1 teaspoon paprika
3/4 cup white wine
2 pinches of salt
2 pinches of black pepper

Boil chicken for 15 minutes. Drain. Let cool and slice into bite-sized pieces.

In a large cast-iron skillet, add olive oil, chicken, mushrooms, chickpeas, tomato, green pepper, garlic, and paprika. Cook for 30 minutes. Add salt, black pepper, and white wine, and cook for a few more minutes, then serve. Serves 4.

Mexican Stuffed Peppers

- 6 large green peppers
- 1 pound lean ground beef
- 1 medium-size onion, sliced
- 2 cups crispy rice cereal
- 1/8 teaspoon minced garlic
- 2 teaspoons chili powder
- 1 teaspoon salt
- 1/8 teaspoon pepper
- 1 teaspoon sugar
- 1 6-ounce can tomato paste
- 1 16-ounce can peeled whole tomatoes, drained
- 1/2 cup (2 ounces) sharp Cheddar cheese, shredded

Wash peppers. Cut off tops and remove seedy portions. Precook in large amount of boiling water about 5 minutes. Drain well. Place peppers, cut side up, in shallow nonstick baking pan sprayed with low-fat cooking spray. Set aside.

Place ground beef and onion in a large skillet. Cook over medium heat, stirring frequently, until ground beef is browned. Drain excess drippings. Stir crispy rice cereal, garlic, chili powder, salt, pepper, sugar, tomato paste, and tomatoes into ground beef mixture, cutting tomatoes into pieces with spoon. Remove from heat. Spoon mixture into peppers, dividing evenly.

Bake at 350°F for about 20 minutes or until filling is thoroughly heated. Remove from oven. Sprinkle tops with cheese. Return to oven, and bake about 5 minutes longer or until cheese begins to melt. Serves 6.

Mixed Chinese Vegetables

- 5 large Chinese mushrooms, dried
- 1 cup lukewarm water
- 3/4 cup green cabbage
- 1/2 cup carrot
- 1/2 cup cucumber
- 1 6-ounce can bamboo shoots
- 2 tablespoons sesame-seed oil
- 1/4 cup frozen peas
- 1/2 cup hot chicken broth
- 2 tablespoons soy sauce
- pinch of sugar

Soak mushrooms in water for 30 minutes. Shred cabbage; cut carrots, cucumber, and bamboo shoots into julienne strips. Cube mushrooms. Heat oil in skillet. Add cabbage and cook for 2 minutes. Add mushrooms, cucumbers, carrots, bamboo shoots, and peas. Pour in chicken broth. Season with soy sauce and sugar. Simmer over low heat for 15 minutes. Serve immediately. Serves 2.

Monkfish Kebabs

1 pound monkfish fillets, cubed
2 tablespoons vegetable oil
2 tablespoons dry white wine
1 clove garlic, peeled and finely chopped
1 tablespoon lemon juice
salt and pepper to taste
1/2 teaspoon thyme
1/2 teaspoon oregano
2 onions, cut into chunks
2 green peppers, cut into 2-inch pieces
8 cherry tomatoes
1 zucchini, sliced

Place monkfish in shallow dish. Combine oil, wine, garlic, lemon juice, salt, pepper, thyme, and oregano in bowl and pour over monkfish. Refrigerate for at least one hour.

Drain monkfish; reserve marinade. Place fish, onions, green peppers, tomatoes, and zucchini on eight skewers. Place skewers in shallow baking dish. Pour reserved marinade over skewers, cover, and refrigerate for three hours.

Preheat broiler. Drain skewers; reserve marinade. Place skewers on broiler pan and broil for 8 to 10 minutes, or until fish and vegetables are tender. Baste with reserved marinade; turn skewers frequently. Place skewers on serving platter; serve on or off skewers. Serves 4.

Pasta Fagioli

- 1/3 cup pinto beans
- 1/3 cup kidney beans
- 1/3 cup Great Northern or white beans
- 3 onions, chopped
- 4 stalks celery, chopped
- 4 teaspoons parsley
- 1 8-ounce can tomatoes
- 1 pound trimmed chuck steak, cut into chunks
- salt and pepper to taste
- Italian seasoning to taste
- garlic powder to taste
- water
- large meat bone
- 1 cup farfalle (bow tie) pasta

Soak beans overnight and drain. Brown meat, onions, and celery. Add tomatoes, meat bone, parsley, salt, pepper, Italian seasoning, garlic powder, beans, and 2 quarts water. Cook at least two hours. Remove bone. Add pasta and cook 10 minutes more. Best if marinated one day before eating. It may need to be thinned by adding 1 cup boiling water and a dissolved bouillon cube. Serves 4.

Quick Jamaican Chicken

- 1 chicken breast, split
- 2 tablespoons crushed corn flakes or cracker meal
- salt (or garlic salt)
- pepper to taste
- 3/4 cup tomato juice
- 4 tablespoons scallions or onions, finely chopped (or 1 tablespoon instant onion)
- 1/2 teaspoon allspice, ground
- pinch of thyme, ground
- pinch of hot pepper

Moisten chicken with water. In a plastic bag, shake chicken with crumbs, salt, and pepper. Place chicken skin-side down in a small nonstick pie pan that has been sprayed with cooking spray for no-fat frying. Place pan, uncovered, in an oven preheated to 450°F. Bake 15 minutes; turn chicken skin-side up and bake another 15 to 20 minutes until skin is golden-crisp and well rendered of fat. Drain and discard fat.

Combine tomato juice with remaining ingredients and pour over chicken. Lower heat to 350°F. Bake, basting often, until chicken is tender and sauce is thick (add water if sauce simmers away). Remove skin before serving. Serves 2.

Shrimp and Asparagus

- 1 pound shrimp, shelled, deveined, and cooked
- 1 6-ounce can medium chestnuts, drained and sliced
- 1 medium onion, sliced
- 1 cup fresh mushrooms, sliced
- 1 cup celery, sliced diagonally
- 1 4-ounce can mandarin oranges, drained
- 1 1/2 pounds fresh asparagus, steamed
- 2 tablespoons oil
- 1/4 teaspoon salt
- 1/2 teaspoon black pepper, freshly ground
- 2 tablespoons sugar
- 2 tablespoons soy sauce
- 3 cups rice, cooked

Prepare shrimp and set aside. Drain and slice water chestnuts. On a large tray arrange shrimp, chestnuts, onion, mushrooms, celery, mandarin oranges, and asparagus.

Heat oil in a wok. Add onion, celery, salt, pepper, and sugar. Stir-fry until vegetables are tender, but still on the crisp side. Add asparagus and shrimp. Place water chestnuts and mushrooms over shrimp. Sprinkle with soy sauce and place orange sections on top. Cover and cook until mixture steams. Serve with rice. Serves 4.

Special Turkey Salad

- 1 14-ounce cooked turkey breast, cut into strips
- 1 1/4 cups celery
- 2 yellow peppers, seeded and cut into strips
- 1 small onion, grated
- 1/4 cup low-fat mayonnaise
- 1 6-ounce container plain low-fat yogurt
- 2 teaspoons hot mustard
- 2 teaspoons maple syrup
- 1/2 teaspoon salt
- 1/8 teaspoon pepper
- green celery tops for garnish

Mix turkey, celery, and yellow peppers together in bowl. Mix grated onion with mayonnaise, yogurt, mustard, maple syrup, salt, and pepper. Toss turkey mixture in dressing, cover, and let stand at room temperature for 10 minutes before serving. Garnish with green celery tops and serve. Serves 4.

Stuffed Zucchini

- 2 zucchini
- 2 cups mushrooms, chopped
- 1 cup onion, chopped
- 2 cloves garlic, crushed
- 2 tablespoons dry white wine
- 1/4 cup parsley, chopped
- 1/2 teaspoon basil or thyme
- pepper to taste
- 1 teaspoon soy sauce
- 1 cup non-fat cottage cheese
- 3/4 cup cooked brown rice (or millet or bread crumbs)

Slice zucchini in half lengthwise. Cut out center with a knife or spoon, leaving about 1/4-inch skin thickness all around. Place zucchini shells in a large pan and add a little water. Steam for 5 minutes. Sauté mushrooms, onion, and garlic in wine in a sauté pan for a few minutes. (Add the zucchini insides if you want.) Add parsley, basil, pepper, and soy sauce, sautéing several more minutes.

Turn off heat, add cottage cheese and rice, and mix well. Let mixture sit a few minutes. Drain mixture through a colander, saving liquid for later. Fill zucchini with vegetable-cheese mixture. Lay zucchini on a baking dish, and bake for 30 minutes at 350°F. Place drained liquid in saucepan, heat. To thicken, add a little cornstarch or arrowroot and cold water to the sauce. Cook sauce lightly to thicken, stirring often. Spoon sauce over zucchini and serve. Serves 4.

Vegetable Lasagna

- 4 medium zucchini, coarsely chopped
- 1 large onion, chopped
- 1 medium green pepper, chopped
- 1 carrot, finely chopped
- 1/2 cup celery, chopped
- 2 garlic cloves, minced
- 1/4 cup olive oil
- 2 16-ounce cans tomatoes in tomato sauce
- 1 8-ounce can tomato sauce
- 1 6-ounce can tomato paste
- 1/4 cup dry white wine
- 2 tablespoons parsley, finely chopped
- 2 teaspoon oregano
- 1 teaspoon basil
- 1 teaspoon salt
- 1/2 teaspoon thyme
- 1/4 teaspoon pepper
- 9 wide curly lasagna noodles, cooked
- 2 cups (1 pound) part-skim ricotta cheese
- 10 ounces skim mozzarella cheese, shredded
- 1/2 cup Parmesan cheese, grated

In a large skillet, cook zucchini, onion, green pepper, carrot, celery, and garlic in oil over medium heat for 15 minutes, stirring frequently. Stir in tomatoes, tomato sauce, and tomato paste; add seasonings. Bring to a boil, stirring to break up tomatoes. Reduce heat, cover, and simmer 30 minutes. Uncover and boil to reduce sauce to about 5 cups.

In an $11\frac{1}{2}$- by $9\frac{1}{2}$-inch baking pan, spread about one fourth of the sauce over bottom of pan. Arrange three noodles on top; dot with one-third of the ricotta; then sprinkle with one-fourth of the mozzarella and one fourth of the Parmesan. Repeat procedure twice. Spread remaining sauce over all; top with remaining mozzarella and Parmesan. Bake at 350°F for 30 to 45 minutes. Let stand 5 minutes before serving. Serves 8.

Delicious Desserts

Apple-Grape Salad

2 medium tart apples, peeled, quartered, cored
1/2 pound blue grapes, halved, seeded
1 stalk garden mint (leaves only)
2 teaspoons sugar
2 tablespoons lemon juice

Cut apples crosswise in thin slices. Arrange grapes, apples, and mint leaves in glass bowl. Sprinkle with sugar and lemon juice. Toss lightly, then cover. Chill one hour before serving. Serves 4.

Cranberry Applesauce

5 pounds red apples (about 25 apples)
3/4 cup water
1 pound cranberries
1 1/4 cups sugar, more or less, depending on sweetness of apples

Wash apples; cut into quarters. (Do not peel or core.) Place water and quartered apples in large Dutch oven (5- or 6-quart size).

Wash cranberries; place on top of apples. Cover; bring to boil over medium heat. Lower heat; cook until apples lose their shape and are tender, about 30 minutes. Stir occasionally to prevent sticking and to allow apples to cook uniformly. When apples and cranberries are cooked, remove from heat. Press through food mill or blend until desired consistency. Sweeten with sugar to taste. Serve applesauce warm or chilled. Extra applesauce can be frozen or canned. Serves 6.

Crocked Acorn Squash

2 acorn squash
1/2 cup apple juice or cider
cinnamon (or pumpkin pie spice)

Cut squash into quarters and scrape away seeds. Place squash in a crock cooker skin-side down. Pour 1/4 -cup to 1/2 -cup apple juice over squashes and sprinkle very lightly with ground cinnamon. Cover and cook on low setting two to four hours. Serves 8.

Lemon Sherbet

1 1/2 teaspoons unflavored gelatin
2 tablespoons cold water
2 cups skim milk
3/4 cup sugar
1/2 cup lemon juice
1/2 teaspoon lemon rind, grated
2 egg whites, stiffly beaten

Soak gelatin in water several minutes. Heat milk. Add sugar and gelatin; stir until dissolved. Chill in refrigerator until just firm. Gradually stir in lemon juice and rind. Pour into freezer-safe tray or bowl and freeze until slushy. Turn into chilled bowl; beat with electric beater until fluffy but not melted. Fold in beaten egg whites. Return to freezer and freeze until firm. Serves 6.

Pineapple-Grape Parfaits

2 1/2 cups seedless green grapes, halved
1 8-ounce can crushed pineapple, drained
1/4 cup brown sugar
dash of ginger
1 cup low-fat vanilla yogurt

Reserve 6 grape halves for topping. Combine grapes and pineapple. In a separate bowl, stir brown sugar and ginger into yogurt. Alternately spoon fruit mixture and yogurt mixture into 6 parfait glasses, starting with fruit and ending with yogurt. Place reserved grape halves on top of each parfait. Chill at least 3 hours before serving. Serves 6.

Three Fruit Sherbet

2 bananas
3/4 cup orange juice
1/3 cup lemon juice
1 egg
1 cup powdered sugar
1 cup skim or evaporated milk

Place all ingredients in electric blender and beat until smooth, about 1 minute. Pour fruit mixture into ice cube tray and freeze until firm. Serves 6.

Variation: Instead of bananas, use 4 to 5 medium-sized peeled pears or 1 medium melon.

Refreshing Beverages

Apple-Pineapple Cooler

3 cups unsweetened apple juice
2 cups unsweetened pineapple juice
1 cup orange juice
2 tablespoons freshly squeezed lime or lemon juice
orange slices to garnish

Combine juices and orange slices; chill. Garnish glasses with orange slices. Serves 6.

Fruit Tea Punch

- 2 cups boiling water
- 4 black-tea bags
- 1/4 cup lemon juice
- 2 cups orange juice
- 1 tablespoon honey
- 1 lemon
- 2 oranges
- 2 cups fresh strawberries
- 1 bottle soda water

Pour boiling water over tea bags. Steep 3 minutes; remove tea bags. Blend in lemon and orange juice; sweeten with honey. Cut peel from lemon and oranges; section fruit. Remove all membranes. Add to tea. Wash and hull strawberries; cut in half; add to tea. Cover and refrigerate punch at least six hours to blend flavors. Just before serving, add bottle of soda water. Serves 10.

REFERENCES

Barnard, Neal. *Food for Life*. New York: Harmony Books, 1993.

———. *Foods That Can Cause You To Lose Weight*. McKinney, Texas: The Magni Group, 1992.

Bennion, Lynn, Edwin L. Bierman, and James M. Ferguson. *Straight Talk About Weight Control*. New York: Consumer Reports Books, 1991.

Bricklin, Mark, and Claire Gerus. *Prevention's Lose Weight Guidebook*. Emmaus, Pennsylvania: Rodale Press, 1994.

Bricklin, Mark, and Sharon Stocker. *Prevention's Medical Healing Yearbook*. Emmaus, Pennsylvania: Rodale Press, 1991.

Brody, Jane. *Jane Brody's Nutrition Book*. New York: W. W. Norton & Co. Inc., 1981.

Consumers Guide, ed. *Cholesterol: Your Guide for a Healthy Heart*. Lincolnwood, Illinois: Publications International Ltd., 1989.

MacDonald, Helen Bishop, and Margaret Howard. *Eat Well, Live Well: The Canadian Dietetic Association's Guide to Healthy Eating.* Toronto: MacMillan, 1990.

Moquette-Magee, Elaine. *Fight Fat & Win!* Minneapolis: CHRONIMED/DCI Publishing, 1990.

Ornish, Dean. *Stress, Diet & Your Heart.* New York: Henry Holt & Co., 1982.

Schwartz, Rose. *The Enlightened Eater.* Toronto: Stoddart Publishing Co. Ltd., 1989.

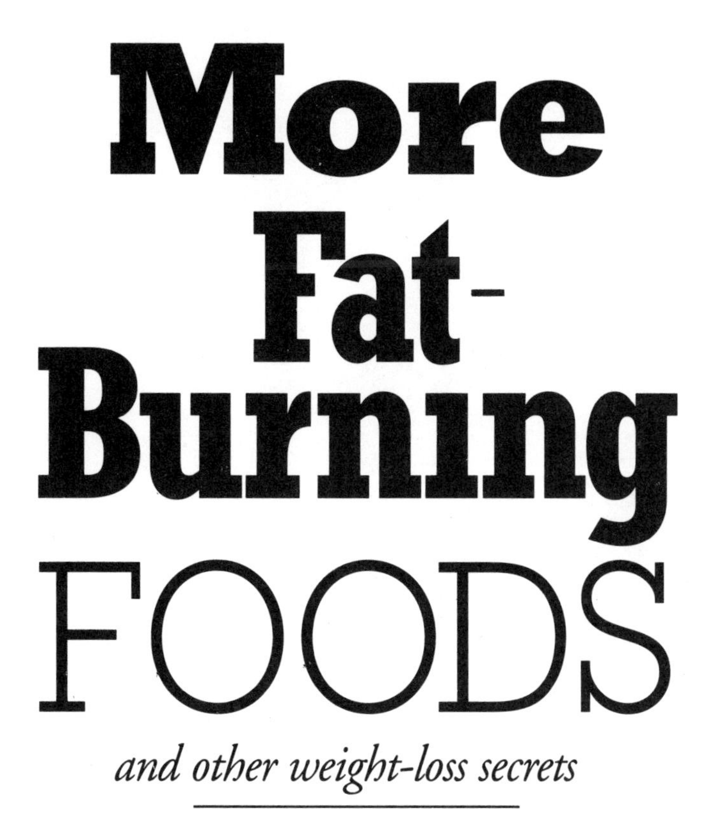

More Fat-Burning FOODS

and other weight-loss secrets

By Porter Shimer
Recipes edited by Betty Bianconi, R.D.

5 Park Center Court, Suite 300
Owings Mills, Maryland 21117 USA

Printed in the United States of America
HE007 M L K J I H G F E D C B A

CONTENTS

INTRODUCTION
193

CHAPTER 1
YOUR FULL—AND FLAT!—STOMACH
197

CHAPTER 2
TIPS FOR A LEANER LIFESTYLE
239

CHAPTER 3
HOW FITNESS FIGHTS FAT
281

CHAPTER 4
VITAMINS AND MINERALS: BEST FOOD SOURCES
311

CHAPTER 5
NICE AND EASY FAT-BURNING RECIPES
319

INTRODUCTION

Hello—and welcome to the end of your struggles to lose weight.

No matter how many times you have tried before, this time you're going to succeed! The reason: You're going to learn how to live *with* food rather than without it.

If food was your enemy before, it will soon be your friend. No longer will you fear it, or feel guilty about eating it, or have to endure the pain of doing without it. The truth is, the fatal flaw of your previous weight-loss efforts probably has been that you've been trying to eat too little!

No way, you say? It's those second helpings and midnight trips to the refrigerator that are your downfall?

Well, while it's true that those activities certainly won't help you lose weight, have you ever asked yourself why you feel the need for that extra food? Hunger, perhaps? Feelings of deprivation? Or could your body be telling you that it's not happy skipping breakfast, or eating just a salad for lunch, or pouring "dinner" from an eight-ounce can?

Fact: Any weight-loss effort that deprives us is going to fail. That's a rule engraved in the very genes that have gotten us where we are today. Our ancestors who lived in caves survived because they were able to feed their hunger, not ignore it. Why should we be any different?

We aren't, as the latest surveys make painfully clear. During the past 40 years, when "dieting" has become so popular, we've not only not lost weight, we've gained an average of 10 pounds. That's right: We're fatter today than we were back when we buttered our white bread clear to the edges, went to the malt shop instead of the gym, and ate our cheeseburgers guilt-free!

The "Dieter's" Dilemma

Our diets have failed not just because they ask us to accept feeling hungry but because they undermine the very biochemical processes on which fat-loss depends. Studies now show that to burn fat most effectively, our bodies need energy—something that's in very short supply when dinner is little more than a salad or a cup of broth. Think of the excess fat on your body as something like a log in a fireplace: Without energy from the right "kindling"—that is, food—your body cannot generate enough heat to get the fat "burning" as energy.

In fact, the less we eat, the more stubborn our body fat becomes. This is because cutting calories forces our bodies into what scientists call their "starvation response"—a holdover from prehistoric times when we learned to burn fewer calories as a way of preserving body fat to help us survive times of famine. The consequence of this response for us today, unfortunately, is that the fewer calories we consume, the more inclined our bodies are to store these calories as fat.

Making matters even worse is what low-calorie diets do to our metabolism in the long run: By causing the loss of muscle tissue, which is the best calorie burner we have, diets make us even more prone to gain weight when the diet is over.

The end result is a "Catch-22" you may know all too well. You are haunted by hunger pangs and cravings when you're on a low-calorie diet, and whatever you do eat becomes even more fattening because your metabolism has slowed to a crawl. Worse yet, *you* slow to a crawl. Out of calories and "out of gas," you're left with barely enough energy to go about your day. You certainly don't feel like engaging in any fat-burning or muscle-building exercises.

Fat-Burning Foods to the Rescue

There is a solution to the dilemma—and it's a surprisingly simple and appetizing one: To keep your fat-burning fires adequately "stoked," you've got to eat!

But before you call your local pizzeria or head to the nearest ice cream parlor, be aware that you can't eat just anything you want. If you fill up on foods that are high in fat or that contain too much refined sugar, you'll be feeding your fat cells instead of starving them. What you will have to do is stoke your body's fat-burning fires with the foods it will use directly and immediately for energy.

We'll be looking at these foods and the biology behind their fat-burning powers shortly, but let it suffice to say that not all foods are created equal when it comes to weight gain. Calorie-for-calorie, some foods are better at burning fat while others are more chemically suited for becoming fat. A lifetime of successful weight control, therefore, can become a simple matter of consuming more of the former foods and less of the latter.

Fat-Burning for the Health of It

Weight control aside, there's another reason fat-burning foods should be on your table every day: They can be your "meal ticket" to better health. Studies by such prestigious organizations as the American Heart Association, the American Cancer Society, and the Centers for Disease Control and Prevention in Atlanta now show that a diet centered around these foods can help reduce risks of virtually every major illness we face today, including heart disease, high blood pressure, strokes, diabetes, osteoporosis (softening of the bones), and cancers of the prostate, cervix, and breast.

That these foods also are economical and among the most tasty on the planet is simply icing on the cake.

At the end of this book, you will have learned about foods that will help you live not only leaner but longer! So make yourself comfortable and get ready to say goodbye to your fat.

Get ready, too, to learn about the right ways to exercise to give these foods an even greater fat-burning effect. Exercise—by bringing oxygen into the body like a strong breeze to a brush fire—has been shown to turn up the metabolic "heat" of fat-burning foods even more. Exercise also can help maintain and build the muscle tissue that is your body's greatest ally for making weight loss last.

Encouraged? Good. You should be. You're about to embark on the weight-loss venture that will be your last!

CHAPTER 1

YOUR FULL—AND FLAT!—STOMACH

Have you ever noticed how your appetite can be like a bar of wet soap: The more you try to control it, the more it's apt to slip away? You can be good for a while, but then whammo: out come the butter pecan ice cream and the chocolate marshmallow cookies.

There's a reason for this, and it goes as far back as we do—back to when a full stomach was a goal and not a source of guilt. "Severe calorie restriction runs counter to a very basic human instinct," says Yale University psychologist Judith Roden, Ph.D., "which is to perceive hunger as a threat."

In other words, our aversion to hunger is in our genes. We endured the rigors of our evolution by eating what we could, when we could. Survival of the fittest meant survival of the fullest, and to a degree we are genetically programmed to think of food in these same terms today.

F.Y.I.

Number of Americans currently on a diet:	48 million
Percentage increase in overweight Americans over the past 10 years:	28
Weight the average American gains between the ages of 25 and 55:	30 pounds
Amount of muscle that converts to fat during this time:	15 pounds
Percentage of Americans who exercise irregularly or not at all:	58
Number one excuse given by the average American for not exercising more:	Lack of time
Minutes per day the average American watches TV:	240
Estimated yearly cost associated with health complications caused by obesity:	$68.8 billion

Diets Teach Fat to Fight Back

We go head-to-head with Mother Nature when we try to starve ourselves thin, and it's a battle Mother Nature wins nearly every time. As we saw in our introduction, severely restricting calories not only slows the rate at which our bodies burn calories, it robs us of the very muscle tissue on which fat-burning depends! This is why nine out of ten dieters who attempt to reduce their caloric intake fail.

Reducing calories is a trap that has snared dieters by the millions. In fact, many nutritionists feel that our attempts to lose weight have been a major reason we've put on so much weight. Low-calorie diets teach our bodies to hold on to the very fat we're trying so desperately to lose.

"Diets teach fat cells to defend themselves," explains nutritionist Debrah Waterhouse. "Fat cells evolved to keep us alive during times of famine, and they interpret low-calorie diets as just that—a famine. They respond by holding onto the fat they already have, and by becoming even more aggressive at taking in new fat once the diet is over. The result is a system of fat protection that can be very hard to break, especially since the system gets stronger each time a new diet is tried."

Eating Less But Weighing More

Now we understand that drastically cutting calories can actually make fat cells more stubborn. The average woman today, despite consuming 200 fewer calories a day, weighs six pounds more than the average woman did 30 years ago. Might it be because she has been on an average of ten diets in her lifetime?

Witness, moreover, the bodily "inflation" we've suffered in the last 10 years alone, a decade during which dieters have joined weight-loss programs in record numbers. The National Center for Health Statistics reports that while 41 percent of women and 51 percent of men exceeded acceptable weight limits in 1987, both of those figures are up by nearly 20 percent today.

Dieting is so damaging to the body's ability to burn fat, some doctors actually put their underweight patients on low-calorie diets, followed by periods of normal eating, to give their bodies a fat-gaining boost!

Weighty Matters

Average yearly cost of participating in a commercial weight-loss program:	$608
Number of people participating in commercial weight-loss programs who maintain their weight loss for at least seven years:	One out of 250
Average cost of liposuction (surgical removal of fat):	$5,000 per pound!
Percentage of liposuction patients who experience a regrowth of their fat:	29

Satisfaction Guaranteed

Are you afraid that hunger might be a problem on a low-fat diet? Then feast on this fact. To get the same amount of fat in just one fast-food super burger, such as a Whopper or a Big Mac (approximately 60 grams), you would have to eat all of the following:

- *half a pound of broiled chicken*
- *four ounces of a low-fat fish*
- *six scallops*
- *an entire head of lettuce*
- *one onion*
- *one cup of kidney beans*
- *one cup of brown rice*
- *one pound of string beans*
- *one sweet potato*
- *one ear of sweet corn*
- *one cup of raisins*
- *one orange*
- *two red beets*
- *four spears of asparagus*
- *one half pound of peas*
- *one cup of air-popped popcorn*
- *one cup of cooked spaghetti*
- *two slices of whole wheat bread*

Now that's a sandwich!

Race Not Always to the Swift

Wait a minute? No miraculous overnight results? You were hoping to squeeze into that size eight by the weekend?

Sorry, but fat loss—true fat loss—cannot be rushed. Most experts now agree that losses of approximately one pound a week are best to assure that the majority of the weight lost will be from actual fat. Any diet that has you losing weight faster than that is going to be cheating you in either of two ways: It's going to have you losing mere water weight, which you can gain back with one trip to the water cooler, or it's going to cost you the muscle tissue needed to make your weight loss last.

Sure, when you lose weight fast, you can weigh less according to your bathroom scale. But not because you've actually lost any appreciable amounts of fat and not because you've done anything to improve your chances of maintaining a desirable weight in the future. There's a rule of thumb regarding weight loss in this regard that you might consider posting on your refrigerator door:

The Longer Weight Loss Takes,
The Longer It's Going To Last!

Losing weight is a race won by the tortoise rather than the hare. You've got to learn to get comfortable with the foods that are not just going to get you thinner, but that will keep you that way for the rest of your life.

Fat-Burning Foods under the Microscope

And just what sort of foods might these be? Lots of lettuce and celery, perhaps? There's certainly not a lot of fat-making potential there, right? Or will it be some bizarre combination like vinegar and ice cream? (Now there's a combo sure to limit your caloric intake!)

Relax. Not only are the best foods for burning fat surprisingly "normal," they are tasty, nutritious, and filling. They're foods you see in your supermarket every time you shop. If there's anything "unusual" about these foods, it's that they have a biochemical inclination for helping your body get rid of fat rather than store it. They're fat "breakers" not fat "makers."

FAT-BURNING FACT:

Percentage of people able to stop taking high blood pressure medication after losing just 10 pounds: 60.

If that sounds a little too good to be true, it's not. Research shows that certain foods, with one or more of the following components, are capable of waging war against fat:

- **Complex Carbohydrates:** Capable of fighting fat by providing the energy needed to step up the body's basic metabolic (fat-burning) rate. Complex carbohydrates are found in starchy foods such as breads, potatoes, cereals, pasta, and rice. They are not to be confused with the faster-digested simple carbohydrates (sucrose, glucose, and fructose) found in sweet-tasting foods such as candies, cookies, soft drinks, and sugary desserts. Because simple carbohydrates contain virtually no nutrients or fiber, and because they fail to provide feelings of fullness as complex carbohydrates do, they should be eaten sparingly as part of a fat-burning diet.

- **Fiber:** Capable of fighting fat by controlling insulin levels (and hence the ease with which calories can be stored as fat) and by providing feelings of fullness. Fiber also helps to send fats through the intestines before they have time to be fully absorbed. Fiber is most abundant in fruits, vegetables, beans, and whole-grain cereals and breads.

- **Low-Fat Protein:** Capable of fighting fat by building and maintaining fat-burning muscle tissue and by preventing other foods (including carbohydrates) from being digested too quickly. Best sources are low-fat varieties of fish and seafood, lean meats, low-fat dairy products, and beans.

- **Healthy Fats:** Capable of fighting fat by providing feelings of fullness and by controlling cravings. Research also shows that healthful fats—the monounsaturated fat found in olive oil, for example, and the polyunsaturated omega-3 fatty acids found in fish—can help keep the heart and blood vessels healthy by lowering levels of harmful (LDL) cholesterol levels in the blood. The type of fat to avoid is the saturated fat found in beef, pork, the skin of chicken and turkey, and full-fat dairy products such as whole milk, ice cream, and cheese.

Your Top Fat-Burning Foods

The following types of foods should make up the bulk of your diet if you're really serious about achieving and maintaining a healthy weight for the rest of your life. The list is by no means complete. Many other fruits, vegetables, complex carbohydrates, and low-fat proteins also can act as valuable weight-control allies. Consider this list of foods as a foundation for getting your lifelong weight-control program off to a healthful—and delicious!—start.

Fruits	Vegetables	Complex Carbohydrates	Low-Fat Proteins
Apples	Asparagus	Bagels	Chicken breast
Blueberries	Beets	Beans (all types)	Egg whites*
Citrus fruits	Broccoli	Couscous	Low-fat cottage cheese
Kiwi fruit	Brussels sprouts	Oatmeal	Low-fat fish
Melons	Carrots	Pasta	Low-fat yogurt
Peaches	Eggplant	Rice	White meat turkey
Strawberries	Green beans	Whole-grain breads	
	Onions		
	Potatoes		
	Yams		

* or non-fat egg substitutes

The Importance of Balance

Potatoes! Pasta! Bagels! You'll be in high-carbohydrate heaven!

But wait! Let's not forget that your ideal fat-burning diet should be a balance of these fat-burning foods. Don't make the mistake of concentrating too heavily on one type. That could be the reason past weight-loss programs have failed. Diets that focus too narrowly on a single food group miss the forest for the trees, sacrificing health and/or flavor along the way.

High-protein diets, for example, achieve weight loss primarily through reducing the water in your body, and diets that allow only limited types of foods (the "ice cream diet" or the "grapefruit diet") usually wind up being simply low-calorie regimens because the monotony of the menu causes dieters to lose their appetites. Even diets too high in otherwise healthful carbohydrates can backfire by causing high levels of insulin in the blood, which results in seemingly insatiable hunger.

Not so if you eat the right foods in the right balance. Most nutritionists now agree that the most healthful diet consists of the following:

- 60 percent of calories from carbohydrates (preferably complex)
- 15 percent from protein
- 25 percent from fat (no more than 10 percent saturated)

FOOD GUIDE PYRAMID

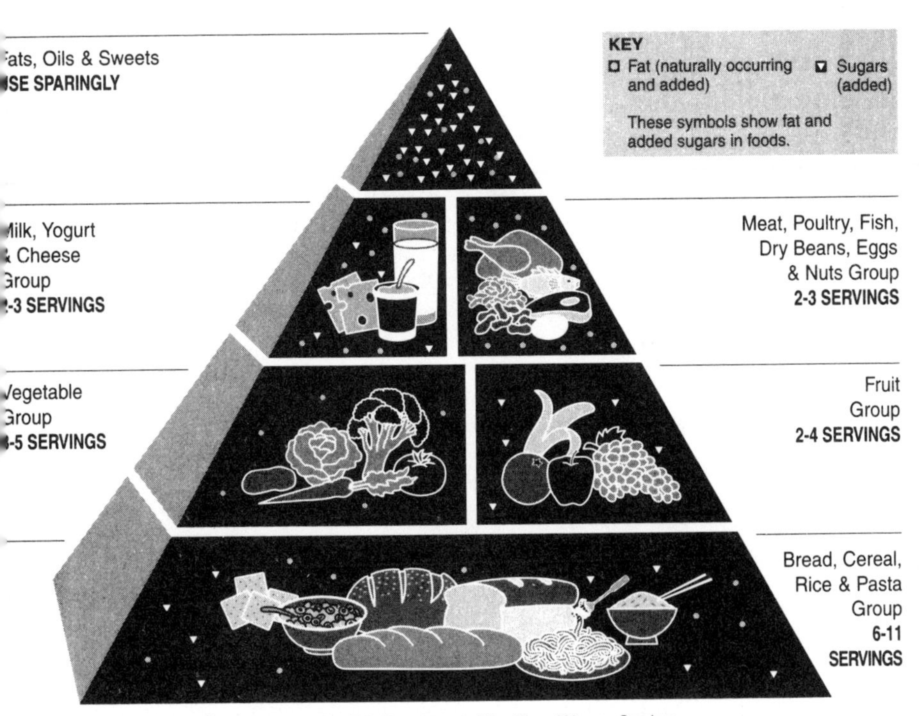

Source: U.S. Department of Agriculture/U.S. Department of Health and Human Services

Climb the Food Pyramid to Better Health

If those numbers confuse you, take a look at the food "pyramid" on the previous page. It was created by the U.S. Department of Agriculture (USDA) to make it easier for Americans to get a clearer "picture" of what a healthful diet should include.

Grain-based Foods *(6 to 11 servings daily):* This is the food group that should make up the bulk of your diet. It includes breads, rice, cereals, and pastas—all important for adding fat-burning complex carbohydrates to your diet.

Fruits *(2 to 4 servings)* **and Vegetables** *(3 to 5 servings):* This is the second most important food group. It is vital for adding important vitamins, minerals, and fiber to your diet.

Protein Foods—Dairy Products *(2 to 3 servings)* **and Meats, Beans, and Eggs** *(2 to 3 servings):* This group makes up the third level of the pyramid. Protein foods are important for maintaining healthy muscle tissue—the best fat-burning tissue your body has.

Fats and Sweets: This is the least important food group and includes butter, margarine, cooking oils, and foods high in refined sugar such as candies and rich desserts. Foods from this group should be eaten sparingly.

Some Facts About Fat

A Fair Shake for Fat: A Little Dab Will Do

But what is any kind of fat doing on a weight-loss program? Doesn't that stuff serve up nine calories per gram compared with only four for carbohydrates and proteins? And isn't fat a major cause of heart disease? And hasn't new research shown that fat's calories are actually more fattening than those from carbohydrates or proteins because, once digested, they turn more easily into fat?

Yes to all of the above. But that doesn't mean that limited amounts of the right kinds of fat can't help grease the wheels of a successful weight-loss program. Research now shows that certain amounts of fat may be needed to slow the rate at which carbohydrates are metabolized. This helps put the brakes on hunger. In fact, some fats are now being recognized as actually lowering cholesterol levels in the blood, which is good for the blood vessels and the heart.

Learn What Kinds of Fat You're up Against

Before you refill your butter dish, understand that we're not talking about a lot of fat—approximately 25 percent of total calories—and that not all types of fat are worthy of inclusion. The most healthful fats are monounsaturated and polyunsaturated fats (for best sources, see below). The fats to avoid are saturated fats, which are found principally in full-fat dairy products, such as butter, and in hydrogenated oils, beef, and pork. Studies show that these fats, in addition to piling on the calories, are without a doubt the primary contributors to the build-up of LDL cholesterol (the bad kind) and other fatty substances in the blood.

As proof, witness one study that found no decreases in cholesterol levels for people on a diet that contained just 25 percent fat but all of it saturated. When these same people were switched to a low-fat diet with unsaturated fat, their cholesterol levels quickly fell by an average of 20 percent.

But cholesterol aside, all fats, regardless of type, are high in calories (approximately 120 calories per tablespoon). Therefore they should be consumed sparingly as part of your fat-burning diet. Keep that in mind as you make that oil and vinegar salad dressing, or prepare to sauté vegetables. Whether it's "good" or "bad" oil, use as little as possible!

FAT-BURNING FACT:

Studies show that for every one percent drop in serum cholesterol levels, the risk of heart disease drops by two percent.

Good Fats

Monounsaturated:

Olive oil	(75%)*
Canola oil	(60%)
Peanut oil	(50%)

In Between Fats

Polyunsaturated:

Safflower oil	(75%)
Sunflower oil	(70%)
Corn oil	(60%)
Cottonseed oil	(55%)

Bad Fats

Saturated:

Coconut oil	(90%)
Butter fat	(65%)
Beef fat	(50%)
Palm oil	(50%)
Chicken fat	(30%)

*Percentages refer to the amount that each oil or fat is comprised of the type of fat represented.

Why Fat Is So Fattening

But please don't be lulled into a sense of false security about the advisability of a certain amount of fat in your weight-control plans. Given our current average intake (approximately 38 percent of calories according to most estimates), the fat in our diets remains the number one contributor to the fat on our bodies. Until we accept that fact—and do something about it—our best weight-loss efforts are going to be exercises in futility.

If your diet is like most people's, you're going to have to cut back on fat to encourage your body to burn more fat. (You may consider that another cardinal rule of weight loss worthy of being displayed prominently on your refrigerator door!)

Why Is Fat Such a Dieter's Waterloo?

Because in addition to containing more than twice as many calories as carbohydrates and proteins per gram, food fat becomes body fat quite easily. While carbohydrates and proteins require considerable "work" from our digestive systems before they are converted to body fat, food fat turns into body fat quickly and easily—within hours of ingestion, in fact. The reason, not surprisingly, is that dietary fat and body fat are chemically very similar. Therefore, very few biochemical steps are needed to make the dietary fat to body fat conversion.

Not so with carbohydrates and proteins. Studies show that nearly one quarter of the calories from carbohydrates and proteins go directly to revving up the body's fat-burning engines. The rest will be stored for later use.

Consider, for example, the following numbers: If you were to eat 100 calories from fat, only 3 of those calories would boost your body's metabolic (calorie-burning) rate. But eat 100 calories in the form of carbohydrates or proteins and whammo: 23 of those calories go toward stoking your body's fat-burning fires.

Fat Really Does "Stick to the Ribs"

If that sounds like much ado about nothing, it's not. A difference of 23 calories for every 100 calories consumed can begin to add up quickly, as people taking part in a study reported in the *International Journal of Obesity* several years ago found out. The people were put on one of two very high-calorie diets—one high in fat, the other low in fat but high in carbohydrates. The purpose of the experiment was to see if there might be a difference in how long it would take for people to gain weight on each diet. There was a difference—a huge one.

"We need to start thinking of the fat we eat as the fat we wear."

Peter Vash, M.D, Professor of Medicine,
University of California

While the people on the low-fat diet took a little over seven months to gain 30 pounds, those assigned to the high-fat regimen amassed their 30 pounds in less than half that time, even though their diet was slightly lower in calories. (Not surprisingly, the people on the high-fat diet, more so than the low-fat group, gained weight primarily in the stomach area.)

So yes, the old saying that fatty foods "stick to the ribs" may be truer than we've known.

Trimming Fat Can Make "Cents," Too!

But aren't low-fat and calorie-reduced foods costly?

Yes, fat-reduced versions of some foods can be more expensive than their regular counterparts, but many foods that are naturally low in fat tend to be cheaper than fattier alternatives. Potatoes, beans, rice, and pasta are fantastic food bargains.

Researchers from Columbia University monitored the food costs of 291 people on low-fat diets for a period of nine months. The food bills of these people averaged approximately a dollar a day less on their low-fat regimens, which researchers calculated could save the average family of four approximately $1,000 dollars a year.

Now that's a nice bonus for eating healthfully. By thinning your waist, you fatten your wallet!

Less Fat for More Muscle

The process by which dietary fat becomes body fat is simple and direct because the two are chemically similar in the first place. Carbohydrates and low-fat proteins, by comparison, prefer not to be turned into fat at all. They're chemically more suited to being consumed by muscle cells for the production of energy. Better yet, some research has suggested that eating carbohydrates and low-fat proteins may encourage muscular growth even without additional exercise.

This was demonstrated in an experiment conducted by researchers from the University of Illinois in which women on low-fat, high-carbohydrate diets not only lost substantial amounts of body fat, they actually boosted their muscle mass by a surprising 2.2 percent. That might not sound like a lot, but the increase occurred without the women engaging in any exercise outside their normal routines. How was that muscle "born"?

The researchers speculated that the high-carbohydrate diet may have increased the women's energy levels to a point where they had become more active without realizing it!

Runners have been aware of the energizing effects of carbohydrates for years. Carbohydrates do well at fueling exercise because they turn into glucose, your body's favorite muscle fuel, so quickly after ingestion. Michael Yessis, Ph.D., exercise physiologist and author of *Body Shaping* (Rodale Press, 1993), puts it this way: "Carbohydrates make you feel most like exercising, they provide the best fuel for that exercise, and they do the best job of replenishing muscles with the fuels that exercise uses up."

Fat Cells: "Fitter" Than Muscle Cells for Regrowth

It doesn't seem fair, but it's a fact of life, nonetheless. While the number of muscle cells we have is fixed at birth (exercise can only make them larger; it cannot increase their number), fat cells can begin to split and multiply any time we eat enough to allow them to become "too big for their britches."

To make matters worse, "The number of fat cells we have can always go up, but never come down," says Dr. Glenn Gaesser, a professor of exercise physiology at the University of Virginia and the author of *Big Fat Lies* (Ballantine Books, 1996). "Once we've got them, they're ours to keep."

"Exercising with a friend gives many people a surge of energy on days when they otherwise wouldn't feel like working out."

Johathan Robison, Ph.D., Executive Co-Director of the Michigan Center for Preventative Medicine

This is not the case with muscle cells, unfortunately, which can wither and die if we don't give them enough to do. This is why it is so important to avoid obesity, which is caused by overeating and lack of exercise. It trades muscle cells for fat cells in a "deal" that can never be fully undone.

The Satisfaction Factor

Okay, so a low-fat, high-carbohydrate diet can be great for providing energy and burning fat. But will such a diet be able to keep visions of cheesecake from dancing in our heads? There's not an apple on earth, after all, that can satisfy like a hot fudge sundae with jimmies.

Try telling that to the group of students who took part in an interesting study done recently at the University of Sydney in Australia. The students were asked to eat 240-calorie portions of dozens of different foods, after which they were measured for degrees of fullness at 15-minute intervals for a period of two hours. Much to everyone's amazement—including the students'—apples satisfied twice as long as ice cream. A bowl of oatmeal satisfied three times longer than a doughnut. A potato six times longer than a croissant.

So, no, foods do not have to be high in fat to satisfy. Other factors are more important. Things such as the sheer weight and volume of a particular food, which signal feelings of fullness within the digestive track. And how long it takes to chew a food—the longer the better so that feelings of fullness can have time to occur before too many calories have been consumed. (How long, after all, does it take to scarf down a 400-calorie piece of cheesecake?) Critical, too, is the amount of fiber in the food. In addition to having the weight-control advantage of sweeping fats through the intestines undigested, fiber gives us a feeling of fullness by absorbing water.

Bottom line: Some of the best foods for weight loss also can be the most satisfying, and if you don't think so, just take a look at the following list. These are the foods that scored the highest, and the lowest, in the "satiation contest" mentioned above.

The numbers that follow these foods refer to the food's "satiation index," that is, the food's ability to quell hunger for as long, and for as few calories, as possible. (Incidentally, virtually all of the "best" foods appear prominently on the list of fat-burning foods that we recommend as the key players in your fat-burning diet!)

Foods To Fill You UP, Not OUT

Best:		**Satiation Index**
	Potatoes:	323
	Fish:	225
	Oatmeal:	209
	Oranges:	202
	Apples:	197
	Pasta (whole wheat):	188
	Lean beef:	176
	Grapes:	162
	Popcorn (air-popped):	154
	Bran cereal:	151
Worst:		
	Ice cream:	96
	Potato chips:	91
	Peanuts:	84
	Candy bar (chocolate):	70
	Doughnut:	68
	Cake:	65
	Croissant:	47

Getting Your Taste Buds in Shape

Low-fat foods can satisfy your stomach, but what about your taste buds? Won't a low-fat diet leave you craving the taste of high-fat foods even though your tummy might be content?

"People who switch to low-fat diets sometimes experience a short period of mild withdrawal in the beginning," says Bryant Stamford, Ph.D., director of the Center for Health Promotion at the University of Louisville, who recently overhauled his own less-than-lean diet. "But within several weeks, the body adjusts and people often find that fats actually become uncomfortable to digest because their bodies begin producing less fat-digesting enzymes. In my own case, the kind of breakfast I used to be able to eat without any problem now would leave me feeling quite ill."

FAT-BURNING FACT:

Percentage of people who have ever lied about their weight: 33.

The enzyme most responsible for the digestion of fats is called lipoprotein lipase (LPL), and it can work much to our disadvantage when we eat fats regularly, says Dr. Stamford. "This is because LPL helps break fats down into molecules small enough to be absorbed by fat cells, and the more fat we eat, unfortunately, the more active this enzyme becomes. Worse yet, this enzyme also becomes more active the fatter we become, so a doubly fattening momentum can begin to build when fatty foods become a regular part of a person's diet."

Sweets Double the Trouble

Worse yet, a preference for sweets can make the fat in our diets even more "fattening," Dr. Stamford explains, because sugar boosts the fat-storing power of LPL to an even higher level. "This is why most junk foods are such dietary disasters. They tend to contain both sugar and fat in very large amounts."

What this means is that junk foods not only swing the doors of fat cells wide open, they also assure that molecules of fat make themselves all-too comfortable once inside.

Try to stay away from particularly harmful "sweet and fatty" combinations to keep your fat-burning fires burning most brightly.

CAUTION: High Risk Area

Buttered toast with jam	Donuts
Cake	Ice cream (except low-fat or sugar-free)
Candy bars (most)	Pancakes or waffles with butter and syrup
Chocolate	Pastries
Cookies	Pies (fruit as well as custards)
Croissants (filled)	Puddings

Lower Fat, Higher Spirits

But let's face it, there's more to life than just a flat tummy. Will reducing the fat in your diet also reduce your fun? Will life without your favorite high-fat sweets turn sour?

Not if the conclusions of a recent study by the University of Washington in Seattle are any indication. That study monitored the moods of 555 women who cut the fat in their diets in half for a year. The women reported a significant lift in their spirits—and not just because they lost an average of nine pounds. In fact, they said they felt more energetic and upbeat than they had when "comforted" by their high-fat diets of old.

Why?

Feelings of accomplishment were a factor, no doubt, but some hard-core physiology may also have been at work. Studies show that eating less fat results in greater oxygen flow and hence more energy for every cell in the body, including those of the "mood center" we call the brain.

FAT-BURNING FACT:

Once a fat cell has been created, it cannot be destroyed. Muscle cells, on the other hand, will wither and die if not exercised adequately.

The Top Ten Reasons Dieters Fail

Why do nine out of ten dieters fail to maintain their weight loss for more than a few months, with many putting on even more weight when their diets are over? Weight-loss experts cite the following reasons:

1. **They bite off less than they can chew.** Reducing caloric intake to near starvation levels slows the fat-burning process on which long-term weight control depends. It also sets dieters up for binges, as it robs them of the energy needed for fat-burning exercise. For weight loss to be safe and effective, your diet should include no fewer than 1,200 calories a day.

2. **They lose too fast.** Any diet that produces rapid weight loss risks "throwing the baby out with the bath water." Such a diet reduces valuable calorie-burning muscle tissue, not just fat. Most experts agree on a weight loss of no more than one pound a week.

3. **They assume that all calories are created equal.** New research shows that calories from dietary fat convert more easily to body fat than calories from carbohydrates or protein. A diet high in fat can be "fattening," even though its caloric content may be relatively low.

4. **They break rather than bend.** Too often dieters allow minor slips to become major falls. "Just one" becomes more like one dozen. The key to permanent weight control is learning to be good, not perfect.

5. **They underestimate the value of exercise.** Not only is exercise a fantastic calorie burner while in progress, it can burn calories for as long as several hours afterward. It's also an effective muscle builder, appetite suppressant, and mood elevator and therefore deserves to be a daily "main course."

6. **They get out of "balance."** Relying too heavily on any one type of food to lose weight is shortsighted and potentially dangerous. Effective weight loss requires a healthy and energetic body, not a sick one.

7. **They aspire to the impossible.** No weight-loss effort in the world is going to alter basic body type. Any diet trying to convert a Rosie O'Donnell type into a Cindy Crawford is more likely to result in loss of self-esteem than weight.

8. **They lack support.** Losing weight is a tough enough job on your own; lack of support from family members and friends can make it even tougher. Studies show that chances for success increase with the support of loved ones and peers.

9. **They succumb to advertising.** It's a fattening world we live in, made even more so by the advertising expertise of the food industry. It's a fact that weight loss and frequent TV-watching make for a counterproductive relationship.

10. **They don't really try.** Sorry, but some studies suggest that real commitment may be one of the highest weight-loss hurdles of all. Millions of people say they want to lose weight, only to find that their stomachs speak louder than their hearts—and brains!

"Mind Games" for Taming Your Appetite

Yes, there are some ways to satisfy hunger that go beyond the stomach. Research shows that we can help put our appetites to rest by soothing our brains as well. Here are some hunger-taming "tricks" worth trying:

- *Dim the lights.* Studies by The Johns Hopkins University in Baltimore show that people tend to eat more in environments where lighting is bright and colors are vibrant. Try dimming the lights for your next evening meal, or go one better and break out the candles!

- *Dine from plainer plates.* Research shows, too, that plates with busy patterns tend to be appetite stimulants, so go plain, Jane. You might also want to switch to smaller plates, as they can trick our tummies into feeling fuller on less.

- *Develop a taste for tepid tunes.* The faster the music, the faster we eat, so make your stereo selections accordingly. Better to dine to Julio Iglesias than Nine Inch Nails. (Save your punk rock favorites for your exercise class.)

FAT-BURNING FACT:

There's more fat in a single teaspoon of butter than in 10 pounds of potatoes.

The Problems with Protein—and How to Solve Them

Where does protein fit into a fat-burning diet?

Intimately, but with one critical provision. While protein is essential to a fat-burning diet to maintain fat-burning muscle tissue, the protein must be low in fat, which is not true of many of our most popular protein foods. The average hamburger patty, for example, is approximately 65 percent fat. The average hot dog is about 70 percent fat. Even a seemingly low-fat broiled chicken breast (including skin) is in the neighborhood of 40 percent fat. To be fat-burning, our proteins need to be put on a "diet."

"If a high-fat meal is followed by inactivity or, worse yet, going to bed, it takes fat cells only four to eight hours to absorb most of the fat that's been taken in."

Ronald M. Krauss, M.D., Chairman of the Nutrition Committee for the American Heart Association

This can be done with proper cooking techniques in some cases, trimming off skin and visible fat in others, or simply opting for low-fat versions of such foods as milk, yogurt, and cheese. We'll be looking more closely at how to buy and prepare fat-burning foods, but we offer now the following list to get you at least thinking in the right direction. These are high-protein foods that do not come in the company of lots of fat. Most are less than 20 percent fat and therefore within permissible (edible) limits.

Food	**Percent of Calories from Fat**
Egg whites (and most egg substitutes)	0
Yogurt, non-fat	3
Skim milk	5
Low-fat (one percent fat) cottage cheese	13
Low-fat fish and shellfish:	
Tuna (packed in water)	3
Cod	5
Haddock	5
Lobster	5
Scallops	8
Shrimp	10
Clams	12
Flounder	12
Snapper	12
Sole	12
Perch	16
Monkfish	18
Halibut	19
Trout	26
Turkey (light meat, no skin, roasted)	8
Chicken (white meat, no skin, broiled)	19
Pork (tenderloin, broiled)	26
Beef (top round, broiled)	28

Fiber: Different Types For Different Gripes

When you think of fiber, what comes to mind? The indigestible roughage in foods such as wheat bran that "passes right through you"?

Congratulations for being half right. That sort of fiber is known as "insoluble" fiber and it does, in fact, pass through the digestive tract essentially unchanged. This type of fiber fights constipation and hemorrhoids and reduces the risks of colon cancer by keeping the intestines clean of potentially cancer-causing compounds. This sweeping action also has been shown to help escort fats through the intestines before their calories have time to be fully absorbed, thus making insoluble fiber an invaluable addition to a weight-loss program.

But fiber comes in a "soluble" form, too, principally in fruits, vegetables, beans, and whole grains. Its area of impact is not so much the bowels as the blood. Studies show that soluble fiber can help lower cholesterol levels and keep levels of insulin stable. This helps control hunger and how readily calories can move into fat cells to be stored. Consequently, soluble fiber is as essential to weight loss as its insoluble cousin, but it's the two types working together that make a truly dynamic, fat-fighting duo.

Studies show that our current intake of fiber (of both types) averages approximately 10 to 15 grams a day, a far cry from the 25 to 30 grams nutritionists say we should be getting for overall health and weight control.

View the following list with 25 to 30 grams in mind and try gradually to include more of these foods in your diet. (For the beginner, high-fiber foods can cause flatulence and bloating, so go slow if these foods have yet to become a regular part of your diet.)

Food	Serving Size	Fiber (Grams)
Apple	1 medium	7.9
Barley (cooked)	1/2 cup	12.3
Blackberries	1 cup	7.2
Broccoli	medium stalk	7.4
Corn bran	2 tablespoons	7.9
Oat bran	2 tablespoons	3.0
Rice bran	2 tablespoons	2.3
Wheat bran	2 tablespoons	1.8
Chick peas	1/2 cup	7.0
Currants	1/2 cup	4.9
Figs, dried	3 figs	5.2
Kidney beans	1/2 cup	6.9
Lentils	1/2 cup	5.2
Lima beans	1/2 cup	6.8
Navy beans	1/2 cup	4.9
Peas	1/2 cup	4.2
Potato	1 medium	3.9
Raspberries	1 cup	6.0
Spinach	1/2 cup	5.7
Succotash	1/2 cup	5.2

(Note: Although not on the list due to slightly lesser levels, virtually all fruits, vegetables, beans, and whole-grain cereals, and breads are good fiber sources and should be part of a fat-fighting diet.)

Know Your Daily Fat "Budget"

The following chart can help you keep your fat intake in the healthful neighborhood of 25 percent of the calories you consume. Simply locate your desired weight in the column at the left and find the corresponding number of grams of fat in the column at the right. This is the amount of fat you should not exceed per day to achieve that desired weight.

Women		Men	
Desired Weight:	**Daily Fat Limit (In Grams)**	**Desired Weight:**	**Daily Fat Limit (In Grams)**
110	37	130	51
120	40	140	54
130	43	150	58
140	47	160	62
150	50	170	66
160	53	180	70
170	57	190	74
180	60	200	78

Butter vs. Margarine: Both Losers

Is their a pat answer to the butter vs. margarine debate?

Yes: It's best to avoid them both. According to experts, both serve up a monstrous 11 grams of fat in a single teaspoon, and both have other unhealthful effects, especially margarine. That might come as a surprise, given margarine's "healthier" reputation. However, researchers at the Harvard School of Public Health and at the George Washington University Medical Center recently have completed studies that should have you thinking twice about margarine in your refrigerator.

Butter is loaded with saturated fat (the kind that increases risks of heart disease by raising levels of LDL, the bad cholesterol). Margarine is full of "trans-fatty acids," which are created when vegetable oil has been "hydrogenated" to make it firm enough to spread. Trans-fatty acids also have been shown to elevate LDL levels.

The bad news doesn't stop there, however. In addition to raising bad (LDL) cholesterol, trans-fatty acids have been shown to lower good (HDL) cholesterol—the kind that can reduce heart disease risks. Saturated fat, by comparison, has been found in some studies actually to raise levels of LDL.

So sorry, "oleo" fans. By raising the bad cholesterol and lowering the good, the type of fat found in margarine wins the dubious distinction of being the most hazardous to be found, proving perhaps that it really isn't nice to fool Mother Nature after all.

If, however, your taste buds *demand* butter or margarine, butter appears to be the more healthful—or the least harmful—of the two. But because butter is a saturated fat, it should be used in very small amounts.

(Note: Hydrogenated fats are found in other products as well. Learn to avoid them in vegetable shortening and many commercially prepared baked goods such as cookies, cakes, pastries, and pies. Always check a food's label to be sure.)

The Tortoise vs. The Hare: The Case of Linda

They shook hands precisely at midnight on New Year's Eve. The contest was to last one year, with a prize of $50 to the winner for every pound marking the margin of victory. Linda at 5'5" weighed 165, while Barbara, one inch taller, tipped the scales at 172.

Barbara decided to blast off from the start like a rocket and get a lead she could hang on to until the finish. Linda planned to go slow and easy and lose just half a pound a week.

Two weeks into the contest, Barbara announced that she had lost "10 big ones" by restricting herself to a salad and one diet milkshake a day. Linda, whose typical lunch was a bowl of bean soup and homemade whole wheat bread, had lost just two pounds.

Because they worked for the same company, the two saw each other often. Barbara would poke her head into Linda's office each Monday morning and hold up her fingers to show the new total of her losses. But one Monday Barbara phoned in sick—"sick" as in totally demoralized. She had succumbed to a major "binge" over the weekend. The weight she so agonizingly had lost began to return almost visibly. Worse yet, she had lost so much muscle tissue during the course of her nearly four-month-long "fast," she had trouble losing any more weight despite limiting herself to 800 calories a day.

Linda, meanwhile, had stayed true to her half-pound-a-week plan, losing 8 pounds painlessly over the four months the contest had lasted.

Moral of the story: Patience may be your greatest weight-loss ally. Go slow if where you're going is a place you plan to stay.

The Calories in Cocktails: Nothing to Celebrate

Where does alcohol fit into an effective weight-loss picture?

As more of a road block than many of us realize, says Dr. John P. Foreyt, of the Nutrition Research Clinic at the Baylor College of Medicine. Foreyt believes that drinking alcohol has essentially the same effect on body weight as does eating fat. "Alcohol may not show up as a layer of oil on top of a glass of water, but in terms of how it's metabolized, it's a lot more like fat than it is a carbohydrate."

Alcohol's calories alone argue this point: 7 calories per gram (fat has 9) as compared with 4 calories per gram for carbohydrates and protein. The higher a drink's alcohol content, the higher the calorie count, as the following chart shows:

Beverage	Portion	% of Alcohol	Calories by Volume
Beer (regular)	12 oz.	5	146
Beer (light)	12 oz.	4	99
Liquor *(bourbon, gin, rum, scotch, vodka)*	1.5 oz.	40	97
Wine (dry)	3.5 oz.	11.5	73
Wine *(sweet fortified, such as port, sherry, and sweet vermouth)*	3.5 oz.	18-19	140

Making alcohol's calories even more "fattening," moreover, is their lack of patience when it comes to being metabolized. When you eat an 800-calorie meal along with a couple of glasses of dry wine (about 150 calories), it's the calories in the wine that are first digested. What this does to the 800 calories in the meal is make them that much more available to be stored as fat rather than burned as energy.

Then, too, alcohol has a tendency to reduce inhibitions—including those responsible for portion control. Studies show that people are more likely to overeat when they've been "primed" with a couple of cocktails. Not surprisingly, they tend to overindulge in fatty foods especially.

"Pub Grub" Packs on the Pounds, Too

But it's not just the calories in our drinks that can give rise to a beer belly. The calories in those "can't have just one" bar snacks add to the swell, too.

	Calories	Grams of Fat	% of Calories from Fat
1 cup peanuts	1,146	72	76
5 buffalo wings	860	55	58
30 corn chips (about 1 oz.)	155	9	53
30 potato chips (about 2 oz.)	315	21	61

Better choices: Air-popped, unbuttered popcorn (12 percent fat) and pretzels (10 percent fat).

10 Commandments For Making Weight Loss Last

Today's leading nutritionists believe that the following are the ten most important strategies for losing weight, not just permanently but painlessly—without hunger, without cravings, and without weakness or fatigue.

1. **Avoid getting hungry.** That's right—no meal skipping allowed. That might sound like weight-loss heresy, but it's not. Your body will adjust its metabolic rate to burn fewer calories if you allow yourself to be chronically famished. You're also likely to overcompensate when you do eat, thinking you "deserve" it, and thus negate any benefit from your misery.

2. **Nibble, don't gorge.** Ever noticed how some people can snack constantly but can still maintain a desirable weight? It's not a mirage. It's been proven that eating small meals produces less of an insulin response from the pancreas. This is good news for the waistline because the job of insulin is to help calories get stored as fat.

3. **Limit, but do not eliminate, dietary fat.** Some fat is necessary to absorb fat-soluble vitamins, such as vitamins A, D, and E. Some fat also is needed to slow down the rate at which carbohydrates and proteins are metabolized, thus helping to stave off hunger. Notice that we said "some." All of the benefits of dietary fat could be achieved with levels as low as 10 percent of total calories,

but that's a level that most people would find severe. Dietary fat levels in the 20 to 30 percent range are more acceptable.

4. **Know your "good" carbohydrates from your "bad."** If all carbohydrates were nutritiously equal, a bowl of table sugar would be as healthful as a baked potato. But while sugar is a "simple" carbohydrate (meaning it digests quickly and has no significant nutrients or fiber), the potato is a "complex" carbohydrate that delivers a wide range of energizing nutrients the body digests more slowly.

5. **Learn to slim down your proteins.** Protein is critical to your fat-burning diet because it helps maintain muscle cells, which burn fat for energy. Equally important, protein helps block fat storage by keeping insulin levels low, and it provides feelings of fullness by preventing carbohydrates from being metabolized too quickly.

6. **Fill up on fiber.** Because fiber does not fully digest, it tends to be exceptionally filling, despite being very low in calories and virtually free of fat. Better yet, insoluble (cannot be dissolved) fiber acts like a janitor by grabbing onto fats in the intestines and sweeping them out of the body before they can be fully absorbed. Diets high in insoluble fiber can reduce caloric absorption by as much as 3 percent—enough, on a 2,000-calorie diet, to allow you 60 calories absolutely "free." Soluble (dissolvable) fiber, which quells hunger by stabilizing insulin levels in the blood, is no fat-fighting slouch either.

7. **Impound your bathroom scale.** The loss of true body fat, which is lighter in weight than either muscle tissue or water, might not be evident when you step on your scale. Some people even wind up weighing more when they lose body fat, especially if they exercise, because they gain muscle in place of the lost fat.

8. **Exercise, don't agonize.** Exercise is critical to long-term weight loss, as we'll be seeing in more detail in Chapter 3. But the only exercise that's going to work is the exercise you're going to do consistently. Engage in activities you enjoy and involve friends or family members whenever possible. Research shows that exercising within approximately 30 minutes of eating can boost calorie burning by as much as 10 percent.

9. **Don't let small slips become major slides.** Maybe you know the scenario all too well: One chocolate chip cookie becomes two, becomes three, becomes a bowl of ice cream. Suddenly, with weeks' worth of work down the drain, you figure you should pack in your weight-loss effort and try again another day. But don't panic. By sticking to a low-fat diet, you can afford such misdemeanors. In fact, one study found that people on low-fat diets experienced no ill effects despite eating "splurge" meals (a ham and cheese sandwich and a milkshake) as often as once every other day.

10. **Eat light at night.** Sorry, midnight snackers, but studies show that calories consumed shortly before bed will more than likely become fat because there simply isn't enough competition from your body's muscle cells when you're in dreamland to encourage them to do much else. Many weight-loss experts recommend putting a padlock on your appetite after about 7:00 PM. If you find that you need a before-bed snack to help you sleep, make it as low in fat as possible: a glass of skim milk, some nonfat or low-fat yogurt, a small bowl of cereal, or a piece of fresh fruit.

CHAPTER 2

TIPS FOR A LEANER LIFESTYLE

Of course there's more to permanent weight loss than just knowing the right foods to eat. First, you must actually eat the food—both consistently and enthusiastically. The more a diet asks you to deprive yourself, after all, the more likely it is to fail.

Then, too, there are the challenges of dealing with issues other than food. Less than supportive family members ("why can't we call for pizza?"). Or undeniable cravings for sweets. Or those times when life's stresses weigh on your weight-loss efforts with the force of a giant pound cake.

Relax. If you've got the will, we've got the way. In this chapter, you'll learn the "nuts and bolts" of what it takes to get a successful weight-control program going—and keep it going. The secret to sticking to any weight-loss program lies in being determined but also in being flexible—in learning to bend, not break. Just because you slip doesn't mean you have to fall.

So What Should You Weigh, Anyway?

The $64,000 question is: What is my ideal weight?

More and more, doctors are beginning to realize that it's not an easy question to answer. Until recently it was thought that our weight should be within the standards established by insurance companies based on what is average for most Americans. However, the fallacy of this approach now is being understood because it says nothing about why we weigh what we do. A football player who exercises strenuously and eats a healthful low-fat diet could be considered overweight purely by virtue of being heavily muscled. A "couch potato" who is primarily bones and flab, on the other hand, could be considered at a healthy weight despite having a terrible diet and getting no exercise at all.

FAT-BURNING FACT:

Four out of ten adults currently weigh at least 20 percent more than they should. This computes to be 2.5 billion pounds of excess body fat—the weight of approximately 300,000 adult hippos.

Nor do the "ideal" weight charts say anything about where our extra pounds are located, which research is now showing to be very important. People who tend to carry their extra weight in their abdomens appear to be at greater risks for heart disease, diabetes, and certain forms of cancer than people who carry their surplus poundage on their hips, buttocks, and thighs. It's riskier to be shaped like an apple, in other words, than a pear.

But why should people shaped like apples be at a greater health risk than people shaped like pears?

The reason has to do with the difference in the metabolic activity of what doctors have recently identified as two distinctly different types of fat. People with large, apple-shaped midsections usually have a high percentage of what is known as "visceral" fat—fat located inside, as opposed to outside, the abdominal wall. Because this type of fat is close to vital organs such as the liver, gallbladder, and pancreas, it's thought to influence risks of diabetes and heart disease by adversely affecting levels of fat, cholesterol, and insulin in the blood.

This is not the case, however, with the other more visible type of fat called "subcutaneous" fat, which lies underneath the skin but outside the abdominal wall. Because it is not as close to vital organs as visceral fat, subcutaneous fat appears not to have similar health risks. This is ironic given that subcutaneous fat is the type we most despise because of its greater visibility. People with this type of fat usually are pear-shaped.

Are both types of fat equal in terms of the efforts needed to lose them?

Thankfully, no. Because of its greater metabolic involvement, visceral fat appears to be more responsive than subcutaneous fat to diet and exercise. When you begin following the recommendations given in this book, therefore, you may take comfort in knowing that you'll be burning fat where it counts most. Yes, the unwanted fat on your hips and thighs also will be diminished, but your most dangerous, internal, fat will be the first to feel the brunt of your efforts.

Your Best "Fighting" Weight: One You Don't Have to Fight

This brings us to an important point that you should keep in mind as you begin to incorporate fat-burning strategies into your life. By eating a nutritious low-fat diet and getting at least 30 minutes of physical activity each day, you'll achieve a weight that is "ideal" because it will be the weight best suited for helping you achieve ideal health. If the figure you achieve is not the one of your dreams, blame your genes. Some of us are simply born to carry more body fat than others, and new research shows this does not necessarily have to be unhealthful.

What does matter are the lifestyle factors responsible for our weights. Someone who keeps his or her weight down by skipping meals, taking diet pills, or smoking is going to be less healthy than someone who may be plump despite eating well and being physically active. As Dr. Steven Blair of the Cooper Institute of Aerobics Research said, "Healthy bodies come in all shapes and sizes. We need to stop hounding people about their weight and encourage them to eat well and exercise."

How Healthful Is Your Diet?

Take This Test and Find Out

Before we go further, we need to know what your current eating habits are. If you're like most Americans, they probably need some work. While we've begun to make some progress in our efforts to cut down on fat—by reducing our average food intake from 38 percent of calories from fat down to 34—we still have a way to go to reach the level of 25 percent that most nutritionists now recommend. Considering that we've actually gotten heavier in recent years despite making this cutback, it's clear that we may need to reduce our calorie intake overall. Take the following test and see how you fare.

1. **My usual pattern of eating is to:**
   a. eat a healthful breakfast, ample lunch, and a small dinner interspersed with healthful snacks in between
   b. sit down to three fairly traditional "square" meals a day
   c. skip breakfast or lunch and have a big dinner
   d. skip breakfast *and* lunch and have a huge dinner

2. **In an average day I will have the following number of servings of vegetables:**
   a. four or more
   b. two or three
   c. one
   d. I despise vegetables and eat them rarely, if ever

3. **In an average day I will have the following number of servings or pieces of fresh fruit:**
   a. four or more
   b. two or three
   c. one
   d. usually none

4. **The type of bread I usually eat is:**
   a. whole-grain bread that I make myself with no added fat
   b. whole-grain bread I buy at a bakery
   c. whole wheat, pumpernickel, or rye from the supermarket
   d. white bread from the supermarket

5. The breakfast that most closely resembles my usual one is:

a. a high-fiber, vitamin-fortified cereal with skim milk and a piece of fresh fruit
b. frozen waffles with butter and syrup and a glass of juice
c. eggs with bacon or sausage and buttered toast
d. a piece of pastry and coffee or no breakfast at all

6. The way I most often eat potatoes is:

a. baked, with yogurt or a tiny bit of butter as a topping
b. mashed, with butter and/or a gravy topping
c. French-fried, with ketchup
d. French-fried, with a melted cheese topping

7. Most of the protein in my diet comes from:

a. chicken or turkey (skinless) and/or fish, usually baked or broiled
b. beef and pork
c. cheese and other full-fat dairy products
d. fast-food entrees such as hamburgers and hot dogs

8. The milk I usually drink or use on my cereal is:

a. skim
b. 1% fat
c. 2% fat
d. regular

9. When pan-frying, I'll use:

a. a non-stick pan so that I won't need to use any fat at all
b. a little bit of olive or vegetable oil
c. a little bit of butter
d. a lot of butter or lard

10. The amount of water I drink in an average day is:
a. six eight-ounce glasses, or more
b. four to six eight-ounce glasses
c. two to four eight-ounce glasses
d. fewer than two glasses

11. The number of times in an average week I eat at a fast-food restaurant is:
a. I avoid eating at fast-food restaurants
b. one
c. two or three
d. four or more

12. My favorite between-meal or TV-time snacks are:
a. fresh vegetable crudités and/or fresh fruit
b. saltless pretzels, rice cakes, or popcorn
c. potato or corn chips
d. cookies, pastry, or candy

13. The number of cans or bottles of non-diet soda I'll have in an average day is:
a. zero
b. one or two
c. three or four
d. more than four

14. I give into the urge to have a really decadent dessert:
a. rarely
b. about once a month
c. about once a week
d. I am having a really decadent dessert right now

SCORING:

Give yourself a one for every "a" answer, a two for every "b," a three for every "c," and a four for every "d."

15–22: High Honors. Congratulations! Your diet is truly a fat-burning marvel that is giving your body every health advantage it deserves.

23–30: Honors. Good work. Your diet is to be commended, although there still are improvements you could make.

31–38: Honorable Mention. Your diet is fair, but nothing special. You could be leaner, healthier, and enjoy more energy by making the changes suggested in this book.

39–46: Less Than Honorable Mention. Careful. Your diet borders on the risky and could affect your health adversely. You owe it to yourself to make the changes suggested in this book.

47 **and above: Dishonorable Mention.** Shame on you. Your diet is a disgrace and is definitely bad for your health. You had better hurry up and change your eating habits.

FAT-BURNING FACT:

A small, steady supply of food during the day keeps insulin levels steadier, so that your brain doesn't turn up your appetite and send signals to fat cells to store more fat.

In The Bag:

Best Strategies for Fighting Fat in the Supermarket

Now that you have a pretty good picture of your present eating habits, it's time to do something about them.

Let's start where every weight-loss effort should start—at the supermarket. You can't eat what you haven't bought. By buying the right food, you can avoid those showdowns with your willpower that occur when you're tired and stressed and that cheesecake in your refrigerator looks awfully good. Shop smart and you will prevent the "enemy" from entering your home and tempting you. Following are some strategies to help you do precisely that:

Do not shop when you're hungry. Shopping on an empty stomach can lead to a heaping shopping cart faster than you can say, "But the sticky buns were on sale!" Try to shop as close after eating a satisfying meal as possible. That way, your brain will dictate your purchases, not your stomach.

Always shop with a list. This, too, can discourage unwise food choices spurred by impulse buying. Compile your list when you're feeling comfortable and have time to concentrate on the consequences of what you'll be buying. Do you really need that half gallon of mint chocolate chip ice cream? Better to be safe than sorry.

Try not to shop with your children. Nothing against the little ones, but they can "fatten" up a shopping cart in the blink of an eye. Get a babysitter if you have to; the cost will be covered by the cupcakes and marshmallow cereal you won't be pressured to buy.

Do not be swayed by food coupons or by special money-saving bargains. It certainly can be tempting to put thriftiness ahead of health, but is anything really a bargain if it's bad for you? Think about that the next time the bags of potato chips or chocolate donuts are two-for-one. Your goal should be maximum nutrition for your food dollar, not just calories.

Buy fresh or frozen foods rather than canned. This applies to meats and fish as well as vegetables and fruits. Not only will you get better taste and in many cases superior nutrition, you'll get less sodium. This is a plus for the estimated 20 percent of the population for whom too much salt can result in high blood pressure.

Buy in quantity if you're also getting quality. If you come across a special on particularly healthful foods—low-fat meats, fish, poultry, fruits, or vegetables (fresh or frozen)—stock up, by all means. Not only will you be saving money, you'll be assuring that these healthful foods eventually will end up on your table.

Know your best low-fat bargains. Have you ever noticed how little a 10-pound bag of potatoes costs—or dried beans, rice, or pasta? These are fantastic food bargains. Your low-fat diet also can be a low-cost diet, so don't pass these foods by.

Avoid the "enemy." Just as there are foods tailor-made to burn fat, there also are those that will very easily become fat. The best way to avoid being tempted by the latter is not to allow them into your home in the first place. Foremost among these foods are butter, shortening, margarine, regular mayonnaise, hard cheeses, whole milk, sour cream, salad dressings (except for low and non-fat), ice cream, bacon, sausage, luncheon meats (except for sliced turkey or chicken breast), creamy soups, corn and potato chips, and high-fat cuts of beef, poultry, and pork. (See next page.)

Learn the fine art of substitution. Acting in response to the concerns of today's health-conscious consumers, the food industry has come up with non-fat or low-fat versions of everything from soup to nuts. Add to these the low-fat foods offered by Mother Nature, and it quickly becomes clear that your supermarket offers a tremendous variety to choose from when putting together low-fat meals.

FAT-BURNING FACT:

Research shows that by reducing the fat in their diets, most people can lower their blood cholesterol levels by 10 to 15 percent—enough to reduce their risks of heart disease by 20 to 30 percent!

The following are healthful substitutes for unhealthful staples:

Head right for:	**Pass on by:**	**Grams of fat saved per serving**
Air-popped popcorn (12%)*	Potato chips (61%)	6.8
Beef, top round roast (26%)	Ground chuck (66%)	16.0
Canned tuna, in water (3%)	Canned tuna, in oil (45%)	5.5
Fresh flounder (12%)	Flounder filets, breaded and fried (49%)	26.0
Fresh fruit (2–10%)	Cookies, chocolate chip (40%)	10.5
Low-fat cheese (36%)	Regular cheese (77%)	7.0
Low-fat mayonnaise (40%)	Regular mayonnaise (98%)	10.0
Non-fat egg substitute (0%)	Eggs (61%)	5.0
Non-fat frozen yogurt (0%)	Ice cream (54%)	11.5
Non-fat yogurt (3%)	Regular yogurt (48%)	7.0
Pork tenderloin (26%)	Pork chops (51%)	7.6
Skim milk (6%)	Whole milk (49%)	8.3
Skinless chicken breasts (19%)	Chicken legs (40%)	5.0
Sliced turkey breast (13%)	Sliced ham (52%)	5.3

*Percentage indicates fat content.

Best and Worst Picks

Beef

Best	Worst
Top Round (29% fat)	Ribs (75% fat)
Eye of Round (30% fat)	Chuck Blade Roast (72% fat)
Top Sirloin (36% fat)	T-Bone Steak (68% fat)
Filet Mignon (38% fat)	Porterhouse Steak (64% fat)

Pork

Best	Worst
Center Loin Pork Chops (26% fat)	Loin Blade Steaks (50% fat)
Tenderloin (26% fat)	Ribs (54% fat)
	Shoulder Blade Steaks (51% fat)

Poultry

Best	Worst
Turkey—light meat (19% fat without skin; 38% with skin)	Turkey—dark meat (35% fat without skin; 47% fat with skin)
Chicken—light meat (23% fat without skin; 44% fat with skin)	Chicken—dark meat (43% fat without skin; 56% fat with skin)

Slim Cookins'

Once nutritional low-fat food has been purchased, we must make sure it stays that way. What happens to that food in your kitchen can make or break low-fat fare. How healthful, after all, is a 12-percent-fat flounder filet if it's been breaded, deep-fried, and smothered in tartar sauce?

At about 50 percent fat—even without the 98-percent-fat tartar sauce!—not very. Even the foods that are most healthful can become little better than "junk" food if the preparation is too "heavy-handed."

That said, the following are the best methods for keeping your cooking "lite:"

Best fat-fighting cooking techniques

- *Broiling.* Broiling is a good fat-fighter—especially if done on a rack or in a pan that allows fat to drain away from what's being cooked.

- *Baking.* Also a good fat-fighter, but, as with broiling, it's best done in a pan with a slightly raised rack to allow the fat to drain.

- *Poaching.* Another good low-fat technique (especially for fish) because fat has a tendency to leach into the poaching liquid.

- *Grilling* (outdoor barbecues included). A fat-fighter extraordinaire, as fat drains into and helps fuel the very fire doing the cooking!

- *Steaming.* Your best fat-free way to cook vegetables.

- *Microwaving.* A very good fat-free way to cook practically anything.

Note: The cooking methods you should avoid are pan-frying, deep-frying, and braising or sautéing in butter or oil.

Best fat-fighting "weapons"

To employ the best fat-fighting cooking techniques, it can help immensely to have your kitchen "armed" with the right fat-fighting equipment. Following are the utensils that can best serve you:

- non-stick frying pans and bake ware
- a ridged grill pan for cooking burgers, chops, and fish
- steaming baskets for steaming vegetables
- a fat-skimmer for skimming the surface fat from soups and gravies
- a fat-free (hot-air style) popcorn popper
- a blender (for making low-fat soups, sauces, and shakes)
- a set of good knives (for chopping fresh vegetables and trimming all visible fat from meats)
- a microwave oven (a great low-fat cooking method)
- plastic storage bags (for freezing low-fat foods purchased in bulk)
- a good collection of low-fat cookbooks

Mealtime Tips for a Trimmer You

Even the most healthful foods can lead to weight gain if we grossly overindulge. So it's important to practice a certain restraint at mealtime. This does not mean depriving yourself, but it does mean learning how to stop eating when you've had your biological fill, something many overeaters fail to do. Here are some helpful strategies if a runaway appetite sometimes poses a problem for you:

Eat slowly. Studies show that it takes approximately 20 minutes for your stomach to tell your brain it's full, so pace your eating accordingly. Take small rather than large bites and chew each bite thoroughly before swallowing. What you want to avoid is the "I can't believe I ate the whole thing" syndrome that happens when you eat too quickly.

Serve meals piping hot. Not only will this slow down the rate at which you eat, hot foods tend to be more satisfying because the heat accentuates their flavors.

Pay attention when you eat. Eating while doing other things, such as watching TV or reading, can have you stuffed in no time. Arrange to have your meals in a calm, relaxing atmosphere and concentrate totally on what you're eating.

Take breaks to breathe. By stopping periodically during a meal to take five or so deep breaths, you'll not only interrupt the mindless "cruise control" approach to dining, you'll help arrest your hunger because your expanding diaphragm will help you get a better "feel" for the amount of food you've actually put into your stomach.

Put leftovers away quickly. The longer leftovers linger, the more likely you'll be to pick at them, so the sooner you can get them out of sight and into your refrigerator, the better.

Drink lots of water with your meals. It's a great way to fill up and 100 percent fat- and calorie-free.

"Eat" lots of water with your meals. We're talking about low-calorie vegetables and salads—great ways to munch and crunch without a lot of caloric dues to pay.

Don't desert dessert. Satisfy post-meal sweet cravings with a low-fat sherbet, low-fat frozen yogurt, Jell-O, or a serving of fresh fruit.

Pay attention to portions. Research has demonstrated that most people underestimate the amount of food they eat in a day, primarily because they have no clear understanding of how large a "serving" actually is. To assist you in this regard, we suggest that you think of servings in the following, visual terms:

- One serving of meat or fish usually constitutes two to three ounces, a portion roughly the size of a deck of cards.

- One serving of cheese usually refers to about 1 1/2 ounces, a piece approximately the size of three dominoes.

- One serving of pasta, rice, vegetables, or mashed potatoes usually constitutes 1/2 a cup, a portion about the size of half a baseball.

Eating Light When Eating Out

But will following a fat-burning diet mean you'll have to curb your appetite when eating out—especially at your favorite fast-food restaurant?

The answer to that depends on you. If you insist on having it truly "your way" when you eat out, restaurant dining needn't be a problem. However, you will need to be knowledgeable and assertive about which dishes you should avoid.

The following are some fat-fighting strategies worth remembering, whether you're eating beneath the Golden Arches or at a four-star restaurant in Paris.

- ***Try to avoid smorgasbords or all-you-can-eat buffets.*** Not only do these formats encourage you to overeat, they allow you little opportunity to request changes in the way the food is prepared.

- ***Order a la carte.*** You benefit from greater variety this way, and you avoid the temptation to overeat when served a meal that is larger than you might like.

- ***Call ahead.*** This is especially advisable if you're not sure about the healthfulness of the food a restaurant serves or about its willingness to make changes.

- ***Don't be afraid to be assertive.*** It can be easy to worry about sounding "picky" when you request changes to a menu, but one simple fact can help make you bold: Most restaurants want your business and usually will do anything reasonably possible to get it.

- ***Don't be afraid to be inquisitive.*** A cheeseburger is easy, but when dishes become more complex and are given names in a foreign language, confusion can reign. This needn't be a problem if you're willing to ask your waitress or waiter what ingredients go into the dish and how it's prepared. If all you get is shrugged shoulders, don't be afraid to ask if you can talk with the chef.

- ***Be wary of appetizers.*** They can seem like a good idea as "just a little something to tide you over," but many are high in fat as well as brimming with enough calories to qualify as an entree. If you do need to nibble on something, stick to bread or order a cup of low-fat soup.

- ***Order sauces and salad dressings on the side.*** Whether it's gravy for your roast beef, Hollandaise sauce for your broccoli, or blue cheese dressing for your salad, you'll have a lot more control if *you* decide the amount.

- ***Know your friendly from your "fiendish" pastas.*** Pasta in a tomato sauce is one thing, but pasta smothered in a creamy cheese sauce is another story entirely. If you have questions about a pasta sauce, be sure to ask how it's made.

- ***Forego rich desserts.*** Unless a fresh-fruit dish or sherbet is being offered, you could be looking at more fat and calories than were in your entree.

Food Labels In Focus

Learn how to read—and understand—nutritional labels. Nearly all foods now have them, and they're a dream come true for the health-conscious and the weight-conscious alike. Following are the most important things to look for:

The amount of fat a serving contains. This will be presented to you in two ways: the number of grams of fat the food has and the number of calories that fat contains. (If this latter figure computes* to be more than about 25 percent of the food's total calories, consider it a high-fat food that you either should not buy or should eat in moderation only.)

The amount of fiber the food contains. This will be listed in grams and also as "% of daily value." Because you should be getting between 25 and 35 grams of fiber in your diet daily, any food with a fiber content of approximately three grams or more per serving (or 10% of your daily value) should be deemed a wise fiber choice.

The percentages of vitamins and minerals the food contains. These will be listed toward the end of the label and, as with the food's other nutrients, will reflect the degree to which the food satisfies your daily needs as expressed by "% of daily value."(If a vitamin or mineral is not listed, it will be because the food's "daily value" is less than two percent.)

** To make this calculation, divide the food's total number of calories per serving by the number of its calories that come from fat. As mentioned, any food that turns out to be approximately 25 percent fat or above should be excluded from your diet or eaten sparingly.*

FAT-BURNING FACT:

Skim milk gets 5 percent of its calories from fat, while whole milk gets 51 percent from fat. More than 30 percent calories from fat increases risks of heart disease, obesity, and cancer.

Taking the Fat out of Fast food

If you're like most American families, 40 percent of your food budget gets spent on eating out, and a whopping portion of that goes toward the burgers and fries. Should you avoid fast-food restaurants?

That depends on what you order and how much. While many of the items offered at these eateries could blow your entire daily fat budget in just one serving—a Double Whopper with cheese from Burger King, for example, serves up a mammoth 55 grams of fat in addition to nearly 900 calories—other fast-food entrees are actually quite lean. Wendy's grilled chicken sandwich, for example, has only 7 grams of fat and a modest 290 calories.

It helps to know what you're biting into at fast-food restaurants. The following fast-food-eating tips and the nutritional chart should help you make fast food, fit food.

Think small. Avoid entrees labeled "jumbo," "giant," or "deluxe." As these adjectives imply, the number of calories and grams of fat in these monstrosities are astronomical.

Think plain. The sauce on the featured sandwich may be "gourmet," but it's not without a price. These sauces are largely mayonnaise, which is nearly 100 percent fat. If it's a burger you want, have it plain or piled with fat-free lettuce and tomato.

Fear the deep-fryer. The chicken or fish sandwich might seem to be a healthier choice than a burger, but not if it's been in the fryer first. Burger King's broiled chicken sandwich has only 10 grams of fat and 280 calories, for example, while its deep-fried fish cousin has 32 grams of fat and 620 calories.

When ordering chicken, think of "extra crispy" as extra crumbly. It's hard to believe, but the crispier the coating, the higher its fat content. If you want chicken and fried is the only way it's offered, put manners aside and remove the coating before eating. Your heart as well as your waistline will thank you.

Chase down the chili. Most chili dishes at fast-food restaurants are less than 30 percent fat and loaded with heart-healthy fiber, thanks to the beans.

Know your friends from your enemies at the salad bar. All those greens and vegetables are great, but don't make the mistake of sabotaging them with salad dressings that easily add as many as 200 calories per tablespoon. Use vinegar or low-calorie dressings instead. Try to avoid the mayonnaise-based potato salads and coleslaws; choose instead vinegar-based red beets, three-bean salad, or chow-chow. Other healthful, low-fat choices include bean sprouts, chick peas, cottage cheese, and hard-boiled eggs (providing you can avoid the yolk).

Pick low-fat toppings for your pizza. While a single slice of regular pizza without any trimmings has only about 10 grams of fat, piling on the pepperoni and extra cheese can double that. If it's toppings you must have, choose veggies such as mushrooms, green peppers, and onions.

Visit at mealtimes only. With the average fast-food meal coming in at 685 calories, it's important to consider it just that: a meal, not a snack. But if you do go a bit overboard, don't panic. Just be all the more careful about the fat and calories you consume in your other meals that day.

Fast Food Entrees:
The Good, The Bad, and the Abominable

The above are some general guidelines for having both your good health and your fast food. Now for some specifics. Here's a quick rundown of entrees containing ten or fewer grams of fat per serving. Any entree not on this list is too high in fat to be recommended as part of a fat-burning diet.

Arby's	Light Roast Chicken Deluxe
	Light Roast Turkey Deluxe
	Light Roast Beef Deluxe
	Roast Chicken Salad
Burger King	Broiler Chicken Sandwich
	Hamburger (small)
Dairy Queen	Beef Barbecue Sandwich
	Grilled Chicken Filet Sandwich
Domino's	Pizza (plain)
Hardee's	Real West Beef Barbecue Sandwich
	Grilled Chicken Breast Sandwich
	Turkey Sub
	Roast Beef Sub
	Ham Sub
	Combo Sub
Jack-in-the-Box	Chicken Fajita Pita
Long John Silver's	Baked Fish With Lemon Crumb
	Chicken Light Herb
	Gumbo with Cod
	Seafood Chowder

McDonald's	Hamburger (small)
	McLean Deluxe
	Chicken Fajitas
Pizza Hut	Thin 'N Crispy Pizza (plain)
	Veggie Lovers Pizza
Subway	Turkey Breast Sub
	Ham and Cheese Sub
	Veggie and Cheese Sub
Taco Bell	Chicken Taco (soft)
	Chicken Fajita
Wendy's	Grilled Chicken Sandwich
	Hamburger (junior)
	Chili

A word about those "sides." It's hard to believe but it's true: Most French fries served at fast-food restaurants are higher in fat than the hamburgers they accompany. The same is true of those seemingly innocent onion rings. At Burger King, for example, a small burger serves up 10 grams of fat and 260 calories while a medium serving of fries is good for 20 grams of fat and 372 calories. An order of Burger King onion rings: 19 grams of fat and 339 calories.

Olé! Eating Lean When Eating Ethnic

Do you enjoy "stretching" your palate by trying various ethnic dishes from time to time?

Good. Variety is the spice of a good diet, as well as of life. To keep your ethnic excursions as healthful as possible, however, it can help to know something about the items being offered. While some ethnic dishes can be very low in fat, others can be nutritional disasters. Here's a quick guide to help you separate the former from the latter.

Chinese: Many Chinese dishes are low in fat thanks to the predominance of rice and vegetables. Do be wary, however, of appetizers such as egg rolls, which usually are deep-fried. Stir-fried dishes generally are a good, low-fat choice—especially if you ask your chef to go easy on the oil. "Moo goo gai pan"—a combination of stir-fried mushrooms, bamboo shoots, water chestnuts, and chicken or seafood served over rice—is a particularly good choice. To be avoided: Peking duck with 30 grams of fat in just one 3 1/2 ounce serving.

Mexican: Mexican fare also can be healthful and low in fat providing you avoid dishes smothered in cheese or sour cream. Also to be avoided is guacamole (made from high-fat avocados), refried beans (usually made with coconut oil or lard), and any entree that has been deep-fried or features beef or pork. Set your sights instead on vegetable and bean burritos, fresh-fish dishes, salsas, salads, unfried corn tortillas, beans, and rice.

Italian: Italian food is a case of Dr. Jekyll and Mr. Hyde: Many great low-fat dishes are available (any pasta dish served with a tomato-based marinara sauce, for example), but so are high-fat fiascoes such as "fettucini alfredo," made with cheese, heavy cream, and butter. Other good low-fat choices are vegetarian lasagna (providing you scrape off some of its surface cheese), "pollo cacciatore" (a boneless chicken breast served with a tomato and mushroom sauce), and "shrimp al vino blanco" (shrimp cooked in white wine). As for pizza, it can be as healthful as its toppings. Avoid extra cheese, pepperoni, and olives, opting instead for low-fat vegetables such as mushrooms, green peppers, and onions. High-protein foods like chicken, turkey, and shrimp also are fare game.

Indian: Like Italian food, Indian dishes also have their villains and heroes. Try to avoid dishes made with coconut oil or "ghee," a clarified butter. Look instead for entrees featuring ample amounts of beans, rice, onions, tomatoes, and bell peppers. One especially healthful dish is "murg jalfraize," made with plenty of spices, fresh vegetables, and skinless chicken.

"Haute" But Healthful: Low-Fat Fine Dining

Step up in the dining world, unfortunately, and you've often entered high-fat country. The reason is that costlier cuisines often borrow their cooking techniques from the French, who have never been stingy with butter and heavy cream. By learning the vocabulary associated with French cooking, however, you can avoid the most fat-filled offerings. Here's a list of terms you're most likely to encounter when choosing from a "four-star" menu:

The Vocabulary of Haute Cuisine

"ail"	garlic
"au gratin"	with cheese and bread crumbs
"beurre"	butter
"boeuf"	beef
"canard"	duck
"caneton"	duckling
"champignons"	mushrooms
"creme"	cream
"farci"	stuffed
"frit"	fried
"gigot"	lamb
"gratine"	baked with bread crumbs
"grille"	broiled
"jambon"	ham
"legumes"	vegetables
"mousse"	thickened with cream
"nouilles"	noodles
"oeufs"	eggs
"pané"	breaded

"pocé"	poached
"pommes de terre"	potatoes
"porc"	pork
"poulet"	chicken
"quiche"	anything in a pie crust
"riz"	rice
"sauté"	cooked in small amount of oil quickly
"souffle"	with egg whites added
"veau"	veal
"vin"	wine

The most healthful entrees at French-based restaurants are seafood or poultry dishes that have been poached, baked, or broiled. If a sauce is offered, ask that it be served on the side.

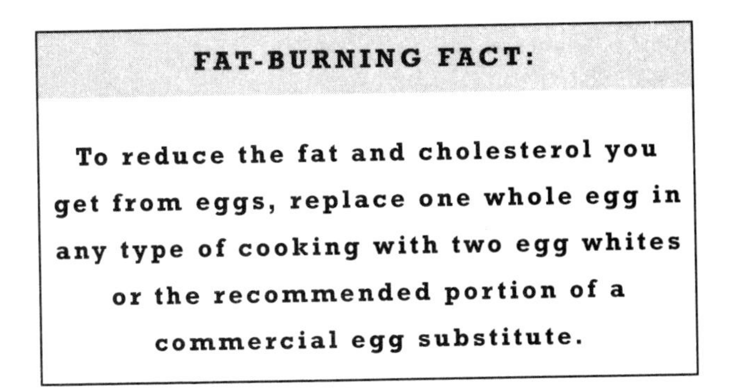

FAT-BURNING FACT:

To reduce the fat and cholesterol you get from eggs, replace one whole egg in any type of cooking with two egg whites or the recommended portion of a commercial egg substitute.

Dining Low-Fat with the Family

There is more to eating healthfully than what goes into your own tummy, of course. If you have a family, you've got their dietary preferences to worry about. How do you prepare a dinner of low-fat poached fish for yourself when everybody else is clamoring for meatloaf and macaroni and cheese? Here are some ideas from nutritional experts.

- *Have a family pow-wow.* It's important that you make clear to your family the importance of your dietary efforts, says Laurie Meyer, R.D., a spokesperson for the American Dietetic Association. Explain why you're making those efforts and suggest ways they can help. If they want nothing to do with your attempts at reform, warn them that they may have to do more cooking for themselves.

- *Try winning them over gradually.* A "cook-for-yourself" policy would not work for young children, of course, so your approach to them—and to an apprehensive spouse—might be to compromise. So go ahead and make the meatloaf, but use ground turkey instead of beef. And make that macaroni dish but use low-fat cheese. Also, try other especially tasty low-fat meals, such as spaghetti in marinara sauce or herb-baked chicken, to help convert your family to a healthful way of eating. By proving that low-fat foods can be satisfyingly delicious, you could have them "on your side" before you know it.

Consider "yours" and "theirs." If family members are not willing to compromise, then you may need to get tough, Meyer says. Tell your spouse he has to do his own cooking, as well as shopping, and inform your children that they either lean your way or settle for prepackaged convenience meals. A steady diet of canned ravioli can speak louder than words.

Give your family the same "pep talk" you give yourself. Explain all the advantages of a low-fat diet—for reasons of health and weight control, for example—and follow up by asking for rational objections. If taste is all they can come up with, counter by whipping up a delicious low-fat version of a family favorite.

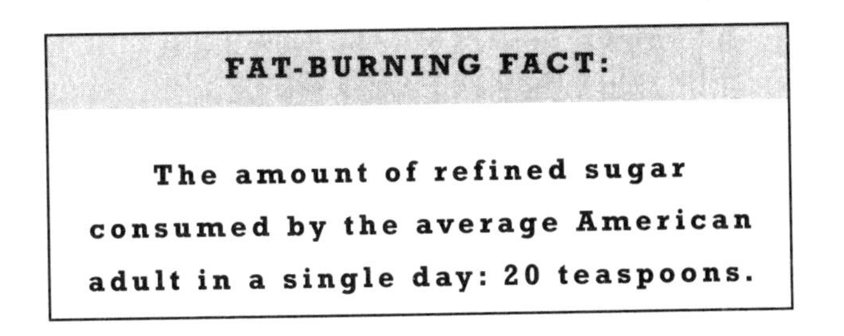

FAT-BURNING FACT:

The amount of refined sugar consumed by the average American adult in a single day: 20 teaspoons.

If You Can't Beat Them, Involve Them: The Case of Susan

Susan felt like she was fighting two battles. Not only was she having her own difficulties sticking to a low-fat diet, the resistance she was getting from her two hot-dog-and-hamburger-loving children, ages 7 and 10, was doubling her trouble.

So she decided to try a little "game." She invited her kids to help make a Chocolate-Banana Thick Shake (see recipe, p. 183). She then told them they could have a shake for dessert providing they peacefully ate whatever she served as the main course. To sweeten the deal even more, she invited her children to assist in the preparation of the main course whenever possible.

"I didn't have them wielding any sharp knives, that's for sure, but I did let them get involved with things like washing vegetables, stirring batters, and hand-forming tuna and turkey burgers," she says.

How'd it work out? "Actually a lot better than I expected," Susan says. "Granted, it meant more work for me—I had to come up with different low-fat desserts!—but it's been worth it because it's given us a chance to interact in ways we didn't before. We talk about school and their friends. We even talk about the importance of nutrition, which I've actually gotten them pretty interested in. They now picture fat as these greasy little creatures that like to hide in the blood vessels and join together to form dams to stop the flow of blood. My husband overheard us one night, and in all honesty I don't think he's had the same passion for fried foods since.

It's Not Just What You Eat, But How You Eat

Whether you're eating at home, at your local diner, or at a restaurant with linen tablecloths, cutting fat from your diet should be the primary goal of your weight-control efforts. But in addition to watching what you eat, you should be careful how you eat—and not just to avoid unwanted pounds. Studies show that eating "mini" meals frequently throughout the day—as many as six a day—can produce some decidedly "maxi" health benefits.

"Mini meals could well be one of the easiest and most effective healthy lifestyle changes that people can make," says Murray Mittleman, the director of the Institute for the Prevention of Cardiovascular Disease at Deaconess Hospital in Boston.

Dr. Mittleman points to research showing that eating small meals encourages the following important health benefits:

Weight control. As the size of a meal goes up, so does the proportion of calories stored as fat—the result of an verproduction of the fat-storing hormone called insulin. Infrequent eating also tends to produce overeating, as hunger often becomes hard to control. (One study of overweight people found that fully 80 percent were taking in fewer calories than people of normal weight, but they were making the "one-big-meal-a-day" mistake.)

Lower cholesterol. Eating small meals seems to create a more favorable environment for the digestion of dietary fats, cholesterol included. One experiment found that eating six small meals a day resulted in cholesterol reductions of 8 percent, which is enough to reduce risks of heart disease by 16 percent, according to David Jenkins, M.D., director of Clinical Nutrition and Risk Factor Modification at St. Michael's Hospital in Toronto.

Reduced risks of heart attacks and strokes. It's not imaginary that hospital emergency rooms experience a marked increase in the number of heart attacks on "feast" days such as Christmas and Thanksgiving. By demanding huge increases in the circulation of blood to the stomach, "very large meals can put the heart through a kind of digestive stress test," says Dr. Mittleman. In one study, a 280-calorie meal required an average of 21 gallons of blood from the hearts of test subjects, while a 720-calorie meal demanded 86 gallons—a difference large enough to fill the gas tank of the average car five times over! Large meals, and especially fatty ones, also can heighten the risks of heart attacks (and strokes) by increasing the danger of artery-clogging clots in the blood.

Prevention of heartburn. The smaller a meal, the less likely it is to "overflow" back into the esophagus—good news for heartburn sufferers. Eating smaller meals is the standard medical advice for victims of this condition, says Dr. Mittleman.

Greater energy and mental alertness. Small meals keep your body and brain supplied steadily with energy-producing glucose. This is not the case with large meals, which can produce drowsiness by drawing inordinate amounts of blood to the stomach, or skipping meals, which allows glucose (blood sugar levels) to drop too low.

Mastering the "Mini Meal"

Wait a minute. Six meals a day? If you're like most dieters, you probably think the best way to lose weight is to skip meals entirely. Get yourself good and hungry and your body will have no choice but to burn fat, right?

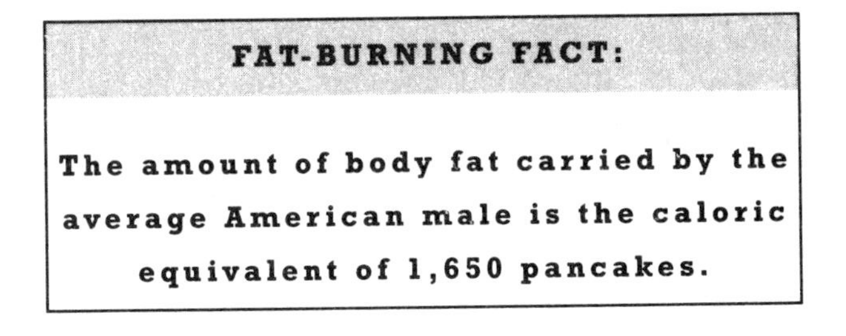
FAT-BURNING FACT:

The amount of body fat carried by the average American male is the caloric equivalent of 1,650 pancakes.

Wrong. As we have seen in Chapter 1, our bodies respond to hunger by attempting to preserve fat, not burn it. Avoiding hunger by eating mini meals, therefore, is actually far superior to starvation as a fat-burning strategy. It gives your body the energy it needs to burn fat the right way, which is through an active metabolism and an increase in physical activity.

Remember, too, that eating three meals a day is a relatively recent custom considering the estimated 50,000-year history of our species. For thousands of years we ate when we were hungry and not according to any predetermined plan. Some nutritionists argue that the convention of "three squares" is one of the reasons we've become so "round."

Fine, you say, but isn't it still a three-meal-a-day world?

Probably, but it doesn't have to be. Here are some tips for breaking free of the "three squares" pattern:

- *Divide before you devour.* The simplest way to turn three meals into six is to divide your breakfast, lunch, and dinner into two meals each. For breakfast, for example, have cereal with skim or low-fat milk, while saving a bagel and piece of fresh fruit for a mid-morning snack. For lunch, have your sandwich while reserving a cup of soup or a serving of low-fat yogurt for an afternoon treat. Dinner? Have your usual low-fat entree and side dishes, while saving your low-fat dessert for a snack an hour or so before bed.

- ***Stock up on healthy snacks to eat at work.*** Don't rely on the company vending machine. If you work at a desk, use it to store low-fat snacks such as individually packaged breakfast cereals, fresh or dried fruits, rice cakes, bagels, or slices of whole-grain bread. If your lunchroom has a refrigerator, use it to keep fresh vegetables, fruit juices, and containers of low-fat yogurt or cottage cheese. If you have access to a microwave, fire it up to make low-fat popcorn or instant soups.

- ***Order appetizers rather than entrees when eating out.*** This is an especially good idea if the entrees being offered could feed King Kong. Don't be afraid to order a more manageable appetizer and perhaps a salad or soup instead.

- ***Pack healthful snacks for the road.*** Why stop for over-priced junk food when you can pack healthful sandwiches, fresh fruits, carrot and celery sticks, saltless pretzels, rice cakes, bagels, and air-popped popcorn?

Mini Meals And Exercise: The Dynamic Duo

Perhaps the greatest advantage of eating small meals is that they don't bloat you and cause paralyzing fatigue. After a feast, you're lucky if you can keep your eyes open, much less engage in any sort of calorie-burning activity.

Not so with small meals, which can actually leave you feeling energized and therefore likely to do something a little more physical than collapsing in front of the TV.

This important but often overlooked point touches on something critical to the weight-loss process. Large meals encourage the inactivity that allows calories to be stored as fat. Small meals, on the other hand, energize you and stimulate the physical activity needed to burn calories for energy.

Better yet, studies show that physical activity within 30 minutes of eating is an especially good way to burn calories—in fact it's 10 percent better than exercising on an empty stomach. The scientific term for this phenomenon is the "thermal effect of food," which can amount to a sizable weight loss advantage over time. Simply by taking a short walk after just one mini meal a day, you could make significant progress in reaching your weight-loss goals.

When "Life" Weighs Too Much: Can Too Much Stress Make You Fat?

If you think it's only too much food combined with too little exercise that makes us fat, you might want to think again. According to research presented in 1994 at the International Conference on Obesity, stress can be fattening and for reasons that use to save lives. During times of stress—whether during a traffic jam or an argument with a co-worker—your body produces adrenalin, which causes molecules of fat to be released into your bloodstream. This gives you the energy needed to deal with the stressful situation.

So what do we do instead?

Instead of getting physical, we get frustrated and begin to "stew." This causes our bodies to produce another hormone called cortisol, which acts as a kind of peacemaker to help the fighting-mad fat molecules get reabsorbed. Unfortunately, cortisol helps other fat molecules get absorbed, too, specifically in the stomach area. It seems unfair and illogical, but numerous studies have proven that it does happen. In a study at Wake Forest University in Winston-Salem, North Carolina, monkeys subjected to chronic stress had significantly more fat in the area of their abdomens than monkeys allowed to live stress free.

"Chronic stress plays a role in abdominal fat distribution," remarked Robert K. Cooper, Ph.D., in his book *Low-Fat Living* (Rodale Press, 1996). "The more minutes of each day you are frustrated, impatient, or angry, the more likely that stress is contributing to fat-making in your body."

Add the overeating we tend to do when we're stressed—usually high-fat junk foods—and the "fret more, weigh more" picture becomes all too clear.

Try These Techniques to Reduce Stress Instantly!

The experts recommend combating stress immediately. The sooner the better, in fact, because the faster stress is defused, the less it's apt to accumulate in ways that can become physically harmful. Here are some clinically proven techniques for reducing stress the moment it strikes.

Breathe stress away. When stress strikes, our first reaction is to halt our breathing entirely for several seconds or more, and then to breathe quickly and shallowly. This reduces oxygen to the brain, which makes us feel stressed even more. To prevent this, it's important to make a conscious effort to breathe deeply and slowly at the first signs of stress. Inhale slowly but deeply through your nose so that your abdomen expands first, then your chest. Then exhale slowly through your mouth, imagining the stress leaving your body as you do.

Think relaxing thoughts. Most stressful situations are beyond our control, which is precisely why we find them stressful. It can be helpful, therefore, to divorce yourself as much as possible from the cause of your stress, thinking totally unrelated and pleasant thoughts, instead. If you're caught in a traffic jam, for example, or find yourself waiting in what seems like an endless line, think of your favorite vacation spot, or a romantic encounter with your sweetheart!

Sharpen your sense of humor. Often the only difference between a stressful situation and a humorous one lies in how we view it. The trash bag that breaks and spills its contents on your newly waxed kitchen floor. The sweater that your daughter converts from a size 12 to a 6 by mistakenly putting it in the dryer. Whether such events are tragedies or comedies is entirely up to you, and the sooner you realize that, the less stressful they're going to be.

Don't take things personally. The stock market takes a plunge. The price of gasoline goes up. It's only natural to view such events in terms of how they affect us personally. But to do so is not only highly stressful, it's self-centered and inaccurate as well. Life's inconveniences affect us all, so we should stop feeling persecuted when they occur.

Get physical. Research shows that physical activity can help stop stress the moment it strikes. In addition, people who are physically active are better at coping with stressful events in the first place. So take a walk, play tennis, go for a jog, or ride a bike the next time life's burdens seem too heavy to bear. The "strength" you gain will lighten your load, both immediately and in the long run.

Open up to loved ones or friends. When stress mounts, it needs an outlet or it will fester and grow. Talk with the people who are closest to you when you're feeling stressed. Not only will this make you feel better, it will tighten your bond with these people, thus ensuring an emotional oasis for the future.

Cook a healthful, low-fat meal. Just because stress is often accompanied by an urge to eat doesn't mean this urge has to be bad. If you can get your mind off your problems by preparing a fantastic, four-star, low-fat feast, that urge to eat can be decidedly healthful!

FAT-BURNING FACT:

Lunch meats are among the fattiest meats and one of the top sources of fat in the American diet. The most healthful choices are boiled ham, honey loaf, and turkey breast.

CHAPTER 3

HOW FITNESS FIGHTS FAT

So where does exercise fit into the fat-burning picture?

Smack dab in the middle. In fact, exercise is essential to the fat-burning process because it infuses our bodies with the very component that fat-burning relies on most: oxygen. This is especially true of aerobic exercise, which "fans the flames" of the fat-burning process. Aerobic exercise can increase your body's uptake of oxygen by as much as 20 times—enough to create quite a fat "bonfire." The more fit you become, moreover, the better your body gets at making sure fat cells become the target of this oxygen rush.

But as great as aerobic exercise is, its appetite for calories can actually be increased if combined with exercises like strength training. Strength training not only exercises your current muscle cells, it helps create new ones, resulting in more "cylinders" in your fat-burning engine. Better yet, muscle tissue is metabolically active even at rest. By adding strength training to your exercise routine, you increase the rate at which you burn calories—not just as you're exercising but as you're sleeping or watching TV!

This is why study after study has shown what every couch potato hates to hear most: People who are the most successful at losing weight and keeping it off are the ones who include at least some form of exercise in their weight-control efforts.

Exercise is crucial to successful weight loss, not just because of the number of calories it burns but because of the *type* of calories it burns. If done regularly and in the right ways (which we'll be seeing shortly), exercise can actually teach your body to burn calories from fat even more so than from carbohydrates. Exercise does this by encouraging the formation of enzymes that make fat more available as fuel for muscular activity. Once these enzymes begin to work their fat-burning "magic," you'll begin to have more energy. You'll start burning more calories at everything you do, whether it's vacuuming the living room or spending an afternoon in the park with your kids.

Give Yourself a Break:
Take It Easy

Exercise is a fat cell's worst nightmare, and that's great. But there are barely enough hours in your day as it is, and you're supposed to find time to work out?

Relax. Exercise need not be as torturous or time-consuming as some fitness experts would like us to believe. In fact, the latest research has found that substantial health benefits can be gained by moderate activities adding up to as little as 150 calories worth of energy expenditure a day.

And please notice we said "add up." Contrary to the belief that exercise must be continuous for at least 20 to 30 minutes to do any good, research shows that you can exercise for shorter periods of time and still reap the benefits. In one study at the University of Pittsburgh, for example, researchers found that women who walked for 40 minutes a day in separate 10-minute sessions enjoyed the same health benefits and actually lost more weight than women who walked for 40 minutes continuously. "The greater flexibility associated with exercising in short bouts evidently had helped the women to be more consistent in their exercise participation," remarked the researchers in their report in the *International Journal of Obesity*.

FAT-BURNING FACT:

A study by the YMCA found that people who lifted weights three times a week for just 20 minutes gained 6 pounds of muscle and lost 15 pounds of fat in just seven weeks.

So, yes, you can be fit and keep a busy schedule, too! All you need to do is find ways to get your exercise in manageable "nibbles" rather than in those inconvenient (and easily skipped) half-hour chunks. A short walk here, a quick bike ride there, and maybe some gardening or housework in between. As long as these activities add up to at least 150 calories of energy expended each day, you're giving your body's metabolism the fat-burning boost that long-term weight control requires.

This is not to say that more exercise cannot burn more calories and therefore more unwanted fat, but an energy expenditure of approximately 150 calories a day is a healthful and reasonable start—especially if you're relatively new to the fitness game. If you choose to pursue an exercise program more avidly, fine. Just be sure to check first with your doctor, and consider consulting a licensed fitness expert on how best to proceed to achieve your desired goals.

Strength Training: Burning Fat by Building Muscle

The key to burning calories is movement. The good news is that the movement doesn't have to be continuous or so strenuous that you find yourself gasping for breath. Studies now show that exercise that's too strenuous—by putting the body into a state of oxygen deficit—can actually shut fat-burning down. You need plenty of oxygen, which is what you will get when you exercise aerobically, to get the fat "going." By exercising so vigorously that you force yourself into an oxygen shortage, you cause your body to switch from burning fat to burning glycogen. Glycogen is a form of carbohydrate stored in the muscles and liver that the body can use for energy with virtually no oxygen at all.

But as mentioned at the beginning of this chapter, there's another type of exercise that can boost fat burning to an even higher level, and that's strength training—the kind that builds muscle. This isn't to say that aerobic exercise isn't an invaluable weight-control aid, because it most certainly is, as dozens of studies show. But the primary value of aerobic exercise lies in its ability to burn calories as you're actually in the process of doing it, which to a degree limits its weight-control value. This is not the case with strength training, which, because it builds muscle, can make you a better calorie burner 24 hours a day, even as you're talking on the phone or relaxing in a nice warm bath. (Some studies have shown that very long and strenuous aerobic workouts also can be followed by a period of increased calorie burning, but usually this lasts no more than several hours.)

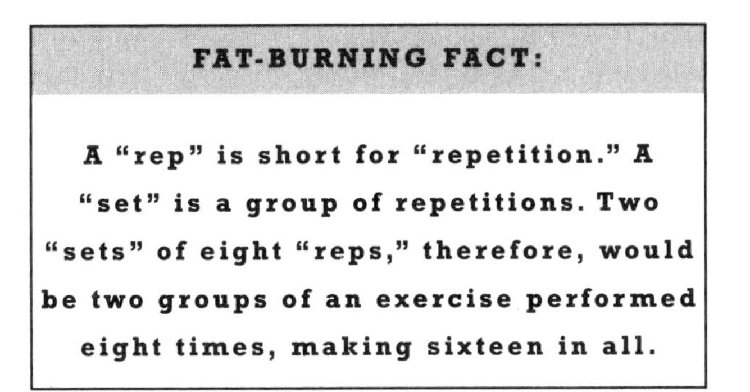

FAT-BURNING FACT:

A "rep" is short for "repetition." A "set" is a group of repetitions. Two "sets" of eight "reps," therefore, would be two groups of an exercise performed eight times, making sixteen in all.

The Proof in the Pudding

As proof of the fat-burning power of strength training, consider the following study done recently with seventy-two men and women at the YMCA in Quincy, Massachusetts. Half of the people worked out aerobically for 30 minutes three times a week, while the other group split their workouts between 15 minutes of aerobics and 15 minutes of lifting weights. Both groups had identical meals (consisting of 60 percent carbohydrates, 20 percent protein, and 20 percent fat), and yet results differed dramatically. The strength-training group had lost an impressive 10 pounds of fat over the course of the eight-week study, while the aerobics group had lost only three.

Sounds great, you say, but you don't want bulky muscles, even if they are such great fat-blasters?

You don't have to have bulky muscles. You can appreciably raise your body's basal metabolism (the rate at which you burn calories at rest) simply by toning and strengthening the muscles you already have. It's important that you do this because studies show that the muscle mass of the average American woman decreases by about a half a pound a year after the age of 35—enough to cause a considerable slow-down in metabolic rate and significant accumulations of unwanted fat.

A Little Goes a Long Way

"This is one of the reasons for the seemingly mysterious weight gain so many of us experience as we get older," says Bryant Stamford, of the Center for Health Promotion at the University of Louisville. "Even though we don't eat any more, and we keep our activity levels basically the same, we gain weight because we lose muscle mass and hence our ability to burn calories at a more youthful rate."

But how much strength training is required to stall this loss of muscle tissue associated with aging? Will you need to be setting up a gym in your garage?

As with aerobic exercise, there's good news here, too. Studies show that age-related muscle loss can be decreased significantly with weight-training sessions or strength-building exercises, such as push-ups and pull-ups, done as infrequently as twice a week. Better yet, many chores around the house also can keep your muscles toned and metabolism perked. Raking leaves, carrying firewood, scrubbing floors, moving furniture, shoveling snow, carrying grocery bags, kneading bread, or toting around a toddler or two. Any activity that pits muscles against some form of resistance—whether it's a barbell or basket of wet laundry—can be an effective way to keep muscle cells functioning at their fat-burning best.

Fitness And Soap Operas

If you're like most Americans, your number one excuse for not getting more exercise is lack of time, yet you still manage to watch an average of 4 hours of television a day. So why not combine the two? By spending just 30 minutes doing some form of light exercise, such as riding a stationary bike or walking on a treadmill while viewing the tube, you could be 20 pounds thinner this time next year.

"I'm convinced that strength training has been the missing link in many peoples' weight-control efforts up to this point, and especially people over the age of about 40," Dr. Stamford says. "Middle age is when muscle-building hormones begin their greatest decline, and yet few of us respond by doing the kind of strength training needed to compensate for it. Usually we'll take up an aerobic activity such as walking or cycling as we age, thus missing out on the opportunity to keep our muscles—and metabolisms—as well toned as they could be."

This is not to say that we can halt the loss of muscle tissue entirely as we age. But take a look at legendary fitness guru Jack LaLanne, who, to celebrate his 65th birthday, swam across a 1 1/2-mile lake pulling 65 rowboats loaded with 65,000 pounds of wood pulp—while handcuffed! It's pretty clear that many of us are letting Father Time take more of our muscle power—and our ability to burn calories—than necessary.

How Active Are You?
Take a Minute to Take This Test

The good news from the Centers for Disease Control and Prevention (CDC) is that we don't have to burden ourselves with continuous 20- to 30-minute aerobic workouts to enjoy the health benefits of exercise. Instead, any combination of moderate activities adding up to an average of at least 150 calories of energy expenditure a day is the new recommendation for helping us avoid the pitfalls (increased risks of heart disease, diabetes, osteoporosis, depression, and certain forms of cancer) of a sedentary lifestyle.

But before you sit down on the couch to celebrate that less exhaustive prescription, you might want to take an honest look at the amount of physical activity your average day actually includes. We offer the following quiz to help you do just that.

1. In an average day, I climb the following number of flights of stairs (12 steps per flight):

a. 0 (0 points)
b. 1–5 (1 point)
c. 6–10 (2 points)
d. more than 10 (4 points)

2. My job requires that I be on my feet and moving for approximately the following number of hours per day:

a. 0 hours (0 points)
b. 1 hour (2 points)

c. 2 hours	(3 points)
d. 3 hours	(4 points)
e. 4 hours or more	(6 points)

3. My job requires heavy labor such as lifting, carrying, shoveling, or climbing for the following number of hours a day:

a. 0 hours	(0 points)
b. 1 hour	(3 points)
c. 2 hours	(5 points)
d. 3 hours	(7 points)
e. 4 hours	(9 points)
f. 5 hours or more	(12 points)

4. I spend the following number of hours a week tending a garden or lawn. (Points assume activity is year-round. Cut points in half if activity is seasonal.)

a. 0 hours	(0 points)
b. 1 hour	(1 point)
c. 2 hours	(2 points)
d. 3 hours	(3 points)
e. 4 hours	(4 points)
f. 5 hours or more	(6 points)

5. I participate in light sporting activities or dancing for the following number of hours a week:

a. 0 hours	(0 points)
b. 1 hour	(1 point)
c. 2 hours	(2 points)
d. 3 hours	(3 points)
e. 4 or more hours	(4 points)

6. I try to walk for the following distance most days of the week:

a. 0 miles	(0 points)
b. 1 mile	(2 points)
c. 2 miles	(4 points)
d. 3 miles	(6 points)
e. 4 miles or more	(10 points)

7. I spend the following number of hours each week doing household chores such as cleaning, dusting, vacuuming, or laundry:

a. 0 hours	(0 points)
b. 1 hour	(1 point)
c. 2 hours	(2 points)
d. 3 hours	(3 points)
e. 4 hours	(4 points)
f. more than 4 hours	(6 points)

8. I engage in some form of aerobic exercise (i.e., jogging, cycling, swimming, fast-walking, aerobic dancing, or working out on a rowing machine or stair-climber) for the following number of hours a week:

   a. 0 hours (0 points)
   b. 1 hour (5 points)
   c. 2 hours (10 points)
   d. 3 hours (15 points)
   e. more than 3 hours (20 points)

9. I participate in strength-building exercise (by lifting free weights, working out on weight machines, or doing strength-building calisthenics such as chin-ups and push-ups) for the following number of hours each week:

   a. 0 hours (0 points)
   b. 1 hour (5 points)
   c. 2 hours (10 points)
   d. 3 hours (15 points)
   e. more than 3 hours (20 points)

10. I am a parent in charge of taking care of one or more preschool-aged children for the following amount of time each day:

a. children home all day (5 points)
b. children home half a day (day-care center the rest) (3 points)
c. children spend all day at day-care center (1 point)

SCORING

15 points or higher: Superb. Congratulations! You're getting more exercise than are approximately 80 percent of your fellow Americans. If you also are eating well, not smoking, avoiding undue stress, and drinking in moderation only, you're doing all you can to live a long and productive life.

10–14 points: Very Good. Nice work. You're doing what's required to satisfy your basic exercise needs. If you're also adhering to the other healthful behaviors mentioned above, your life should be long and prosperous.

5–9 points: Marginal. You're not to be scolded but not commended either. By fitting more activity into your life, you could be slimmer, have more energy, and also improve your chances of living longer.

Less than 5 points: Reprehensible! You're a member of the Couch Potato Hall of Fame and had better check your pulse frequently. Your level of inactivity is hazardous to your health and waistline, too.

Shape Up Your Metabolism in Just 30 Minutes a Week

Strength training can really put a "squeeze" on fat cells. By building and toning muscle tissue, it can make you a better calorie-burner 24 hours a day. Better yet, you don't have to become an iron-pumping fanatic to do it. All you need is to put your major muscle groups up against some form of resistance for approximately 15 minutes at least two to three times a week. Chores around the house and yard can qualify as strength-building exercises (scrubbing floors, moving furniture, digging in the garden, and trimming hedges and trees, for example). If such activities are not available to you, or you'd like something more regimented, try a simple weight-training program (see below) or maybe some strength-building calisthenics, such as push-ups and pull-ups, to give your muscles a major fat-burning boost.

The Six Greatest Fat-burning Muscle Groups— And How To Work Them All In Just 20 Minutes!

The physics principle of calorie burning is this: The larger the muscle group, the more calories it will burn. The key to strength training for weight control is to work the largest muscles you have (listed below). Also listed are the best exercises for getting these muscles into the maximum, fat-burning shape.

And don't think you'll need a lot of expensive equipment, or that you'll have to spend grueling hours at the gym. You can maximize the fat-burning power of all your major muscle groups by using just dumbbells, and you'll only need about 20 minutes, three times a week. Certainly you can find time for that, right?

How Much To Lift

You'll want to do this series of six exercises twice, with a rest period between each series lasting one to two minutes. As for the exercises themselves, do "sets" consisting of 10 repetitions each, using a weight that is heavy enough so that your tenth "rep" is difficult but not torturous. After completing each set of 10 reps, take about a 15- to 30-second rest before moving on to the next set. The entire workout should take only about 20 minutes.

The Muscle Group	The Exercise
Chest	Dumbbell bench presses, or push-ups
Thighs	Squats
Shoulders and Back	Reverse dumbbell "flys" or pull-ups
Biceps	Dumbbell curls
Triceps	Dumbbell presses
Abdomen	Curl-ups

Making The Fitness Fit

Beginning to get the picture? Exercise—a combination of aerobic and strength-building exercise, especially—trains the body to favor fat as an energy source. Better yet, the amount and type of exercise required to do this is well within reach of all of us, even working mothers with barely a minute to spare. "Many of us could get all the exercise we need if we'd simply stop trying so hard to avoid it," says Dr. Bryant Stamford.

But, no, we take elevators instead of stairs, and drive around endlessly to find the most convenient parking spot, and buy every device imaginable to make our household chores and yard work easier. Or worse yet, we'll avoid our physical chores entirely by hiring them out to professionals. A recent Gallup poll showed that we spend an average of over $700 a year per household on lawn-care services alone. We're burning our money when we could be burning calories!

"Exercising with a friend gives many people a surge of energy on days when they otherwise wouldn't feel like working out."

Johathan Robison, Ph.D., Executive Co-Director of the Michigan Center for Preventative Medicine

And compounding this absurdity is the fact that millions of us join health clubs—which we fail to visit—in hopes of getting the very exercise we've gone to so much trouble to avoid! "We've made exercise far more complicated, impractical, and inconvenient than it has to be, so no wonder only about a third of us currently get the amount of exercise we need," Dr. Stamford says. "We need to learn to incorporate exercise into our lives in ways that are more enjoyable and practical."

Exercise For The Health Of It

Exercise is just what the doctor ordered for achieving and maintaining a healthy weight. Exercise also is just what the doctor ordered for achieving a healthy body, something ancient healers have known since the writings of Hippocrates. Studies now show that 30 minutes of moderate exercise a day, in addition to keeping your metabolism in the best fat-burning shape, also can bestow the following important health benefits:

- Improved circulation (achieved through the widening of existing blood vessels plus the formation of new ones) resulting in reduced risks of heart attacks and strokes
- Lower blood pressure resulting in reduced risks of aneurysms (an abnormal blood-filled swelling of a blood vessel), glaucoma, heart attacks, and strokes
- Reductions in "bad" (LDL) and increases in "good" (HDL) cholesterol resulting in reduced risks of clogged arteries leading to heart attacks and strokes
- Reduced risks of adult-onset (type 2) diabetes
- Increased physical as well as mental stamina
- Stronger bones resulting in reduced risks of osteoporosis
- Improved joint mobility resulting in reduced risks of osteoarthritis
- A stronger immune system resulting in reduced risks of colds, flu, and possibly even cancer
- Improved digestion resulting in the best absorption of vital nutrients

- Reduced risks of low-back pain
- An increase in the blood's ability to carry oxygen to cells, plus an increase in the ability of muscle cells to use this oxygen to burn fat
- An increase in the blood's ability to rid the body of carbon dioxide and other cellular waste products
- Greater intestinal regularity resulting in reduced risks of cancer of the colon
- Sounder, more restful sleep
- Healthier skin
- Reduced risks of depression and anxiety disorders
- Protection from stress
- More enjoyable sex

Exercise For A Slimmer Appetite

But with all the calories exercise burns, won't it just make you eat more, thus canceling all the exercise's fantastic weight-control benefits?

No. In fact, just the opposite tends to be true. In addition to burning calories, exercise can actually help reduce your urge to take in calories in the first place. "Many people who embark on fitness programs are surprised to find that it actually helps them eat less, not more," says Dr. Stamford.

As evidence of this, he cites a study done several years ago in which people reported feeling less hungry and more energetic several hours after taking a 15-minute walk than they did after eating a candy bar. "The tendency of exercise to reduce appetite probably stems from its ability to mobilize supplies of blood sugar, called glycogen, which is stored in the muscles and the liver," says Dr. Stamford.

Then, too, there are the psychological benefits of exercise that can help keep runaway appetites in check: improvements in self-esteem and self-control and increased abilities to cope with stress, for example. "When people exercise regularly, they often find they feel more in control of every other aspect of their lives—their work, their relationships, and their diets, especially," says Dr. Stamford. "Exercise can be a very powerful catalyst for all sorts of healthful behaviors. Studies show it can even help people give up smoking."

FAT-BURNING FACT:

The amount of refined sugar consumed by the average American adult in a single day: 20 teaspoons.

Every Little Bit Counts

But what about "no pain, no gain"? Can activities that are fun or useful be strenuous enough to do us any good?

Absolutely. "The latest research now shows that exercise is pretty much a case of anything goes," says Stanford University sports medicine specialist Warren Scott, M.D. "As long as it's bodily movement, it qualifies as exercise, and it's clearly better than no activity at all. We know now, too, that exercise that's gotten in bits and pieces can be as beneficial as exercise gotten in larger and more onerous chunks. Exercise does not have to have you huffing and puffing for at least 20 continuous minutes to do you any good, which is the impression, unfortunately, that many people still have."

Look over the activities on the next page with that in mind. They all burn at least 150 calories, the amount that research now indicates is needed to satisfy our minimum daily exercise requirements. If you've got the time or inclination to do more, that's fine. Just don't make the mistake of doing no exercise because you don't think you have the time to do enough. Remember, the latest research shows that any amount of exercise is vastly better than none at all.

More Gain, Less Pain

50 Fun and Practical Ways to Burn 150 Calories in 30 Minutes or Less

Not the jogging or iron-pumping type? No problem. There are plenty of other more enjoyable and practical ways to burn off unwanted pounds, as the following list shows. Your goal, remember, is to burn at least 150 calories by engaging in any of these activities each day. (Calorie expenditures are for someone weighing 150 pounds. Adjust figures up or down slightly if you weigh more or less.)

Activity	Calories Burned In 30 Minutes
Backpacking	280
Basketball (shooting baskets)	180
Basketball (playing in game)	320
Bicycling (leisurely)	160
Bicycling (vigorously)	400
Canoeing (moderate effort)	280
Dancing (ballroom or disco)	220
Dancing (aerobic, low-impact)	240
Dancing (aerobic, high-impact)	280
Fishing (from stream, in wading boots)	160
Football (touch)	320
Golf (pulling clubs)	200
Hackysack	160
Handball	480
Hockey (field)	320
Hockey (ice)	320
Horseback riding (trot)	260
Horseback riding (gallop)	320

Horse grooming	240
Housework (sweeping, mopping, etc.)	180
Hunting (small game)	200
Ice skating (recreational)	280
In-line skating (moderately fast)	280
Jumping rope (moderately fast)	400
Karate (or other martial arts class)	400
Moving furniture (heavy)	360
Painting (outdoors)	200
Ping-Pong	160
Playing with children (vigorous)	200
Playing drums	160
Rock climbing	440
Scuba diving	280
Skateboarding	200
Skiing, downhill (moderate effort)	240
Skiing, cross-country (moderate effort)	340
Sledding (or tobogganing)	280
Snorkeling	200
Snowshoeing (moderate effort)	320
Soccer	360
Softball (pitching)	240
Squash	480
Swimming (freestyle, moderate effort)	320
Tai chi	160
Tennis (singles)	320
Tennis (doubles)	240
Volleyball (beach)	320
Walking (moderate pace)	150
Walking (brisk pace)	180
Water polo	400
Water skiing	240

Fitness On The Mild Side: The Case of Robert

"I used to really hate my workouts, which might help explain why I was so good at missing them," Robert now confesses. "I'd push myself to the limit every time, thinking I wasn't doing myself any good if I didn't. Then I'd sometimes go a week or more without working out at all, because the whole experience was so dreadful for me."

Not just dreadful but unproductive. Robert was about 20 pounds overweight with high blood pressure and a high serum cholesterol level, but his sporadic workouts were having very little effect.

Not only was he failing to lose weight, his cholesterol level and blood pressure were inching upward, "the result, probably, of all the stress I was subjecting myself to," he now says. "I was under tremendous pressure at work, and I think my approach to exercise was probably only adding to it. Either I was dreading my workouts, or feeling guilty for avoiding them, certainly not a very relaxing situation either way."

But as fate would have it, Robert was "saved" one day by an injury. He tore a muscle in his left calf—"the result of going out too fast without adequately warming up," his doctor told him—and was forced to modify his fitness regime. On his doctor's advice, he started walking. Before long he actually started to like it.

"It was a whole different experience," Robert says. "I stopped worrying about how fast I was going, or how far, and just let my mind wander. I started liking it so much, in fact, that I actually began looking forward to it as a way of unwinding after work. I even started inviting my wife along, and we'd have some really great talks."

Better yet, Robert's weight started to come down, along with his blood pressure and cholesterol levels. "I've even started to take a slightly more relaxed approach to my work," he says. "I don't see things so much as just black or white anymore, and I don't think I'm as impulsive or critical. It's as though I've slowed down the revs of my engine, and yet I actually feel more productive."

How To "Excuse-Proof" Your Exercise Routine

But you already know that exercise is good for you, and you want to do it. The problem you have is sticking to a regular schedule. Something always seems to come up that gets in the way. Then you need to make exercise more of a priority, says Kerry Courneya, Ph.D., of the University of Calgary in Alberta, Canada. Here are some tips that can help:

1. **Choose an activity you enjoy.** The reason you're finding excuses not to exercise is probably because you don't like whatever it is you're doing. As we mentioned earlier in this chapter, exercise does not have to be strenuous to work. So go easy on yourself and have fun with your exercise. Take scenic walks, play tennis, play frisbee with the kids. Remember, anything that gets you moving is going to burn calories. It's sitting around feeling guilty for not doing anything at all that can get fattening.

2. **Try to exercise before you begin your day.** Studies show that people who exercise first thing in the morning are less likely to skip their workouts than people who wait until later in the day, when other obligations pop up and get in the way. Remember, too, that exercise is a great energizer and spirit-lifter, so you'll be all the more ready to face the world by working out before you begin your day.

3. **Involve friends.** Not only is it harder to skip workouts when you involve others, exercising with friends also can make the experience a lot more fun.

4. **Reward yourself.** There's nothing like putting occasional "pots" at the end of your exercise rainbow to keep you going, says psychologist James Prochaska, Ph.D., of the University of Rhode Island. If you've succeeded in sticking to a schedule you've set up for yourself, go ahead and do something nice for yourself periodically, he says. A new dress, a dinner out, some new running shoes, perhaps.

3. **Don't get derailed if you do miss.** It's inevitable that even the most dedicated exercisers get knocked off course occasionally—so why shouldn't you? Just remember that it's the "big picture" that's important and get back on track as soon as you can. The worst thing to do is to become immobilized with guilt.

Look Before You Leap Into A Health Club

Should you join a health club or gym to help solidify your exercise commitment?

That depends on you—and the club. For some people, the structure and camaraderie provided by a fitness facility can be very motivating. For others it can be a source of stress that only makes exercising even more burdensome.

If you think you would be more comfortable with the former than the latter, then by all means go for it. But do some investigating before signing on any dotted lines. Visit the facility, of course, but also ask the following questions of the management:

- **What, exactly, does a membership include?** The facility should offer a free fitness evaluation, plus a session with an instructor, to get you started on a program designed specifically for you.

- **Can your membership be refunded or sold to someone else?** Many clubs will allow this if you are dissatisfied.

- **Are discounts available for using the club during off-hours?** Some clubs offer reduced rates for mid-morning hours and afternoons during the week.

- **What qualifications do the instructors have?** Be wary of a facility whose instructors have no formal training at all.

- **Is the facility's equipment leased or owned?** Leasing is preferable because it means the equipment will more likely be kept up-to-date.

- **Will there be hours when any of the club's facilities are unavailable because of special classes or workouts by local teams?** Swimming pools sometimes get reserved for this reason.

- **Does the club demand a down payment before you've had a chance to read the contract?** If so, take your fitness somewhere else.

Last but not least, visit the facility and chat with some of its members. If they have any gripes, chances are you will, too.

Walking: Possibly The Best Exercise Of All

Nothing against all that new fitness equipment available today—everything from stair-climbers to cardio-gliders—but one of the most effective and practical forms of exercise to burn fat continues to be walking. As Mark Bricklin, the former editor of *Prevention* magazine, says, "No other activity bestows the blessings of exercise as easily, enjoyably, and safely as the simple act of going for a walk."

That might sound like a pretty lofty claim, but there's a lot of research to back it up. Studies show that people who walk for fitness suffer the fewest injuries, have the lowest dropout rates, and continue to exercise later in life more than people who exercise in any other way.

The "Leader Of The Pack" For Weight Control

When it comes to weight control, walking really jumps out ahead of the pack. In one study done at the University of California Medical Center, a group of obese people who repeatedly had failed to lose weight by dieting lost an average of 22 pounds in a year simply by walking for 30 minutes a day. "The key to walking seems to be that it's one of the few activities people will do with the consistency that long-term weight loss requires," Bricklin says. "People usually will exercise more frequently and for longer periods of time when they walk, and that translates into more calories burned."

Could walking be your best fitness and fat-burning route? Why not give it a try and find out for yourself? Here are some general guidelines for getting started:

Wear proper shoes.

And no, this does not mean running shoes. They will do in a pinch, but it's best if you wear shoes specifically designed for walking.

Don't be in too great a hurry.

Your goal should be at least 30 minutes a day, but feel free to take as long as a month to reach that goal if your current fitness level is low.

Put consistency ahead of distance or speed.

You're better off walking a little every day than going for longer or faster walks with several days of rest in between.

Try to walk after meals.

Studies show that this can boost the amount of calories you burn by as much as 10 percent.

Use proper form.

You've been walking since the age of approximately 18 months, so you think you've got it down. But don't be so sure. To obtain the best health benefits from your walks:

1. Walk with your back straight, your chin up, and your arms swinging freely at your sides while bent at a 90-degree angle.
2. Do not walk flat-footed. Push off from the balls of your feet and land on your heels.
3. Lean slightly forward and pump harder with your arms when walking up hills.
4. To walk faster, quicken your movement rather than lengthen your steps.
5. Breathe deeply and with a rhythm that feels comfortably in sync with your stride.

A word on walking with weights: Sorry, but studies show they do not appreciably boost calorie-burning as you walk, although they can help tone the muscles of the arms. (Weights weighing between 2 and 3 pounds but no more than 5 pounds are best.) Ankle weights, on the other hand, are not a good idea. Research shows they can increase risks of injury by altering foot placement and stride.

Patience and Realism

So now you know how to eat and exercise your way to a leaner and healthier body. Two things you should try to remember along the way: (1) The longer your weight loss takes, the longer it's apt to last, and (2) Do not strive for a weight that is unrealistically low. Our best "fighting" weights, research has begun to discover, usually are within a range we don't have to fight.

Good Luck!

CHAPTER 4

VITAMINS AND MINERALS

BEST FOOD SOURCES

There's more to food than just protein, carbohydrates, fat, and calories. Food also contains vitamins and minerals—and it's a good thing, too, because you couldn't live without them! Vitamins work as "catalysts," meaning that they help produce the chemical reactions required for your body to put food to proper use. Minerals, in a slightly different way, help provide the right "environment" so that these chemical reactions can happen as they should. Together, vitamins and minerals—a little like Batman and Robin—work as a "dynamic duo."

VITAMINS

VITAMIN A

Vitamin A is appropriately named because it deserves an "A" for its stellar contributions to good health. In addition to playing a vital role in good vision, it contributes to healthy skin, aids in the production of red blood cells, and helps keep the body's immune system in shape. It may even help prevent cancer. Among other foods, Vitamin A is found in:

- Cantaloupe
- Carrots
- Liver (all types)
- Mangoes
- Pumpkin
- Spinach
- Sweet potatoes
- Turnip greens
- Winter squash

THE B VITAMINS

The B vitamins act as your body's spark plugs. They help derive energy from carbohydrates and can be found most abundantly in the following:

- Beans
- Brewer's yeast
- Brown rice
- Eggs
- Liver
- Meats
- Milk
- Nuts
- Whole grains

VITAMIN C

Vitamin C's most critical function is to help the body ward off not just colds but infections in general. The following are excellent sources of Vitamin C:

- Broccoli
- Brussels sprouts
- Cantaloupe
- Citrus fruits
- Currants
- Honeydew melon
- Kiwi fruit
- Kohlrabi (cabbage turnip)
- Red peppers
- Strawberries

VITAMIN D

Your body manufactures bone-building Vitamin D, called the "sunshine vitamin," when exposed to sunlight. Because this can be a problem during cold weather, which keeps us indoors, it's important to get enough D in your diet. The best way to do that is to drink plenty of Vitamin D-fortified low-fat or skim milk. No other foods, unfortunately, contain the vitamin in appreciable amounts.

VITAMIN E

Think of Vitamin E as your body's "enforcer." It helps other essential vitamins work better at protecting you from everything from the common cold to cancer. Because the best food sources of Vitamin E tend also to be quite high in fat (vegetable oils and nuts, for example), many nutritionists recommend a daily supplement of approximately 100 to 400 International Units (IUs) of Vitamin E. Other sources:

- Blackberries
- Corn oil
- Hazelnut oil
- Mangoes
- Mayonnaise
- Olive oil
- Safflower oil
- Sunflower oil
- Wheat germ

MINERALS

CALCIUM

Calcium is a mineral with several important functions: It helps strengthen our bones, it stabilizes our blood pressure, and it helps maintain a healthy heart. Thankfully, calcium is found in many foods, including:

- Broccoli
- Low-fat and nonfat cheeses
- Low-fat and nonfat milk
- Low-fat and nonfat yogurt
- Salmon
- Sardines
- Tofu
- Turnip greens
- Soybeans

IRON

The primary function of iron—and it's a critical one—is to assure that the body manufactures enough hemoglobin, a protein that helps red blood cells transport oxygen to virtually every tissue of the body. Iron also plays an important role in keeping the body's immune system functioning properly, so it's important that our diets include enough of this mineral. The best source of iron is meat, but it also can be found, in a less absorbable form, in plant foods. Because meat can be high in fat, most nutritionists recommend getting iron from a good mix of both meat and non-meat sources. Iron is found in the following foods:

- Beef
- Blackstrap molasses
- Chicken
- Clams
- Leafy green vegetables
- Liver (all types)
- Oysters
- Pork
- Potatoes
- Soybeans
- Tofu
- Whole grains

MAGNESIUM

Magnesium is another "multi-purpose" mineral, important for the health of bones, blood vessels, the heart, and the immune system. It is present in many foods, the best of which are:

- Almonds
- Brown or wild rice
- Cashew nuts
- Halibut
- Mackerel
- Pumpkin seeds
- Spinach
- Sunflower seeds
- Tofu
- Wheat germ

POTASSIUM

Potassium's main function seems to be to help control blood pressure, but new research shows that it also may help prevent strokes and kidney stones, too. People who exercise heavily may need ample amounts of potassium to prevent muscle cramps. Look to these foods as your best potassium sources:

- Avocadoes
- Bananas
- Cantaloupe
- Clams
- Dried apricots
- Lima beans
- Nonfat yogurt
- Oranges
- Potatoes
- Rainbow trout
- Raisins
- Skim milk
- Yams

ZINC

Zinc is the key to a healthy immune system and to healthy (more wrinkle-resistant) skin. As the following list shows, meat products (aside from shellfish) tend to be the richest source of zinc, so try to get your zinc from the leanest cuts when possible. (Zinc requirements will increase during pregnancy, so moms-to-be, take note.)

- Beans
- Beef
- Clams
- Crabmeat
- Liver (most types)
- Nonfat yogurt
- Oysters
- Peas
- Salmon
- Wild rice
- Wheat germ
- Whole grains

The Sense—And Nonsense—of Supplements

If vitamins and minerals are so important for good health, should you be taking supplements to be even healthier? Unless you're over the age of approximately 60 (when the body's ability to absorb nutrients begins to decline), or you're on a strict, very low-calorie diet (which you shouldn't be without the supervision of your doctor), taking more than the current RDA (Recommended Dietary Allowance) of most vitamins and minerals shouldn't be necessary—and in some cases can even be harmful, the experts say. Only Vitamin E is difficult to get in adequate amounts through food, hence a daily supplement of 100 to 400 IUs often is recommend. "There's no question that nutrients are better absorbed when gotten through foods," says vitamin expert Ronald Watson, Ph.D., of the University of Arizona. "Food also contains a wide variety of micronutrients, the benefits of which we're just beginning to understand."

And there's another reason: Healthful foods beat vitamin pills in the taste department every time!

CHAPTER 5

NICE AND EASY FAT-BURNING RECIPES

Simply Delicious Soups and Salads

Onion-Potato Soup

1 tablespoon canola, corn, safflower, or sunflower oil
2 large onions, chopped
2 teaspoons all-purpose flour
1 cup beef broth or bouillon
1 large potato, peeled, and cut into 1/2-inch pieces
1/4 cup frozen peas
2 1/2 cups skim milk
1/2 teaspoon salt
pepper to taste

Heat oil in Dutch oven or large saucepan over high heat; add onions. Cook 5 to 7 minutes or until onions just begin to brown. Reduce heat to medium. Stir in flour. Gradually stir in beef broth, then add potato and peas. Cover and cook until potatoes are tender, about 15 to 20 minutes, stirring occasionally to get up brown bits. In food processor or blender, puree onion-potato mixture and 1 cup milk until smooth. Return to Dutch oven. Add remaining milk, salt, and pepper. Cook until heated through. Makes 4 servings.

Per serving: 188 calories; 9 g protein; 4 g fat; 20% calories from fat; 3 mg cholesterol; 29 g carbohydrates; 557 mg sodium; 3 g fiber

Carrot Soup

4 cups water
2 pounds carrots, peeled and chopped
1 1/2 teaspoons salt, divided
2 tablespoons butter
1 large onion, chopped
2 cloves garlic, minced
1 can (14 fluid ounces) evaporated skim milk
1 tablespoon sugar
1 tablespoon chopped fresh or 1 teaspoon dried dill
1/2 teaspoon ground allspice
pepper to taste

In Dutch oven or large saucepan, bring to boil water, carrots, and 1 teaspoon salt. Reduce heat to low; cover and simmer 12 to 15 minutes or until fork-tender. Drain, reserving cooking liquid. Set carrots aside. Heat butter in small skillet over medium heat. Add onion and garlic. Cook until onion is tender, about 5 minutes. In food processor or blender, carefully puree onion mixture and carrots in batches with some reserved cooking liquid until smooth. Return to saucepan. Add milk and enough reserved cooking liquid until desired thickness. Stir in sugar, dill, allspice, and remaining salt and pepper to taste. Cook until heated through. Makes 4 servings.

Per serving: 205 calories; 8 g protein; 5 g fat; 22% calories from fat; 15 mg cholesterol; 33 g carbohydrates; 836 mg sodium; 6 g fiber

Hearty Potato and Greens Soup

- 2 large potatoes (about 1 1/2 pounds), peeled and cut into 1/2-inch pieces
- 2 cups water
- 4 ounces fresh greens (escarole, romaine, leaf lettuce, etc.), torn (about 4 cups)
- 1 teaspoon salt
- 1/2 teaspoon curry powder
- 1/2 teaspoon ground cumin
- 1 cup nonfat plain yogurt
- 1 cup skim milk
- 2 teaspoons sugar
- lemon wedges for garnish

In Dutch oven or large saucepan, bring to boil potatoes and water. Reduce heat to low; cover and simmer until potatoes are tender, about 7 to 10 minutes. With slotted spoon, remove 1/2 potatoes and put in food processor or blender; let cool slightly. Put remaining half in bowl. Meanwhile, add greens, salt, curry powder, and cumin to saucepan with potato liquid. Cover and cook until greens are tender, about 7 to 15 minutes, depending on greens. Add yogurt to potatoes in food processor; process until smooth. Add potato-yogurt mixture, along with remaining potato, skim milk, and sugar, to green mixture. Heat through over low heat (do not boil or yogurt will curdle). Serve with lemon wedges if desired. Makes 6 servings.

Per serving: 144 calories; 6 g protein; .5 g fat; 2% calories from fat; 1 mg cholesterol; 30 g carbohydrates; 414 mg sodium; 2 g fiber

Beet, Potato, and Celery Salad

- 1/2 cup nonfat plain yogurt
- 1/2 cup light mayonnaise
- 2 teaspoons lemon juice
- 1/2 teaspoon salt
- pepper to taste
- 1 can (14.5 ounces) whole beets, drained and cut into 3/4-inch pieces
- 4 medium red potatoes (about 1 pound), cooked and cut into 3/4-inch pieces
- 3 celery ribs, chopped (about 1 1/2 cups)
- 1 large dill pickle, chopped (about 1 cup)
- chopped parsley for garnish

In large bowl stir together yogurt, mayonnaise, lemon juice, salt, and pepper. Add beets, potatoes, celery, and pickle; toss until well coated. Cover and refrigerate several hours or overnight. Garnish with parsley, if desired. Makes 6 servings.

Per serving: 175 calories; 3 g protein; 7 g fat; 35% calories from fat; 7 mg cholesterol; 25 g carbohydrates; 744 mg sodium; 3 g fiber

Citrus Soufflé Salad

1 package (4-serving size) lemon-flavored gelatin
1 cup boiling water
1/2 cup cold water
1 tablespoon lemon juice
1/2 cup light mayonnaise
1/4 teaspoon salt
pepper to taste
3/4 cup low-fat cottage cheese
1/2 cup diced grapefruit sections
1/2 cup diced orange sections
1/2 cup shredded carrot
greens for garnish

In medium bowl, stir lemon-flavored gelatin and boiling water until gelatin is dissolved. Add cold water, lemon juice, mayonnaise, salt, and pepper until well blended. Pour into 8-inch square metal baking dish; freeze about 15 to 20 minutes or until firm about 1-inch from edge but soft in center. Transfer to large mixing bowl. Beat with mixer until fluffy. Fold in cottage cheese, grapefruit sections, orange sections, and carrot. Pour into 4-cup mold or four individual 1-cup molds. Chill until firm. Serve over greens, if desired. Makes 4 servings.

Per serving: 251 calories; 8 g protein; 11 g fat; 37% calories from fat; 15 mg cholesterol; 32 g carbohydrates; 574 mg sodium; 1 g fiber

Apple and Red Cabbage Slaw

- 3 medium apples, cored and coarsely shredded
- ½ head (about 1 pound) red cabbage, shredded
- 4 medium celery ribs, coarsely chopped
- ¼ cup raisins
- 2 tablespoons olive oil
- 1 tablespoon honey
- 1 tablespoon lemon juice
- lettuce leaves for garnish

In large bowl, combine apples, cabbage, celery, and raisins. In measuring cup, mix together oil, honey, and lemon juice until well blended. Add to slaw; toss until well coated. Serve on bed of lettuce, if desired. Makes 6 servings.

Per serving: 146 calories; 1 g protein; 5 g fat; 29% calories from fat; 0 mg cholesterol; 27 g carbohydrates; 29 mg sodium; 4 g fiber

Breads and Muffins

Vanilla French Toast

2 cups skim milk
cholesterol-free, fat-free egg substitute, equivalent to 4 eggs
1 tablespoon sugar
2 teaspoons ground cinnamon (optional)
1 teaspoon vanilla extract
8 slices high-fiber multigrain or whole wheat bread

In large baking dish, beat milk, egg substitute, sugar, cinnamon, and vanilla until well blended. Add bread in single layer; cover and refrigerate several hours or overnight, turning once. Spray large nonstick skillet with nonstick cooking spray; place over medium heat. With metal spatula transfer 3-4 slices of egg-soaked bread to skillet. Cook 8 to 12 minutes or until brown and crisp on both sides, turning once. Remove and keep warm. Repeat with remaining slices. Makes 4 servings.

Per 2-slice serving: 193 calories; 10 g protein; 2 g fat; 10% calories from fat; 2 mg cholesterol; 33 g carbohydrates; 300 mg sodium; 3 g fiber

Hearty Cran-Apple Muffins

- 1 cup all-purpose flour
- 1/2 cup whole wheat flour or oat bran
- 3/4 cup firmly packed dark brown sugar
- 1 teaspoon baking soda
- 1 teaspoon ground cinnamon
- 1/4 teaspoon salt
- cholesterol-free, fat-free egg substitute, equivalent to 2 eggs
- 1/4 cup canola, corn, safflower, or sunflower oil
- 1 teaspoon vanilla extract
- 3/4 cup diced, unpeeled tart apple
- 3/4 cup fresh or frozen cranberries

Preheat oven to 350°F. Grease well 6 (2 1/2-inch) muffin cups or line with paper baking cups. In large bowl, mix flours, brown sugar, baking soda, cinnamon, and salt. In separate bowl, blend egg substitute, oil, and vanilla. Add to flour mixture all at once, stirring just until dry ingredients are moistened. Gently stir in apple and cranberries. Spoon into prepared cups. Bake 20 to 25 minutes or until muffins are browned and firm to touch. Makes 6 muffins.

Per muffin: 241 calories; 4 g protein; 7 g fat; 26% calories from fat; 0 mg cholesterol; 41 g carbohydrates; 137 mg sodium; 2 g fiber

Banana-Blueberry Oat Bread

- 1½ cups old-fashioned rolled oats
- 1 cup all-purpose flour
- 1 teaspoon baking powder
- ½ teaspoon baking soda
- ½ teaspoon salt
- 1 cup sugar
- ⅓ cup canola, corn, safflower, or sunflower oil
- cholesterol-free, fat-free egg substitute, equivalent to 2 eggs
- 3 tablespoons buttermilk or plain nonfat yogurt
- 1 cup mashed ripe bananas (about 2)
- ½ cup fresh or frozen blueberries

Preheat oven to 350°F. Grease 9x5-inch loaf pan. Cut 18x5-inch strip waxed paper or foil; place in prepared pan, covering short sides and bottom; set aside. In food processor or blender, process oats until consistency of flour. In large bowl, mix processed oats, flour, baking powder, baking soda, and salt. In separate bowl, blend sugar, oil, egg substitute, buttermilk or yogurt, and bananas. Add to flour mixture, stirring until well blended. Stir in blueberries. Spoon into prepared pan. Bake 50 to 60 minutes or until pick inserted in center comes out clean. Remove from pan to wire rack; cool completely. Makes 1 loaf (16 slices).

Per slice: 78 calories; 3 g protein; .5 g fat; 7% calories from fat; 0 mg cholesterol; 15 g carbohydrates; 128 mg sodium; 1.5 g fiber

Oat and Pumpkin Muffins

- 1 1/2 cups oat bran
- 1/2 cup all-purpose flour
- 2 teaspoons baking powder
- 1 teaspoon pumpkin pie spice
- 1/4 teaspoon salt
- 1 cup canned or fresh mashed cooked pumpkin
- 2/3 cup firmly packed brown sugar
- 1/2 cup skim milk
- 2 egg whites
- 2 tablespoons canola, corn, safflower, or sunflower oil

Preheat oven to 425°F. Grease well 12 (2 1/2-inch) muffin cups or line with paper baking cups. In large bowl, mix oat bran, flour, baking powder, pumpkin pie spice, and salt. In separate bowl, blend pumpkin, brown sugar, skim milk, egg whites, and oil. Add to oat bran/flour mixture all at once, stirring until dry ingredients are moistened. Spoon into prepared muffin cups. Bake 18 to 20 minutes or until muffins are firm to touch. Makes 12 muffins.

Per muffin: 125 calories; 4 g protein; 3 g fat; 18% calories from fat; 0 mg cholesterol; 26 g carbohydrates; 122 mg sodium; 2 g fiber

Pizza Bagel

- 2 tablespoons canola, corn, safflower, or sunflower oil
- 1 medium onion, cut into thin wedges
- 1 large potato (about 6 to 7 ounces), cooked, peeled, and cut into 1/4-inch slices
- 1/2 large green pepper, seeded and cut into strips
- 1 teaspoon dried oregano
- 1/2 teaspoon salt
- 2 bagels (oat bran, pumpernickel, or plain), cut in half
- 1 cup shredded skim-milk mozzarella cheese (4 ounces)

Preheat broiler. Heat oil in large nonstick skillet over medium heat. Add onion, potato, and green pepper. Cook, stirring occasionally, 5 to 8 minutes or until onion is browned. Stir in oregano and salt. Place bagels, cut side up, on broiler pan. Broil until lightly toasted. Top each bagel half with 1/4 onion-potato mixture and sprinkle with 1/4 cheese. Broil until cheese is melted and lightly browned. Makes 4 servings.

Variation: Omit green pepper, oregano, and salt. Cook onion and potato as above. Stir in 1 can (8 ounces) sliced beets, well drained and rinsed. Continue as directed above.

Per serving: 245 calories; 11 g protein; 8 g fat; 32% calories from fat; 16 mg cholesterol; 30 g carbohydrates; 551 mg sodium; 2 g fiber

Apple Gingerbread Scones

- 1/3 cup skim milk
- 1/3 cup light molasses
- 3 tablespoons unsweetened applesauce
- 2 cups all-purpose flour
- 2 teaspoons baking powder
- 1 teaspoon ground cinnamon
- 1 teaspoon ground ginger
- 1/4 teaspoon baking soda
- 1/4 teaspoon ground cloves
- 4 tablespoons cold butter, cut up

Preheat oven to 425°F. In small bowl or measuring cup, mix milk, molasses, and applesauce; set aside. In large bowl, combine flour, baking powder, cinnamon, ginger, baking soda, and cloves. With pastry blender or fingers cut in butter until mixture resembles fine granules. Pour in milk mixture and stir with fork to form a smooth, soft dough. On lightly floured surface, knead dough 10 to 12 times. Cut dough in half. Knead each half into ball. On ungreased baking sheet, pat each piece into 5-inch circle. Cut into 6 wedges; separate slightly. Bake 10 to 12 minutes or until crusty and hollow-sounding when tapped. Serve warm. Makes 12 scones.

Per scone: 132 calories; 2 g protein; 4 g fat; 28% calories from fat; 10 mg cholesterol; 21 g carbohydrates; 109 mg sodium; trace g fiber

Main Dishes: Poultry and Fish

Jalapeño Turkey Bake

1 cup uncooked long-grain brown rice
3 cups, 3/4-inch cubes, cooked turkey breast (about 12 ounces)
1 can (10 ounces) enchilada sauce
2 fresh jalapeño peppers, seeded, chopped (about 1/4 cup)
1 1/2 cups frozen or canned (drained) whole kernel corn
1/4 cup chopped green pepper
3/4 teaspoon salt
1 cup nonfat sour cream
additional chopped jalapeño peppers and chopped cilantro for garnish (optional)

Preheat oven to 350°F. Grease shallow 1 1/2-quart casserole or 11x7-inch baking dish. Prepare rice according to package directions. In large bowl stir cooked rice, turkey, enchilada sauce, chopped jalapeño peppers, corn, green pepper, and salt until well blended. Spoon into prepared casserole. Cover and bake 25 to 30 minutes or until heated through. To serve, spoon sour cream over top and sprinkle with jalapeño peppers and cilantro, if desired. Makes 6 servings.

Per serving: 346 calories; 26 g protein; 2 g fat; 7% calories from fat; 55 mg cholesterol; 52 g carbohydrates; 1,083 mg sodium; 3 g fiber

Moroccan-Style Chicken and Couscous

- 1 whole chicken breast (about 1½ pounds), split, skinned, and cut in half
- 1 medium onion, sliced
- 2 medium carrots, cut into 1-inch pieces
- 1 teaspoon turmeric
- 1 teaspoon salt
- ¼ teaspoon pepper
- 2 cups cooked chickpeas
- 2 medium zucchini, cut into ½-inch pieces
- 2 cups shredded cabbage (about 4 ounces)
- 1 large tomato, chopped
- 2 tablespoons chopped parsley
- 2 tablespoons chopped cilantro
- 1 package (10 ounces) plain couscous

In Dutch oven or large saucepan, bring to boil 3 cups water, chicken, onion, carrots, turmeric, salt, and pepper. Reduce heat to medium-low; cover and cook 30 minutes. Add chickpeas, zucchini, cabbage, tomato, parsley, and cilantro. Cover and cook 15 to 20 minutes more or until chicken and vegetables are fork-tender. Meanwhile, prepare couscous according to package directions. To serve, place ¼ couscous in shallow bowl; top with ¼ chicken-broth mixture. Makes 4 servings.

Per serving: 382 calories; 29 g protein; 4 g fat; 11% calories from fat; 43 mg cholesterol; 57 g carbohydrates; 415 mg sodium; 6 g fiber

Turkey Tabbouleh

1½ cups warm water
1 cup uncooked bulgar
2 tablespoons olive oil
3 cups coarsely chopped, cooked turkey breast (about 12 ounces)
3 green onions with tops, sliced
1 large Granny Smith or Winesap apple, cored and chopped
1 celery rib, finely chopped
1 clove garlic, minced
½ cup finely chopped parsley
¼ cup finely chopped red onion
1 cup nonfat plain yogurt
½ teaspoon salt
pepper to taste
2 tablespoons sliced almonds for garnish

In large bowl, place water, bulgar, and olive oil; let stand at least 30 minutes or until all liquid has been absorbed. Add chopped turkey, green onions, apple, celery, garlic, parsley, red onion, yogurt, salt, and pepper; toss to combine. Chill at least 30 minutes to blend flavors. To serve, sprinkle with almonds, if desired. Makes 8 servings.

Per serving: 227 calories; 20 g protein; 6 g fat; 25% calories from fat; 37 mg cholesterol; 22 g carbohydrates; 196 mg sodium; 5 g fiber

Summer Chicken Salad

3 cups, 3/4-inch cubes, cooked chicken breast (about 12 ounces)
3 cups 3/4-inch melon balls or cubes (cantaloupe, honeydew, cassava, etc.)
1 large celery rib, chopped
1/3 cup light mayonnaise
1/4 cup chopped walnuts
1/2 teaspoon salt
lettuce leaves for garnish

In large bowl place chicken cubes, melon, celery, mayonnaise, walnuts, and salt; toss until well blended. Serve over lettuce, if desired. Makes 4 servings.

Variation: If desired, omit melon balls and substitute 3 cups fresh or drained canned peach slices.

Per serving: 273 calories; 24 g protein; 14 g fat; 46% calories from fat; 65 mg cholesterol; 13 g carbohydrates; 478 mg sodium; 2 g fiber

Chicken and Rice Cajun-Style

- 2 cups, 3/4-inch cubes, cooked chicken or turkey breast (about 8 ounces)
- 1 cup cooked brown rice
- 1 can (16 ounces) stewed tomatoes, undrained
- 1 medium onion, chopped (about 1/2 cup)
- 1 medium celery rib, finely chopped
- 1/2 cup finely chopped green or red pepper
- 1 small yellow squash, cut into 1/2-inch cubes
- 1 clove garlic, minced
- 1/4 teaspoon dried thyme
- 1/4 teaspoon crushed hot red pepper, or to taste
- 1/4 teaspoon ground cloves
- 1/4 teaspoon ground allspice
- 1/3 cup Italian seasoned bread crumbs

Preheat oven to 350°F. Place all ingredients except bread crumbs in lightly greased 2-quart casserole. Stir until well blended. Top evenly with bread crumbs. Bake 35 to 40 minutes or until heated through. Makes 4 servings.

Per serving: 253 calories; 25 g protein; 4 g fat; 15% calories from fat; 59 mg cholesterol; 27 g carbohydrates; 304 mg sodium; 3 g fiber

Asparagus, Mushroom, and Chicken Stir-Fry

- 1 tablespoon cornstarch
- 1 tablespoon chicken bouillon granules
- 3 tablespoons soy sauce
- 1 cup water, divided
- 4 tablespoons canola, corn, safflower, or sunflower oil, divided
- 12 ounces boneless, skinless chicken breast, cut into 2x1-inch strips
- 1 pound fresh asparagus, cut diagonally into 2-inch pieces
- 4 ounces fresh mushrooms, sliced
- 6 green onions, cut into 1-inch pieces
- 1/2 cup sliced canned water chestnuts
- 1 1/2 cups halved cherry tomatoes
- cooked brown rice (optional)

In small bowl or measuring cup, stir cornstarch, bouillon granules, and soy sauce into 3/4 cup water until well blended; set aside. Heat 2 tablespoons oil in large skillet or wok over medium-high heat. Add chicken; cook, stirring constantly, 2 minutes or until chicken is white. Remove chicken; keep warm. Add 1 tablespoon oil to skillet. Add asparagus. Stir to coat with oil. Add remaining 1/4 cup water; cover and cook 3 minutes. Remove cover; add remaining tablespoon oil, mushrooms, green onions, and water chestnuts. Cook, stirring constantly, 4 minutes or until asparagus is tender-crisp.

Add reserved chicken and tomatoes and then cornstarch mixture. Cook, gently stirring constantly, 2 minutes or until sauce thickens, bubbles, and tomatoes are heated through. Serve over hot cooked brown rice, if desired. Makes 4 servings.

Per serving: 245 calories; 25 g protein; 10 g fat; 37% calories from fat; 54 mg cholesterol; 14 g carbohydrates; 1,109 mg sodium; 4 g fiber

Chicken and Peanut Stir-Fry

- 2 whole chicken breasts, split, boned, skinned, and cut into bite-size pieces
- 1/2 cup dry sherry
- 1/2 teaspoon minced fresh ginger
- 2 tablespoons canola, corn, safflower, or sunflower oil
- 1 medium onion, chopped
- 1 small carrot, cut diagonally into thin slices
- 1 medium green pepper, cut into strips
- 1/2 cup sliced fresh mushrooms
- 1/2 cup broccoli florets
- 1/4 cup unsalted dry-roasted peanuts
- 1/2 teaspoon salt
- pepper to taste
- 2 cups hot, cooked brown rice

In small bowl, toss chicken, sherry, and ginger; let stand 2 hours to marinate. Heat oil in large skillet or wok over medium-high heat. Add onion; cook, stirring constantly, 2 minutes or until onion is tender-crisp. Remove chicken from marinade, reserving marinade, and place in skillet or wok. Cook, stirring constantly, 5 minutes or until chicken turns white. Add carrots and green pepper; cook, stirring constantly, 3 minutes. Add mushroom, broccoli, and peanuts. Add reserved marinade, salt, and pepper. Cook, stirring constantly, 1 to 2 minutes or until sauce thickens and vegetables are tender-crisp. Serve over hot cooked brown rice. Makes 4 servings.

Per serving: 492 calories; 40 g protein; 16 g fat; 31% calories from fat; 95 mg cholesterol; 35 g carbohydrates; 369 mg sodium; 3 g fiber

All-in-One Fish Dinner

1 pound boneless, skinless, fresh or frozen (thawed) fish fillets (cod, haddock, or pollack), cut into serving pieces
1/2 teaspoon salt
pepper to taste
1 tablespoon canola, corn, safflower, or sunflower oil
1 large onion, thinly sliced
1 small clove garlic, minced
1 can (8 ounces) tomato sauce
1 cup hot water
1/4 teaspoon dried fennel or dill
dash cayenne pepper
2 medium potatoes, peeled and thinly sliced
1/2 cup frozen or canned (drained) peas

Preheat oven to 350°F. Grease 2 1/2-quart shallow casserole or baking dish. Sprinkle fish with salt and pepper. Heat oil in medium skillet over medium heat. Add onion and garlic; cook 5 minutes or until onion is tender. Stir in tomato sauce, water, fennel, and cayenne pepper. In prepared casserole, layer fish, potatoes, and peas, ending with potatoes. Pour tomato-onion sauce over fish and vegetables. Cover and bake 40 minutes. Remove cover and cook 10 to 15 minutes longer or until fish flakes easily when tested with fork. Makes 4 servings.

Per serving: 245 calories; 24 g protein; 4 g fat; 17% calories from fat; 48 mg cholesterol; 27 g carbohydrates; 676 mg sodium; 4 g fiber

Sesame-Ginger Haddock

- 1 pound boneless, skinless, fresh or frozen (thawed), haddock fillets
- 1/2 teaspoon salt
- 1 1/2 tablespoons butter
- 2 tablespoons minced green onion with tops
- 2 tablespoons toasted sesame seeds
- 1/2 teaspoon grated fresh or 1/4 teaspoon ground ginger

Preheat oven to 350°F. Grease shallow 2 1/2-quart casserole or baking dish. Sprinkle fish with salt; place in single layer in casserole. Melt butter in small skillet over low heat. Add green onion, sesame seeds, and ginger; cook 2 minutes. Spoon evenly over fish. Bake 15 to 25 minutes or until fish flakes easily when tested with fork. Makes 4 servings.

Per serving: 165 calories; 24 g protein; 7 g fat; 41% calories from fat; 74 mg cholesterol; trace g carbohydrates; 379 mg sodium; 0 g fiber

Flounder with Fresh Orange Sauce

- 1 pound boneless, skinless, fresh or frozen (thawed) flounder fillets
- 1/2 teaspoon salt
- pepper to taste
- 1/4 teaspoon ground ginger
- 1/2 cup orange juice
- 2 tablespoons lemon juice
- 1 green onion with top, thinly sliced
- 1 medium tomato, peeled and chopped
- 1/4 medium green pepper, chopped
- 1 tablespoon butter, melted
- 3 oranges, peeled and thinly sliced

Preheat oven to 350°F. Grease 2 1/2-quart shallow casserole or baking dish. Sprinkle fish with mixture of salt, pepper, and ginger and place in shallow dish or bowl. Add orange and lemon juice to fish; let stand 20 minutes. Lightly drain fish, reserving remaining marinade; place in prepared casserole. Top with green onion, tomato, and green pepper. Drizzle evenly with butter. Bake 10 minutes. Pour reserved marinade over fish; top with orange slices. Bake 15 minutes more or until fish flakes easily when tested with fork. Makes 4 servings.

Per serving: 199 calories; 23 g protein; 4 g fat; 20% calories from fat; 62 mg cholesterol; 17 g carbohydrates; 386 mg sodium; 3 g fiber

Onion-Dill Halibut

- 4 halibut steaks (4 ounces each), fresh or frozen (thawed)
- 1/2 teaspoon salt
- pepper to taste
- 2 large onions, thinly sliced
- 1 tablespoon butter
- 1 tablespoon olive oil
- 1 tablespoon fresh chopped or 1 teaspoon dried dill

Preheat oven to 400°F. Season halibut steaks evenly with salt and pepper. In 9-inch square baking dish, place onions, butter, oil, and dill. Bake 10 to 15 minutes or until onions begin to brown. Remove 1/4 onions; place steaks in baking dish and top with reserved onions. Bake 10 to 15 minutes or until fish flakes easily when tested with fork. Makes 4 servings.

Per serving: 176 calories; 18 g protein; 8 g fat; 44% calories from fat; 35 mg cholesterol; 6 g carbohydrates; 338 mg sodium; 1 g fiber

Easy Turkey Lasagna

9 lasagna noodles
1 pound raw, ground white meat turkey
1 small onion, chopped
1 jar (28 ounces) spaghetti sauce with mushrooms (or your favorite sauce)
1 cup part-skim ricotta cheese
2 tablespoons chopped parsley
2 tablespoons grated Parmesan cheese
2 tablespoons skim milk
1/8 teaspoon ground pepper
3 ounces part-skim-milk mozzarella cheese, shredded (3/4 cup)

Preheat oven to 350°F. Grease 11x7-inch baking dish; set aside. Cook lasagna noodles according to package directions; drain and rinse. Meanwhile, in medium nonstick skillet over medium-high heat, cook ground turkey and onion until turkey is brown. Drain off fat. Remove from heat; stir in spaghetti sauce. In small bowl, mix together ricotta cheese, parsley, Parmesan cheese, milk, and pepper. In prepared dish, arrange 3 lasagna noodles in single layer; top with 2/3 turkey-sauce mixture, then with 1/2 cheese mixture; repeat. Top with remaining noodles, remaining turkey-sauce mixture, then mozzarella. Bake 40 to 50 minutes or until bubbly and heated through. Let stand 5 minutes before serving. Makes 8 servings.

Per serving: 355 calories; 24 g protein; 12 g fat; 30% calories from fat; 71 mg cholesterol; 37 g carbohydrates; 635 mg sodium; 3 g fiber

Main Dishes: Vegetarian

Spinach-Garlic Fettuccine

- 8 ounces uncooked fettuccine
- 3 tablespoons olive oil
- 3 large cloves garlic, minced
- 3/4 pound fresh spinach, trimmed, washed, and torn into bite-size pieces (about 8 cups)
- 1/3 cup grated Parmesan cheese
- 1/2 teaspoon salt
- pepper to taste
- dash ground nutmeg

Cook fettuccine according to package directions. Meanwhile, heat oil in Dutch oven or 12-inch skillet over medium heat. Add garlic; cook 2 to 3 minutes or until lightly brown. Add spinach; cook, stirring occasionally, 5 minutes or until spinach is limp and tender. Drain fettuccine. In large serving bowl, toss fettuccine, spinach mixture, cheese, salt, pepper, and nutmeg until well blended. Serve immediately. Makes 4 servings.

Per serving: 305 calories; 10 g protein; 12 g fat; 37% calories from fat; 5 mg cholesterol; 38 g carbohydrates; 448 mg sodium; 5 g fiber

Green Vegetable Spaghetti Sauce

2 tablespoons canola, corn, safflower, or sunflower oil
2 green onions with tops, sliced
1 clove garlic, minced
1 cup vegetable broth, divided
3 medium tomatoes, chopped
1 package (10 ounces) fresh or frozen (thawed) Brussels sprouts, cut into quarters
10 ounces fresh or 1 package (9 ounces) frozen (thawed) whole green beans, cut into 1-inch pieces
1 teaspoon dried basil
1 teaspoon dried oregano
1/2 teaspoon salt
pepper to taste
2 teaspoons cornstarch
1/4 cup fresh or frozen peas
1/4 cup chopped fresh or 2 tablespoons dried parsley
6 ounces spaghetti, cooked and hot

Heat oil in large skillet over medium heat. Add green onions and garlic; cook 1 minute. Add 1/2 cup broth, tomatoes, Brussels sprouts, green beans, basil, oregano, salt, and pepper. Cook, covered, about 8 to 12 minutes or until Brussels sprouts are tender. Stir cornstarch into remaining 1/2 cup broth. Add to skillet with peas and parsley. Cook, stirring occasionally, until thickened and vegetables are tender. Serve over hot spaghetti. Makes 4 servings.

Per serving: 275 calories; 9 g protein; 8 g fat; 24% calories from fat; 0 mg cholesterol; 45 g carbohydrates; 307 mg sodium; 8 g fiber

Tomato-Onion Stuffed Eggplant

- 2 small eggplants (about 3/4 pound each)
- 1 tablespoon olive oil
- 1 tablespoon butter
- 2 medium onions, thinly sliced
- 2 cloves garlic, minced
- 3 medium tomatoes (about 1 pound), peeled, seeded, and chopped
- 1/2 cup finely chopped fresh parsley
- 1/2 teaspoon salt
- 1 bay leaf
- 1 stick (2 inches) cinnamon
- pepper to taste
- 8 black olives, coarsely chopped

Grease shallow 2 1/2-quart baking dish. Cut top stem and cap from eggplant. Heat oil in large nonstick skillet over medium-high heat. Add eggplants; cook 5 minutes, or until tender, turning often. Cut in half lengthwise; scoop out pulp, leaving thin shell. Coarsely chop pulp. Set eggplant shells and pulp aside. Heat butter in same skillet over medium heat; add onions and garlic. Cook 5 to 8 minutes or until golden brown. Add tomatoes and reserved eggplant pulp; cook 10 minutes. Preheat oven to 375°F. Add parsley, salt, bay leaf, cinnamon stick, and pepper to skillet; cook 10 minutes. Remove bay leaf and cinnamon stick. Place reserved eggplant shells in prepared baking dish. Place 1/4 tomato-eggplant mixture into each. Top with chopped olives. Bake 10 minutes or until heated through. Makes 4 servings.

Per serving: 165 calories; 4 g protein; 9 g fat; 44% calories from fat; 7 mg cholesterol; 22 g carbohydrates; 381 mg sodium; 9 g fiber

Sesame Vegetable Stir-Fry

- 1 tablespoon canola, corn, safflower, or sunflower oil
- 1 small clove garlic, finely minced
- 1 teaspoon finely minced fresh or 1/2 teaspoon ground ginger
- 3/4 pound broccoli, trimmed and cut into florets
- 3 medium carrots, peeled and thinly sliced
- 3 medium leeks (white part only), thinly sliced
- 2 tablespoons vegetable broth
- 1 tablespoon toasted sesame seeds
- 1 teaspoon soy sauce
- 1 teaspoon Oriental sesame oil

Heat oil in large skillet or wok over medium-high heat. Add garlic and ginger; cook, stirring constantly, 15 seconds. Reduce heat to medium. Add broccoli, carrots, and leeks; cook, stirring constantly, 1 minute. Add broth; cover and cook 3 minutes. Increase heat to high; uncover and cook, stirring constantly, 5 minutes or until vegetables are tender. Add sesame seeds, soy sauce, and sesame oil; toss until well coated. Serve immediately. Makes 4 servings.

Per serving: 123 calories; 3 g protein; 6 g fat; 41% calories from fat; 0 mg cholesterol; 16 g carbohydrates; 131 mg sodium; 5 g fiber

Red Beans and Rice

2 tablespoons olive oil
1 medium onion, chopped
1-2 cloves garlic, minced
1 large celery rib with leaves, thinly sliced
½ cup chopped green pepper
4 cups water or vegetable broth
1 cup uncooked long-grain brown rice
1 teaspoon salt
½ teaspoon dried thyme
crushed red pepper or liquid hot pepper sauce to taste
2 cans (15½ to 19 ounces) red kidney beans, rinsed and drained

Heat oil in Dutch oven or large saucepan over medium heat. Add onion, garlic, celery, and green pepper. Cook 5 minutes or until vegetables are tender. Add water, rice, salt, thyme, and red pepper to taste. Bring to boil over high heat. Reduce heat to simmer; cover and cook 40 to 45 minutes or until rice is almost tender. Stir in beans; cover and cook until beans are heated through and rice is tender. Makes 5 servings.

Per serving: 357 calories; 14 g protein; 6 g fat; 16% calories from fat; 0 mg cholesterol; 62 g carbohydrates; 439 mg sodium; 12 g fiber

Zucchini and Rice Casserole

1 tablespoon canola, corn, safflower, or sunflower oil
1 cup uncooked brown rice
1 teaspoon grated fresh ginger
3 green onions with tops, chopped
3 medium zucchini, sliced
1/2 medium green pepper, seeded and chopped
3 small tomatoes, cored and cut into eighths
2 3/4 cups boiling vegetable broth
1 teaspoon soy sauce
1 clove garlic, minced

Preheat oven to 350°F. Grease shallow 2 1/2-quart casserole. Heat oil in large skillet over medium-low heat. Add rice and ginger; cook, stirring, 5 minutes or until rice is golden brown. Spoon evenly into prepared casserole; top with layers of green onion, zucchini, green pepper, and tomato. Stir together broth, soy sauce, and garlic; pour over vegetable-rice mixture. Cover and bake 1 hour and 15 minutes or until rice and vegetables are tender. Makes 6 servings.

Per serving: 151 calories; 3 g protein; 3 g fat; 18% calories from fat; 0 mg cholesterol; 28 g carbohydrates; 64 mg sodium; 2 g fiber

Barbecued Bean Casserole

- 2 tablespoons canola, corn, safflower, or sunflower oil
- 1 small onion, chopped
- 1 clove garlic, minced
- 1 can (16 ounces) vegetarian baked beans
- 1 package (10 ounces) frozen or 1 can (15½ ounces) drained lima beans (about 2 cups)
- 1 can (15½ to 19 ounces) or 2 cups cooked red kidney beans, rinsed and drained
- ½ cup catsup
- 3 tablespoons apple cider vinegar
- 1 tablespoon brown sugar
- 1 teaspoon salt
- 1 teaspoon dry mustard
- ¼ teaspoon pepper

Preheat oven to 350°F. Heat oil in heat-and-oven-proof 2-quart casserole over medium-high heat. Add onion and garlic; cook 5 minutes or until onion is tender. Stir in remaining ingredients. Bake 45 minutes or until heated through and bubbly. Makes 6 servings.

Per serving: 266 calories; 12 g protein; 6 g fat; 19% calories from fat; 4 mg cholesterol; 44 g carbohydrates; 911 mg sodium; 13 g fiber

Veggie Pockets

- 3/4 cup low-fat cottage cheese
- 1/4 cup crumbled blue cheese
- 1 tablespoon tarragon or apple cider vinegar
- 1/4 teaspoon dried Italian herb seasoning
- 1/2 large cucumber, cut in half lengthwise and then sliced (about 1/2 cup)
- 1 medium tomato, diced
- 1 medium carrot, peeled and shredded
- 1/2 cup broccoli florets, cut into bite-size pieces
- 1/4 cup shelled sunflower seeds
- 4 (6-inch) whole wheat or plain pita breads, cut in half
- alfalfa sprouts for garnish

In large bowl, gently mix cottage cheese, blue cheese, vinegar, and seasoning until well blended. Add cucumber, tomato, carrot, broccoli, and sunflower seeds; toss until well blended. Spoon 1/8 vegetable-cheese mixture into each pita half. Top with alfalfa sprouts, if desired. Makes 4 servings.

Per serving: 295 calories; 16 g protein; 8 g fat; 24% calories from fat; 11 mg cholesterol; 41 g carbohydrates; 595 mg sodium; 3 g fiber

Vegetable Side Dishes

Pineapple and Yam Casserole

- 2 pounds fresh yams (about 2 large), peeled and cut into 1-inch pieces
- 1 cup water
- 1 cup unsweetened pineapple juice
- 2 tablespoons lemon juice
- 2 teaspoons cornstarch
- 1 teaspoon sugar
- 1/4 teaspoon salt
- 1/2 fresh pineapple (about 3 1/2 pounds), peeled, cored, and cut into 1-inch pieces
- 1 green onion with top, sliced
- 1 small celery rib, diagonally sliced (1/4 cup)

In Dutch oven or large saucepan, over medium heat, cook yams in water, covered, about 10 to 15 minutes or until almost tender. Drain. In same Dutch oven, over medium heat, cook, stirring constantly, pineapple juice, lemon juice, cornstarch, sugar, and salt until thickened and bubbly. Add drained yams, pineapple pieces, green onions, and celery. Reduce heat to low; cover and cook until heated through, about 5 minutes. Makes 6 servings.

Per serving: 216 calories; 3 g protein; .5 g fat; 2% calories from fat; 0 mg cholesterol; 51 g carbohydrates; 112 mg sodium; 5 g fiber

Yam Soufflé

- 1 cup mashed yams—fresh cooked, canned, or frozen (thawed)
- 1/2 cup firmly packed brown sugar
- 1/4 teaspoon ground nutmeg
- 1/2 teaspoon grated orange peel
- 1/8 teaspoon salt
- 3 egg whites, at room temperature
- 1/8 teaspoon cream of tartar

Preheat oven to 350°F. Grease 1-quart casserole or baking dish. In medium bowl, stir yams, brown sugar, nutmeg, orange peel, and salt until well blended. In small bowl, beat egg whites and cream of tartar with mixer at high speed until stiff peaks form. Gently fold into yam mixture and then spoon into prepared casserole. Place in pan of hot water. Bake 35 to 40 minutes or until puffed and starts to pull away from sides. Makes 4 servings.

Per serving: 173 calories; 3 g protein; .5 g fat; 1% calories from fat; 0 mg cholesterol; 40 g carbohydrates; 350 mg sodium; 1 g fiber

Garlicky Black Bean Dip

2 cans (15 ounces each) black beans, drained
1 medium onion, coarsely chopped
1 small green pepper, coarsely chopped
2 cloves garlic, chopped
3 tablespoons red wine vinegar
3 tablespoons olive oil
1 teaspoon sugar
1 teaspoon salt
pepper to taste
baked tortilla chips and/or raw vegetable dippers

In food processor or blender, place beans, onion, green pepper, garlic, vinegar, oil, sugar, salt, and pepper. Process until beans are coarsely mashed or of desired consistency. Serve with chips and/or vegetables, if desired. Makes 4 cups, 32 servings (2 tablespoons).

Per serving: 37 calories; 1 g protein; 1 g fat; 32% calories from fat; 0 mg cholesterol; 4 g carbohydrates; 67 mg sodium; 2 g fiber

Asparagus-Cheese Casserole

- 1 1/2 pounds fresh or 2 packages (10 ounces each) frozen asparagus, cooked
- 2 tablespoons canola, corn, safflower, or sunflower oil
- 1 medium onion, chopped
- 1 clove garlic, minced
- 1 can (16 ounces) tomatoes, undrained
- 1 teaspoon salt
- 1/4 teaspoon dried thyme
- 1/4 teaspoon liquid hot pepper sauce
- 1 can (8 ounces) tomato sauce
- 4 ounces part-skim-milk mozzarella, shredded
- 2 tablespoons grated Parmesan cheese

Preheat oven to 350°F. In shallow baking pan or casserole, arrange asparagus; set aside. Heat oil in medium saucepan over medium heat. Add onion and garlic; cook 5 minutes or until lightly browned. Add tomatoes, salt, thyme, and pepper sauce. Reduce heat to low. Cook, uncovered, 20 minutes. Add tomato sauce. Cook 20 minutes or until flavors blend. Pour sauce evenly over asparagus; top with cheeses. Bake 20 to 25 minutes or until asparagus is heated and cheese melts. Makes 8 servings.

Per serving: 119 calories; 7 g protein; 6 g fat; 47% calories from fat; 8 mg cholesterol; 9 g carbohydrates; 630 mg sodium; 2 g fiber

Green Bean and Olive Toss

- 1 package (9 ounces) frozen French-cut green beans
- 1/4 cup sliced pitted black olives
- 1 tablespoon olive oil
- 1 tablespoon red wine vinegar
- 1/4 teaspoon salt
- 1/4 teaspoon crushed dried oregano
- 1/8 teaspoon garlic powder
- pepper to taste

Cook green beans according to package directions. In the meantime, in small saucepan over medium heat, cook olives, oil, vinegar, salt, oregano, garlic powder, and pepper until heated through (about 3-5 minutes). Drain green beans; place on serving platter. Pour olive mixture over beans; toss well. Serve immediately. Makes 4 servings.

Per serving: 59 calories; 1 g protein; 5 g fat; 68% calories from fat; 4 mg cholesterol; 0 g carbohydrates; 195 mg sodium; 2 g fiber

Asian-Style Green Beans

- 2 tablespoons peanut oil
- 1 small onion, finely chopped
- 1 clove garlic, minced
- 2 tablespoons shredded lemon peel
- 1/2 teaspoon dried chili pepper
- 1 pound fresh trimmed, or 2 packages (9 ounces each) frozen (thawed), whole green beans
- 1 teaspoon salt
- pinch sugar

Heat oil in large skillet over medium heat. Add onion, garlic, lemon peel, and chili pepper. Cook, stirring constantly, 3 minutes. Reduce heat to low. Add green beans; toss to coat well. Cover and cook 5 minutes or until barely tender, adding water, if necessary. Makes 6 servings.

Per serving: 73 calories; 2 g protein; 4 g fat; 52% calories from fat; 0 mg cholesterol; 8 g carbohydrates; 360 mg sodium; 2 g fiber

Asparagus Vinaigrette

1 teaspoon dill weed, divided
water
40 thin (1/2-inch thick) asparagus, trimmed and washed
3 tablespoons olive oil
1 teaspoon salt
1/2 teaspoon dry mustard
1/2 teaspoon cracked pepper
3 tablespoons tarragon white-wine vinegar
lemon wedges for garnish

In large skillet over medium heat, bring 1/2 teaspoon dill weed and 2 inches water to boil. Add asparagus; cook 3 minutes or until fork-tender. Remove; run under cold water. Drain well. To make vinaigrette dressing: In small bowl, stir remaining 1/2 teaspoon dill weed, oil, salt, mustard, and pepper until well blended. Add vinegar; stir until well blended. To serve: Toss asparagus with enough dressing to coat lightly. Serve with additional dressing and lemon wedges, if desired. Makes 4 servings.

Note: If desired, use a smaller number of thicker asparagus. Cook 2 to 3 minutes longer. Proceed as directed above.

Per serving: 88 calories; 3 g protein; 7 g fat; 66% calories from fat; 0 mg cholesterol; 5 g carbohydrates; 182 mg sodium; 2 g fiber

Skewered Brussels Sprouts

1	container (10 ounces) fresh Brussels sprouts, trimmed
	water
1½	tablespoons butter, melted
1½	tablespoons lemon juice
	paprika to taste
	pepper to taste

Preheat grill or broiler. In medium skillet over medium-high heat, cook Brussels sprouts in 1 inch boiling water for 7 to 10 minutes or until tender-crisp. Drain. In medium bowl, mix butter and lemon juice. Add Brussels sprouts; toss to coat well. Thread coated Brussels sprouts on skewers. Sprinkle with paprika and pepper. Grill or broil 2 to 3 minutes or until brown, turning once. Makes 4 servings.

Per serving: 66 calories; 2 g protein; 4 g fat; 53% calories from fat; 11 mg cholesterol; 6 g carbohydrates; 44 mg sodium; 3 g fiber

Lemon Dill Beets

8 medium whole fresh beets, scrubbed well with tops removed
1 tablespoon butter
1 tablespoon lemon juice
1½ teaspoons chopped fresh dill

Preheat grill or broiler. Place beets in center of large piece of heavy-duty foil; fold edges up around beets. Add butter, lemon juice, and dill. Seal edges of foil tightly. Place over grill. Cook, turning frequently, 45 minutes or until beets are tender. Makes 4 servings.

Per serving: 57 calories; 1 g protein; 3 g fat; 45% calories from fat; 7 mg cholesterol; 7 g carbohydrates; 73 mg sodium; 2 g fiber

Lemon Broccoli

1 tablespoon cornstarch
1/4 teaspoon salt
1/4 teaspoon pepper
1 cup skim milk
2 tablespoons lemon juice
1 tablespoon butter
1 tablespoon chopped parsley
1 large head broccoli, trimmed, or 2 packages (10 ounces each) frozen broccoli spears, cooked and drained

In 1-quart saucepan, mix cornstarch, salt, and pepper. Gradually stir in milk until smooth. Place over medium heat. Bring to boil, stirring constantly. Boil 1 minute. Remove from heat; stir in lemon juice, butter, and parsley. In shallow serving dish, arrange hot broccoli; top with hot lemon sauce. Makes 8 servings.

Per serving: 48 calories; 3 g protein; 2 g fat; 27% calories from fat; 4 mg cholesterol; 6 g carbohydrates; 112 mg sodium; 2 g fiber

Creamy Broccoli-Rice Casserole

- 2 tablespoons butter
- 1 medium onion, chopped
- 1 package (10 ounces) frozen chopped broccoli, thawed
- 1 can (10 1/2 ounces) cream of chicken soup
- 1/4 teaspoon garlic salt
- 1/4 teaspoon celery salt
- 1/4 teaspoon onion salt
- 2 cups hot cooked brown rice
- 1 ounce Swiss cheese, shredded (1/4 cup)

Preheat oven to 350°F. Grease 1 1/2-quart casserole. Heat butter in medium nonstick skillet over medium heat. Add onion; cook 5 minutes or until tender. Add broccoli; cook 3 minutes. Add undiluted soup, garlic, celery, and onion salt. Cook until bubbly, stirring occasionally. Pack rice in greased 2-cup mold or small bowl; invert into center of prepared casserole. Pour broccoli mixture around rice. Sprinkle with cheese. Bake 10 minutes or until cheese melts. Makes 4 servings.

Per serving: 270 calories; 9 g protein; 10 g fat; 33% calories from fat; 20 mg cholesterol; 37 g carbohydrates; 645 mg sodium; 4 g fiber

Tex-Mex Potatoes

1½ cups water
4 medium potatoes (about 1½ pounds), peeled and cut into ¼-inch-thick slices
½ teaspoon salt
3 tablespoons canola, corn, safflower, or sunflower oil
4 green onions with tops, thinly sliced (½ cup)
1 can (4 ounces) diced green chilies, drained
1 medium clove garlic, minced
4 ounces Monterey Jack cheese, shredded (1 cup)
finely chopped cilantro for garnish

In 10-inch skillet over high heat, bring water to boil. Add potatoes and salt. Reduce heat to medium. Cook, covered, 10 to 12 minutes or until tender; drain.

In same, well-dried, skillet, heat oil over medium heat. Add green onions, chilies, and garlic. Cook, stirring often, 2 minutes. Add potatoes; toss to mix well. Cook 5 to 10 minutes or until potatoes begin to brown, occasionally stirring gently. Sprinkle top with cheese. Reduce heat to low. Cook until cheese melts. Garnish with cilantro, if desired. Makes 4 servings.

Per serving: 265 calories; 11 g protein; 10 g fat; 35% calories from fat; 4 mg cholesterol; 32 g carbohydrates; 826 mg sodium; 3 g fiber

Chinese Eggplant and Scallion

1 large eggplant, stem removed and cut into 6 wedges
water
2 tablespoons canola, corn, safflower, or sunflower oil
1 large green onion, cut into 2-inch pieces
2 tablespoons soy sauce
1/4 teaspoon sugar
pepper to taste

In large skillet or Dutch oven, cook eggplant over medium heat in steamer basket or on rack over boiling water, 20 to 30 minutes or until tender. Heat oil in large skillet or wok over medium-high heat. Add green onion. Cook, stirring constantly, 1/2 minute. Add eggplant, soy sauce, sugar, and pepper. Cook, stirring constantly, 3 minutes or until heated through and well blended. Makes 4 servings.

Per serving: 113 calories; 2 g protein; 7 g fat; 51% calories from fat; 0 mg cholesterol; 12 g carbohydrates; 522 mg sodium; 6 g fiber

Delectable Desserts

Strawberry-Pineapple Crisp

- 12 ounces fresh strawberries (about 2 cups), sliced in half
- 1/2 fresh pineapple (about 3 1/2 pounds), peeled, cored, and cut into 1/2-inch cubes (about 3 cups)
- 6 tablespoons firmly packed brown sugar, divided
- 2 tablespoons cornstarch
- 1 1/4 cups unsweetened pineapple juice
- 1/2 cup regular or quick-cooking rolled oats
- 2 tablespoons all-purpose flour
- 2 tablespoons butter
- 1/2 teaspoon ground cinnamon

Preheat oven to 350°F. In greased 9-inch square baking dish, deep pie plate, or shallow 9-inch round casserole, gently toss strawberries and pineapple until well blended; set aside. In small saucepan, mix 2 tablespoons brown sugar with cornstarch. Stir in pineapple juice. Cook over medium heat, stirring constantly, 3 to 5 minutes or until thickened. Pour over fruit. In small bowl, stir remaining 1/4 cup brown sugar, oats, and flour. With fingers or pastry blender, cut in butter until mixture is crumbly; sprinkle evenly over strawberry-pineapple mixture. Top with cinnamon. Bake 30 to 35 minutes or until bubbly around edges and top is lightly browned. Makes 6 servings.

Per serving: 214 calories; 2 g protein; 5 g fat; 20% calories from fat; 10 mg cholesterol; 43 g carbohydrates; 41 mg sodium; 3.5 g fiber

Chocolate-Banana Thick Shake

2 medium very ripe bananas, cut into pieces
2½ cups skim milk, divided
2 tablespoons unsweetened cocoa powder
2 tablespoons sugar
1 cup fat-free chocolate ice cream

Place bananas, 1 cup skim milk, cocoa powder, and sugar in blender. Process until smooth. Add remaining skim milk and ice cream. Process until thick and foamy. Makes 4 servings.

Per serving: 180 calories; 9 g protein; 3 g fat; 13% calories from fat; 7 mg cholesterol; 33 g carbohydrates; 122 mg sodium; 2 g fiber

Lemon Glazed Tangerines

- 1 large lemon
- 1 large orange
- water
- 1/3 cup sugar
- 4 seedless tangerines or clementines, peeled and segmented

With zester or vegetable peeler, remove peel from lemon and orange (avoid the bitter white pith); reserve peels. Squeeze lemon; reserve juice. Save orange for another use. In small saucepan over high heat, bring to boil reserved lemon and orange peels and enough water to cover. Remove from heat; let stand 5 minutes. Drain. In same small saucepan, place drained peels, lemon juice, 1/2 cup water, and sugar. Bring to boil over medium-high heat. Reduce heat to low; simmer, uncovered, 10 to 15 minutes or until consistency of syrup. Cool, then strain. To serve, place tangerine segments in serving bowl; top with syrup. Toss to coat evenly. Chill 1 to 2 hours. Makes 4 servings.

Per serving: 94 calories; .5 g protein; .5 g fat; 1% calories from fat; 0 mg cholesterol; 24 g carbohydrates; 1 mg sodium; 2 g fiber

Cantaloupe-Strawberry Alaska

- 1/2 cup fresh strawberries, divided
- 1 small cantaloupe (about 1 pound), seeded and cut in half
- 2 tablespoons sweet sherry
- 1/4 cup plus 2 teaspoons sugar, divided
- 2 egg whites, at room temperature
- pinch salt

Place 1/4 cup strawberries into each cantaloupe half. Sprinkle strawberries evenly with sherry and 2 teaspoons sugar. Cover and chill at least 1 hour. Preheat oven to 400°F. To make meringue: In small bowl with mixer at high speed, beat egg whites until foamy. Gradually beat in remaining 1/4 cup sugar until sugar is dissolved and stiff peaks form. Spoon 1/4 whites evenly over each melon half. Place on baking sheet. Bake 5 minutes or until meringue is golden brown. Makes 2 servings.

Per serving: 160 calories; 4 g protein; .5 g fat; 4% calories from fat; 0 mg cholesterol; 36 g carbohydrates; 46 mg sodium; 3 g fiber

Strawberry-Yogurt Treat

1 cup fresh or frozen (thawed) strawberries
1 container (8 ounces) nonfat vanilla yogurt
1 cup club soda

Place all ingredients in blender and process until smooth. Makes 2 servings.

Per serving: 86 calories; 7 g protein; .5 g fat; 5% calories from fat; 2 mg cholesterol; 14 g carbohydrates; 112 mg sodium; 2 g fiber

Peachy-Almond Ice Milk

1 cup skim milk
2 tablespoons instant nonfat dry-milk powder
fat-free, cholesterol-free egg substitute, equivalent to 1 egg
1/3 cup sugar
2 tablespoons amaretto liqueur (optional)
1 teaspoon vanilla extract
1/2 teaspoon almond extract
2 cups fresh (peeled) or frozen (thawed) sliced peaches
1 tablespoon lemon juice

To make custard: In medium saucepan over medium heat cook skim milk, milk powder, egg substitute, and sugar, stirring constantly, 5 to 8 minutes or until mixture is slightly thickened. Remove from heat; cover and chill at least 1 hour or until cool. Stir in liqueur and vanilla and almond extracts. In food processor or blender, puree peaches until smooth. Stir pureed peaches and lemon juice into cool custard. Freeze in ice cream maker according to manufacturer's directions or spoon into shallow metal baking pan and freeze, uncovered, until almost firm. Remove from pan and place in large bowl; beat peach mixture with mixer until slushy; return to chilled pan. Freeze until firm. Scoop and serve immediately. Makes 8 servings.

Note: Canned peaches may be used in the winter.

Per serving: 63 calories; 2 g protein; .5 g fat; 1% calories from fat; 0 mg cholesterol; 34 mg sodium; .5 g fiber

Blueberry and Pudding Parfait

1 cup fresh or frozen (thawed) unsweetened blueberries
2 tablespoons grape jelly
1 teaspoon sugar
1 teaspoon cornstarch mixed with 2 teaspoons water
1 package (4-serving size) cook-and-serve vanilla pudding-and-pie-filling mix
2 cups skim milk

Place blueberries and grape jelly into food processor or blender. Process until smooth. In small saucepan over medium heat, bring to boil, stirring constantly, blueberry-grape puree, sugar, and cornstarch mixture. Cook 1 minute more, stirring constantly. Remove from heat; let cool slightly. Cover and chill at least 30 minutes or until thickened. Prepare pudding according to package directions using skim milk; cool until just thickened. In each of four 6-ounce parfait glasses, layer 1/4 pudding and then 1/4 blueberry mixture, making alternate layers and ending with pudding. Cover and chill at least 1 hour or until set. Makes 4 servings.

Per serving: 114 calories; 4 g protein; .5 g fat; 3% calories from fat; 2 mg cholesterol; 24 g carbohydrates; 101 mg sodium; 1 g fiber

Kiwi-Lemon Sorbet

- 1 cup water
- 1/2 cup sugar
- 1/2 cup light corn syrup
- 4 kiwis, pared and cut in half
- 5 teaspoons lemon juice
- 1/4 teaspoon grated lemon peel

In small saucepan over medium heat, stir water, sugar, and corn syrup. Cook, stirring occasionally, 2 minutes or until sugar is dissolved. In food processor or blender, puree kiwis until smooth. Measure out 3/4 cup. (Save any remaining puree for another use.) In shallow metal baking pan, combine pureed kiwis, sugar syrup, lemon juice, and peel; freeze, uncovered, until almost firm. Remove and place in large bowl; beat kiwi mixture with mixer until light and fluffy; return to chilled baking pan. Freeze about 2 hours or until firm. Scoop and serve immediately. Makes 4 servings.

Per serving: 258 calories; 0 g protein; .5 g fat; 1% calories from fat; 0 mg cholesterol; 67 g carbohydrates; 23 mg sodium; 3 g fiber

Fruity Orange-Sicles

1 envelope unflavored gelatin
1/2 cup water
4 cups orange juice, divided
1/3 cup honey
1/2 cup pureed cantaloupe or peaches
10 5-ounce paper drinking cups

In medium saucepan, sprinkle gelatin over water; let stand 5 minutes or until softened. Stir in 1 cup orange juice and honey. Cook, stirring occasionally, 2 to 3 minutes or until gelatin dissolves. Stir in remaining orange juice and pureed fruit. Place ten 5-ounce paper drinking cups on tray or shallow baking pan. Fill with orange gelatin mixture almost to top and cover tray with foil. Insert wooden stick or plastic spoon in small hole in center of each cup. Freeze 3 hours or until firm. To serve, run warm water over outside and remove paper cup. Makes 10 servings.

Note: For longer storage, store in freezer, once frozen, in tightly closed plastic bag.

Per serving; 81 calories; 2 g protein; .5 g fat; 3% calories from fat; 0 mg cholesterol; 19 g carbohydrates; 3 mg sodium; 0 g fiber

No Bake Blueberry-Peach Pie

Crust

1 cup reduced-fat chocolate-wafer cookie crumbs (about 35 1-inch cookies)
2 tablespoons butter, melted
2 tablespoons honey

Filling

2 cups fresh or 1 package (12 ounces) frozen (thawed) blueberries, divided
1/4 cup water
1/4 cup sugar
2 tablespoons cornstarch
1 1/2 cups fresh, drained canned or frozen (thawed) sliced peaches
1 teaspoon vanilla extract

Preheat oven to 350°F. In medium bowl, mix chocolate cookie crumbs, butter, and honey until well blended. Press crumb mixture evenly on bottom and sides of 9-inch pie plate. Bake 8 to 10 minutes or until set and edges slightly brown. Remove from oven. Meanwhile, in medium saucepan over medium heat stir 1 cup blueberries, water, sugar, and cornstarch until well blended. Cook, stirring constantly, until mixture comes to boil. Boil, stirring constantly, 1 minute. Stir in remaining blueberries, peaches, and vanilla. Spoon into prepared crust. Chill at least 2 hours or until set. Makes 8 servings.

Per serving: 168 calories; 1 g protein; 4 g fat; 21% calories from fat; 8 mg cholesterol; 33 g carbohydrates; 92 mg sodium; 1.5 g fiber

CONVERSIONS

Metric Volume Equivalents

Measuring Cup		
1/4 cup	=	60 mL
1/3 cup	=	75 mL
1/2 cup	=	125 mL
3/4 cup	=	180 mL
1 cup	=	250 mL
2 cups	=	500 mL
3 cups	=	750 mL
4 cup	=	1,000 mL

Tablespoon		
1T	=	15 mL
2T	=	30 mL
3T	=	45 mL
4T	=	60 mL

Teaspoon		
1/4 t	=	1mL
1/2 t	=	2mL
1 t	=	5mL
2 t	=	10mL
3 t	=	15mL
4 t	=	20mL

Metric Weight Equivalents

1 ounce	=	30g
4 ounces (1/4 lb)	=	120g
12 ounces (3/4 lb)	=	225g
16 ounces (1 lb)	=	360g
32 ounces (2 lb)	=	900g

Oven Temperature Equivalents

225°	=	110°
250°	=	120°
275°	=	140°
300°	=	150°
325°	=	160°
350°	=	180°
375°	=	190°
400°	=	200°
425°	=	220°

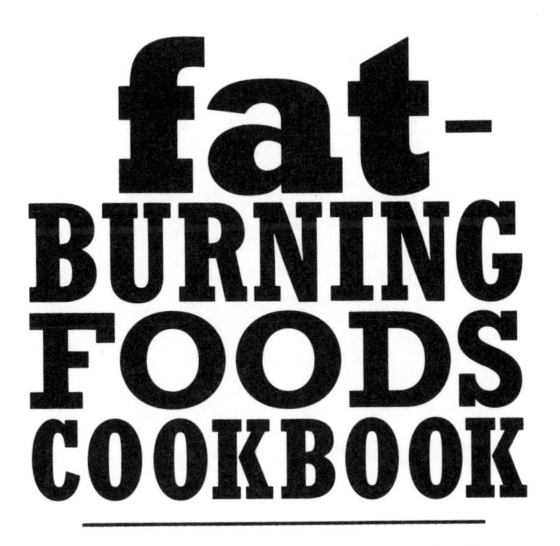

Edited by Betty Bianconi, R.D.

Created and manufactured by Ottenheimer Publishers, Inc.

10 Church Lane
Baltimore, Maryland 21208, USA

Printed in the United States of America
CB731E

CONTENTS

INTRODUCTION 385

HOW TO READ THE NUTRITION INFORMATION 396

SEVEN-DAY MENU 397

SAVORY SOUPS 404

SUPER SALADS 423

BOUNTIFUL BREADS 444

EXCITING ENTRÉES 464

DELECTABLE SIDE DISHES 514

DELICIOUS DESSERTS 549

INTRODUCTION

by Judy Jameson, author of
Fat-Burning Foods and Other Weight-Loss Secrets

THANK YOU, READERS. AND CONGRATULATIONS!

Your support and enthusiasm have turned our book, *Fat-Burning Foods and Other Weight-Loss Secrets,* into a runaway best-seller. Hundreds and thousands of people have now learned that you can be more slender and more energetic than ever before, without hunger.

The amazing discoveries revealed in *Fat-Burning Foods and Other Weight-Loss Secrets* have taught readers that you do not have to travel the road to a slender new you on an empty stomach. **You do not have to be hungry to lose weight!**

Many of you have discovered that the recipes in *Fat-Burning Foods and Other Weight-Loss Secrets* were delicious as well as satisfying. But there was a problem—there weren't enough of them! So here's an entire book of recipes that will help you keep incorporating "fat-burning foods" into your meals. This book is our way of helping you keep your commitment to good health.

Before you begin browsing through these mouth-watering recipes, let's review your program for permanent weight loss.

Why Dieting Doesn't Work

"Fad-of-the-month" dieting causes more harm than good, because every time you starve yourself, your body's survival instinct kicks in and actively tries to preserve its fat stores. And your body becomes more efficient at hanging on to its fat with every successive diet. So when you go off one of these diets—and just about everyone does, because your body eventually wants to start eating normally again—not only do you gain all the weight back, but you likely end up heavier than ever. This is the vicious cycle many dieters know so well: lose 10 pounds, gain back 15, lose those 15 pounds, then gain back 20, and so on.

Eventually, conventional dieting will slow your metabolism down so much that even small portions of food can make you gain weight. **Starvation diets are the problem—not the solution—for overweight people.**

One of the keys to success in this exciting program is that you are never hungry. Your body never thinks it's starving, so you can keep burning off that fat, slowly and steadily.

To get off the "yo-yo-diet" syndrome of weight loss followed by weight gain, you must eat enough food to keep your metabolic rate up. **Your diet must contain at least 10 calories per pound of your ideal body weight.** In other words, if you want to weigh 120 pounds, you should be eating at least 1,200 calories every day.

The best way for you to lose weight permanently is to:

- ➢ eat the fat-burning foods on this program, and
- ➢ raise your metabolic rate through moderate exercise.

Miracle Foods Every Day Keep the Waistline at Bay

"Miracle" foods high in complex carbohydrates are the foundation of the *Fat-Burning Foods* program. These foods, which include fruits, vegetables, legumes, brans, grains, cereals, pasta, rice, potatoes and bread, not only are extremely nutritious, satisfying and inexpensive, but also are extraordinary fat-burning tools.

Here is the list of the 30 amazing fat-burning foods as it originally appeared in *Fat-Burning Foods and Other Weight-Loss Secrets*. These foods are all high in complex carbohydrates and low in fat. They are also the foundation of most of the recipes in this book. Whenever you feel the urge, grab (or cook) one of these miracle foods and eat until you're satisfied.

30 Fat-Burning Foods

- Apples
- Bananas
- Beans (all varieties)
- Bread (plain)
- Broccoflower
- Broccoli
- Cabbage
- Cauliflower
- Celery
- Citrus fruit
- Corn, including air-popped popcorn
- Cranberries
- Grains and grain products
- Grapes
- Jam (sugar-free, low-cal only)
- Leeks
- Lettuce
- Melons
- Mushrooms
- Pasta (low-fat, preferably whole-grain)
- Pears
- Peas
- Peppers
- Pineapple
- Potatoes
- Root vegetables
- Spinach
- Tomatoes
- Waffles and pancakes (frozen, low-fat)
- Zucchini

Why Does This Program Take Off Pounds?

Scientists aren't sure why, but your body seems to handle complex carbohydrates differently than it does other types of food. Meals high in complex carbohydrates appear to raise the metabolic rates of overweight people more than meals containing a comparable number of calories made up mostly of fats or proteins. Furthermore, your body seems to "prefer" complex carbohydrates to fats for energy. A number of studies now indicate that it's "easier" for the body to convert carbohydrates into energy and dietary fat into body fat for future use. Perhaps dietary fat is so similar in chemical composition to our body fat that it just takes less energy to convert it into flab. These foods seem to lose many of their calories just in the process of digestion! **Calories from starch, sugar and other carbohydrates are not stored in your body as easily as calories from fat.**

Although you don't need to count calories on this program, the truth is that complex carbohydrates don't have a lot of calories. Not only will foods rich in complex carbohydrates provide the same energy ounce for ounce as protein, but they have less than half the calories of fat. You can eat as much as you want of these foods to satisfy your appetite. In fact, your appetite is "cued" to tell your body to stop eating during the time your body converts energy from carbohydrates into glucose for energy.

Fortunately, complex carbohydrates are also very good for you. Because they break down easily into glucose (blood sugar), your main source of energy, these foods are like high-octane, clean-burning fuel for your body. Not incidentally, they're also high in dietary fiber and may well reduce your risk of diseases such as cancer. **Your body prefers to fuel itself with carbohydrate calories.**

The two main types of dietary fiber, water-soluble and insoluble fiber, are both excellent for weight control and for your health.

Water-soluble fiber is a type of fiber that can dissolve in water. It's found in foods such as oat bran and in many legumes, fruits and vegetables. In general, these foods help regulate blood sugar levels and may also lower cholesterol levels in your blood. The soluble fiber in apples and oats has also been linked to reduced risk of heart disease.

Insoluble fiber, found in foods like wheat bran, peanuts and many legumes, fruits and vegetables, provides bulk to keep your digestive system in good order. It is the roughage your digestive system needs to stay healthy, acting like a toothbrush on the interior of your digestive tract. It therefore reduces your risk of constipation, hemorrhoids, diverticular disease and possibly some cancers. The insoluble fiber in wheat bran has been linked with reduced risk of colon cancer and possibly breast cancer.

Like other complex carbohydrate foods, fiber helps satisfy hunger and thus helps you resist the temptation to overload on fat. Fiber in your diet adds necessary bulk and is satisfying. It takes a long time to chew most fibrous foods, which gives time for the "I'm full" signal to reach your brain.

All of which leads to two simple conclusions:

- ➢ The bulk of your diet should come from complex carbohydrates.
- ➢ Plan to eat 30 to 40 grams of fiber every day.

Fats: Just Say No

Fats, found in most meats, dairy products, nuts and grain products, are necessary for your health. But the average North American diet comprises a hugely excessive 35% to 40% fat, thanks to our fondness for red meat, fried foods, dairy products and desserts. And all you really need to satisfy your body's minimum requirements is the equivalent of a daily teaspoon of canola oil. You'll get at least that if you eat the minimum protein recommendations of this program.

The problem with too much fat in your diet is that calories from fat are more likely to "stick to your waistline" than calories from carbohydrates and protein. Fat calories are also harder to burn off than carbohydrates and protein. And they're more readily converted to body fat, since your body prefers to use carbohydrate calories for fuel. The more fat you eat, the more likely you are to be overweight—and stay overweight. **Fat consumption is the critical factor in obesity.** You must reduce your fat intake to 20% to 30% of your daily calories, preferably less.

Cutting down your fat intake is also essential for your good health. Studies show that a low-fat diet can make fatty deposits in coronary arteries start to shrink, especially if you also quit smoking, exercise sensibly and keep the stress in your life under control.

All fats are bad for your waistline. Saturated fats (the kind found in red meat and butter) are the most obvious source of fat in your diet. You must cut down your intake of red meat to a maximum of 5 ounces per serving, no more than twice a week. The rest of your meat intake should consist of chicken and fish.

The fat in dairy products is another fat-maker on you. You must switch to skim milk and low-fat cheese products and limit your daily consumption of them to a maximum of 2 cups of skim milk or the equivalent amount of low-fat yogurt or cottage cheese. Avoid butter, whole milk and hard cheese.

Oils, margarine and other "pure" fats, such as those found in most commercial salad dressings, should be avoided as much as possible. And although vegetables are one of the mainstays of this program, some vegetables, such as avocados and olives, are loaded with fat and should also be avoided. **Eat as little fat as possible, from all sources.**

Protein: Too Much, Too Often

You need a new supply of protein every day to repair and build almost all body tissues and to produce virtually every chemical in your body.

The trouble is, most people consume too much meat and cheese and not enough potatoes and bread. A person whose daily intake is 2,000 calories requires only 200 to 400 calories of protein from animals a day, which you can get from 6 ounces of broiled fish and an ounce or two of cottage cheese. Another way of calculating this is to realize that you need only about an ounce of protein for every 18 pounds of ideal body weight. In other words, a 126-pound woman needs only about 7 ounces of protein, and a 162-pound man needs about 9 ounces of protein in a day.

You can easily reduce your overall protein intake by filling up on healthy fat-burning complex carbohydrates instead.

Skim milk, low-fat yogurt, and low-fat cheeses are a good source of calcium and protein and can be consumed in limited quantities. You can also eat small amounts of eggs, beef, pork and chicken and still lose weight.

Plan to eat one or two dinners of lean red meat weekly, one or two dinners featuring chicken, one or two of fish, and *at least* one vegetarian dinner a week. Never eat more than 5 ounces of protein from animal sources in a day. **You need only a maximum of 10% to 15% of your daily calories from protein.**

Exercising: Get a Move On!

Your basal metabolic rate, the speed at which your body burns off calories, is an important factor in your ability to lose weight and keep it off. Food alone won't do the trick. Only regular activity will keep your metabolism high enough to keep the fat-burning action going. Simple, moderate exercise on a regular basis will keep your metabolism high enough to ensure maximum fat burning. Hours after activity, your basal metabolic rate remains raised. **Regular activity will keep your metabolism high enough to keep that body fat burning off.**

Not insignificantly, exercise also makes you feel more energetic and good about yourself. You'll sleep better, cope with stress better, deal with the ups and downs of life more calmly. That feeling of vitality can only help you—and your eating program—in the long run.

What type of exercise is best for weight loss? Believe it or not, you don't have to "go for the burn" to maximize fat-burning potential. In fact, if you work too hard at your workout, your body could stop drawing on your fat stores for food and start depending on your carbohydrate supplies.

Especially if you're older than 45, you should avoid high-impact aerobic activities, like jogging and jumping, which force too much sudden weight onto joints and the lower back. And you must certainly take competitive sports with a grain of salt. They're too hard on your system and not necessary for weight loss. Your victory will be a new slim body, not first prize at the Boston Marathon.

An activity like walking is absolutely the best form of exercise. Find a half-hour a few times a week, mark it down on your calendar and set aside that time in your schedule for the next few months. Your waistline will reap the benefits.

Summing Up: the Basic Rules for This Amazing Weight-loss Program

- Eat as much as you want of the 30 fat-burning foods.
- Enjoy as many complex carbohydrate foods as you need to feel full, such as fruits, vegetables and grains. These foods must provide at least 65% of your daily calories.
- Aim to eat at least 30 to 40 grams of fiber daily. To keep your fiber intake up, read package labels and always buy the higher-fiber product (it's usually lower in fat, too!).

- Consume no more than 20% to 30% of your total daily calories as fat. To keep life simple, avoid fat when possible.
- Up to 10% to 15% of your daily calories can come from animal sources of protein.
- Eat no more than 5 ounces of animal protein in a day and no more than two dinners of lean red meat a week.
- Eat at least one vegetarian dinner a week—preferably two.
- Eat as little hard cheese as possible and even low-fat varieties in moderation.
- Drink up to 2 cups of skim milk a day, or eat the equivalent amount of low-fat yogurt or cottage cheese.
- Enjoy regular activity such as a brisk daily walk; it will keep your metabolism high enough to burn that body fat off.

A Word of Warning

Following this program will improve your health, but before making changes to your diet or activity level, discuss your decision with your physician. This book is designed to enhance your physician's prescribed treatment, not replace it.

Using This Book from Morning to Night

Let's take a quick look at how you can use this book, starting with breakfast.

A good breakfast is essential for weight loss. One Midwestern study showed that overweight people who received their entire allotment of the day's calories at breakfast lost weight, whereas those who took in all their calories at dinnertime gained weight. You wouldn't jump in your car and go on a big trip without filling your gas tank! So why would you even consider starting your day without a good breakfast?

Break away from the expected and eat leftovers from last night's dinner for breakfast. The Garbanzo Bean Salad (page 55), Broccoli Casserole (page 84), Noodles Milanese (page 118), and even Lentil Soup (page 36) in this book are just as nutritious in the morning as they were the night before.

As the day progresses, some of the same people who skip breakfast also think that a quick lunch on the go will help them lose weight. They're wrong. Lunches on the go tend to be long on fat and short on satisfaction. Plan a fat-burning meal that you can relax and enjoy if only for 20 minutes.

Consider fresh fruit, a sandwich of low-fat cheese, turkey or chicken breast, a fillet of fish, with lettuce and tomato, sliced vegetables or leftovers warmed up from dinner. Spice up your sandwiches with low-fat mayonnaise, ketchup, salsa or mustard rather than butter or margarine. If you're in a rush, consider beans on toast or cold rice salad.

If you're a soup fan, the soup recipes (pages 20 to 38) will really provide you with midday satisfaction. A big bowl of chowder will fill you up and keep you going. Dry soup to which you add water is also a good low-fat bet. Whatever soup you choose, stick to clear broths rather than cream soups.

Toward sunset, the temptation to overeat could feel overwhelming. You're relaxed, maybe a little tired after the challenges of your day, and stuffing yourself into oblivion looks like a pretty appealing prospect. Stop!

You can accompany the entrées in this book with relatively large portions of baked potatoes, whole grains, vegetables, salads splashed with low-fat dressing, and fruits. Consult the salad and side dish sections for inspiration. And eat dinner no later than 5 to 6 P.M. to give your body time to digest the meal before bedtime.

Fat-Burning Flavor Boosters

The nutritional information accompanying each recipe in this book is based on its basic ingredients. But don't forget that garnishes or other additions could add fat or calories. You can, however, use the following condiments and sauces to zip up your food:

- Bouillon cubes
- Chili sauce
- Clear broth
- Cocktail sauce
- Cranberry sauce
- Herbs
- Horseradish
- Ketchup
- Lemon juice
- Lime juice
- Low-fat mayonnaise
- Mint sauce
- Mustards
- Pickles
- Relishes
- Salsa
- Soy sauce
- Spices
- Steak sauce
- Sweet-and-sour sauces
- Vinegars
- Worcestershire sauce

Keep in mind that many of these condiments, while low in fat, are high in sodium. Many are available in reduced sodium and lower fat varieties.

Conclusion

As you've already learned, this program is incredibly easy to follow. It involves no calorie counting, no complicated calculations, no specialized foods or food combinations—and no more hunger pangs.

So here is an array of exciting new experiments in eating. These recipes will take you from breakfast to bedtime and to a new, slim, health-conscious you.

HOW TO READ THE NUTRITION INFORMATION

The *Fat-Burning Foods Cookbook* includes another helpful tool to assist you with your meal planning. Each recipe features nutrition information, which includes:

Calories	Consume at least 10 calories per pound of your ideal body weight.
Protein	Only 10% to 15% of your daily calories should come from animal sources of protein. To determine the percentage of calories from protein, multiply the grams of protein by 4, divide that number by the number of calories, and multiply by 100.
Fat	Consume no more than 65 grams a day.
% fat calories	No more than 20% to 30% of your daily caloeries should come from fat. Remember, it's your total consumption over the whole day that's important, not the percentage in one food or meal.
Cholesterol	Consume no more than 300 mg. daily.
Carbohydrates	These are good for you! At least 65% of your daily calories should come from complex carbohydrates. To determine the percentage of calories from carbohydrates, multiply the grams of carbohydrates by 4, divide that number by the number of calories, and multiply by 100.
Sodium	Keep this under 2,400 mg. daily.
Fiber	Eat 30 to 40 grams every day.

SEVEN-DAY MENU

Day 1

Breakfast	1 cup tomato juice 1 orange 1 low-fat frozen waffle 1 Whole-Wheat Date Biscuit (page 68)
Lunch	Green and Yellow Pasta (page 99) 1 sliced tomato Ginger Muffin (page 65)
Dinner	Curried Chicken Salad (page 42) Nutty Brown Bread (page 75) Cranberry Ice (page 165)
Snack	1 banana

Day 2

Breakfast	1 cup orange juice 1 slice cantaloupe melon 1 ounce prepared cereal with ¼ cup skim milk 1 Oatmeal Muffin (page 63)
Lunch	1 Lentil Burger on a whole-wheat pita (page 104) Cucumbers in Dill (page 130) 1 apple
Dinner	Gazpacho (page 26) Mediterranean Baked Fish (page 124) Marinated Vegetables (page 131) 1 slice Peachy Yogurt Pie (page 181)
Snack	1 cup air-popped popcorn

Day 3

Breakfast	1 cup apple juice ½ grapefruit ½ cup cooked oatmeal with cinnamon and raisins 1 slice Banana Bread (page 78)
Lunch	Health Salad (page 46) 1 slice Nutty Brown Bread (page 75) 1 orange
Dinner	Beef and Bean Soup (page 28) Corn Bread (page 73) Small mixed greens salad with fat-free dressing 1 slice Upside-Down Cake (page 172)
Snack	½ cup grapes

Day 4

Breakfast	1 cup orange juice
	1 apple
	1 ounce prepared cereal with ¼ cup skim milk
	1 Applesauce Banana Muffin (page 66)
Lunch	Curried Chicken Salad (page 42)
	½ cup steamed broccoli
	½ cup applesauce
Dinner	Stuffed Squash (page 89)
	Spanish Rice (page 143)
	Whole-Wheat Irish Soda Bread (page 77)
	Frozen Pineapple Yogurt (page 184)
Snack	1 slice Banana Bread (page 78)

Day 5

Breakfast	1 cup pineapple juice ½ cup hot cereal topped with fresh blueberries 1 Ginger Muffin (page 65)
Lunch	Beef and Bean Soup (page 28) 1 slice Nutty Brown Bread (page 75) Frozen Pineapple Yogurt (page 184)
Dinner	Sole with Sweet-Sour Vegetables (page 122) Orange Rice (page 141) Honey Corn Muffin (page 61) Fresh Harvest Pie (page 174)
Snack	1 apple

Day 6

Breakfast	1 cup orange juice 1 low-fat frozen pancake topped with fresh strawberries 1 Whole-Wheat Date Biscuit (page 68)
Lunch	Tomatoes Stuffed with Chicken (page 109) Corn Bread (page 73) 1 Carrot-Date Bar (page 177)
Dinner	Eggplant Italiano (page 86) Spinach Salad Veronique (page 47) Ambrosia (page 171)
Snack	1 cup carrot sticks

Day 7

Breakfast	1 cup tomato juice 1 slice honeydew melon 1 ounce prepared cereal with ¼ cup skim milk, topped with sliced bananas
Lunch	1 All Green and White Sandwich (page 100) Oven French Fries (page 148) Frozen Pineapple Yogurt (page 184)
Dinner	Sweet-and-Sour Cabbage Soup (page 31) Moo Goo Gai Pan (page 111) Steamed Brown Bread (page 71) Orange Sherbet (page 182)
Snack	1 pear

SAVORY SOUPS

Green Pepper Soup

3 tablespoons butter
½ cup chopped green peppers
½ cup chopped onions
2 cups defatted chicken broth or bouillon
¼ teaspoon dried oregano
2 tablespoons flour
¼ teaspoon salt
1 cup skim milk
Chopped green peppers for garnish

Melt 1 tablespoon butter in large saucepot over medium heat. Sauté peppers and onions until onions are golden. Add chicken broth or bouillon and oregano. Reduce heat to low; simmer for 10 minutes. Place in blender; carefully puree for a few seconds.

In same saucepot, melt remaining 2 tablespoons butter; stir in flour and salt. Cook, stirring, until bubbly. Remove from heat. Gradually stir in milk. Return to heat; cook, stirring, until thickened and smooth. Stir in blended green pepper mixture. Serve hot or cold, sprinkled with chopped green peppers. Makes 4 servings.

Per serving: 141 calories; 5 g. protein; 9 g. fat; 61% calories from fat; 24 mg. cholesterol; 8 g. carbohydrates; 626 mg. sodium; trace g. fiber

Puree of Vegetable Soup

- 2 medium onions, sliced
- 2 tablespoons butter or margarine
- 4 cups water
- 1½ pounds beef with bones for soup
- 3 ribs celery, cut into large pieces
- 3 medium carrots, cut into large pieces
- 2 medium potatoes, peeled and cut into large pieces
- 1 large parsnip, peeled and cut into large pieces
- 5 sprigs fresh parsley
- 1½ teaspoons salt
- ¼ teaspoon ground white pepper
- 1 tablespoon snipped fresh dill, or 1 teaspoon dried dill

Melt butter or margarine in large saucepot over medium heat. Sauté onions until golden. Add water, bones, celery, carrots, potatoes, parsnip, parsley, salt and pepper. Bring to boil. Reduce heat to low; cover and simmer for 2 hours or until meat is tender.

Remove meat and bones from broth; reserve for future use. With slotted spoon, remove vegetables and transfer to food processor, blender or food mill. Puree until smooth; return mixture to broth with dill. Heat through. Makes 8 servings.

Per serving: 72 calories; 1 g. protein; 1 g. fat; 19% calories from fat; 3 mg. cholesterol; 13 g. carbohydrates; 442 mg. sodium; 2 g. fiber

Quick Tuna Chowder

1 can (7 ounces) solid white tuna packed in oil
1 large onion, chopped
3 cups water
2 large potatoes, peeled and thinly sliced
½ teaspoon salt
¼ teaspoon pepper
¼ teaspoon dried oregano
1 can (10¾ ounces) condensed tomato soup
1 tablespoon chopped fresh parsley (optional)

Drain oil from tuna; measure 2 tablespoons reserved oil into large heavy saucepan. Flake and reserve tuna. Add onions to oil in saucepan; cook over low heat, stirring often, until soft. Stir in water, potatoes, salt, pepper and oregano. Cover and cook 15 minutes, or just until potatoes are tender. Stir in undiluted tomato soup and flaked tuna. Simmer 5 minutes to blend flavors. Sprinkle with parsley, if desired. Makes 4 servings.

Per serving: 278 calories; 18 g. protein; 8 g. fat; 27% calories from fat; 28 mg. cholesterol; 33 g. carbohydrates; 979 mg. sodium; 2 g. fiber

Vegetable-Burger Soup

½ pound lean ground beef
2 cups water
1 can (16 ounces) stewed tomatoes
1 can (8 ounces) tomato sauce
1 package (10 ounces) frozen mixed vegetables
½ envelope (¼ cup) dry onion soup mix
1 teaspoon sugar

In large heavy saucepan over medium heat, lightly brown ground beef; drain off fat. Stir in remaining ingredients. Bring to boil. Reduce heat; cover and simmer for 20 minutes. Makes 8 servings.

Per serving: 120 calories; 9 g. protein; 5 g. fat; 40% calories from fat; 24 mg. cholesterol; 9 g. carbohydrates; 337 mg. sodium; 2 g. fiber

Minestrone

4 ounces dried white beans, rinsed and picked over
9¼ cups water
2 medium onions, sliced
2 cloves garlic, minced
1 slice bacon, chopped
2 tablespoons olive oil
2 large tomatoes, chopped
½ cup red wine
1 tablespoon fresh oregano, or 1 teaspoon dried oregano
2 medium carrots, peeled and diced
2 ribs celery, diced
2 small potatoes, peeled and diced
1 small turnip, peeled and diced
½ small cabbage (about 8 ounces), shredded
½ cup uncooked macaroni or other small pasta
Salt and pepper to taste
Grated Parmesan cheese (optional)

In large saucepot or Dutch oven, place beans in 1¼ cups water; let stand overnight.

In large skillet over medium heat, sauté onions, garlic and bacon in oil until bacon is cooked. Add tomatoes, wine and oregano. Boil rapidly 5 minutes, or until liquid is reduced. Add bacon mixture to beans; stir in remaining 8 cups water. Bring to boil. Reduce heat to low; cover and simmer 1½ hours.

Add carrots, celery, potatoes and turnip. Cover and simmer 30 minutes. Add cabbage and macaroni. Cover and simmer 15 minutes more, until macaroni is tender. Season with salt and pepper. Top with cheese, if desired. Makes 6 servings.

Per serving: 266 calories; 8 g. protein; 8 g. fat; 28% calories from fat; 0 mg. cholesterol; 39 g. carbohydrates; 89 mg. sodium; 8 g. fiber

Beet Soup

1 can (16 ounces) whole beets
2½ cups water
1 small onion, finely chopped, or ½ teaspoon onion salt
1 teaspoon sour or regular salt
1 teaspoon sugar
Nonfat sour cream (optional)

Drain beets, reserving liquid, and shred coarsely.

In medium saucepan, place beets, reserved liquid, water, onions or onion salt, salt and sugar. Bring to boil. Top with sour cream, if desired. Makes 4 servings.

Per serving: 44 calories; 1 g. protein; 0 g. fat; 3% calories from fat; 0 mg. cholesterol; 10 g. carbohydrates; 832 mg. sodium; 2 g. fiber

Gazpacho

2 cups tomato juice
1 cup finely chopped peeled tomatoes
½ cup finely chopped green peppers
½ cup finely chopped celery
½ cup finely chopped cucumbers
¼ cup minced onions
1 clove garlic, minced
2 tablespoons tarragon vinegar
2 tablespoons olive oil
2 teaspoons chopped fresh parsley
1 teaspoon chopped fresh, frozen or freeze-dried chives
1 teaspoon salt
½ teaspoon Worcestershire sauce
¼ teaspoon pepper

In large bowl or container, stir all ingredients until well blended. Cover tightly; chill at least 4 hours. Stir just before serving. Makes 6 servings.

Per serving: 66 calories; 1 g. protein; 4 g. fat; 59% calories from fat; 0 mg. cholesterol; 6 g. carbohydrates; 667 mg. sodium; 1 g. fiber

Chili Bean Soup

1 package (16 ounces) pink, red or pinto beans, rinsed and picked over
7 cups water
1 teaspoon garlic salt
1 teaspoon onion salt
¼ teaspoon dried thyme
¼ teaspoon dried marjoram
1 can (10½ ounces) condensed beef or chicken broth
1 can (16 ounces) stewed tomatoes
1 package (1⅝ ounces) chili seasoning mix or 1 can (7 ounces) green chili salsa

In large saucepot or Dutch oven, place beans and enough water to cover; let stand overnight.

Add 6 cups water, garlic salt, onion salt, thyme and marjoram. Bring to boil. Reduce heat to low; cover and simmer 2½ to 3 hours, or until beans are tender. Add hot water as needed to keep moist.

Remove 3 cups cooked beans; save for another use. With potato masher or fork, mash remaining beans with their liquid. Add remaining ingredients and 1 cup hot water. Cook 10 minutes, or until heated through. Makes 6 servings.

Per serving: 126 calories; 7 g. protein; 0 g. fat; 6% calories from fat; 0 mg. cholesterol; 23 g. carbohydrates; 476 mg. sodium; 10 g. fiber

Beef and Bean Soup

1½ packages (16 ounces each) dried beans of any combination (lentils, lima, navy, pinto, black turtle, black-eyed peas, red kidney), rinsed and picked over
1 pound beef bones with meat for soup
4½ quarts water
2 cloves garlic, minced
1 tablespoon dried basil, or to taste
2 teaspoons dried thyme, or to taste
2 teaspoons lemon pepper, or to taste
3 large potatoes, cut into bite-size pieces
1 can (28 ounces) crushed tomatoes
Salt to taste

In large saucepot or Dutch oven, place beans in enough water to cover; let stand overnight.

If desired, brown bones in large skillet over medium heat. Add bones to undrained beans. Stir in water, garlic, basil, thyme and lemon pepper. Bring to boil. Reduce heat to low; cover and simmer 1½ hours, or until beans are just tender.

Stir in potatoes and tomatoes. Cook 15 to 25 minutes more, or until potatoes and beans are fully tender. Remove bones. Season with salt. Makes 24 servings.

Per serving: 116 calories; 7 g. protein; 1 g. fat; 8% calories from fat; 5 mg. cholesterol; 20 g. carbohydrates; 61 mg. sodium; 6 g. fiber

Mushrooms in Broth

1½ cups sliced dried mushrooms
2 cups chicken broth or stock
1 green onion
1 slice (½ inch) fresh ginger
¼ cup soy sauce
1 tablespoon cornstarch, mixed with 2 tablespoons cold water
1 teaspoon sugar
1 teaspoon salt

In medium saucepan, place mushrooms and broth or stock; let stand 30 minutes.

Add onion and ginger. Bring just to boil. Reduce heat to low; cover and simmer 1 hour. Remove and discard onion and ginger. Stir in remaining ingredients. Cook over medium heat, stirring constantly, until smooth and slightly thickened. Makes 5 servings.

Per serving: 100 calories; 5 g. protein; 0 g. fat; 6% calories from fat; 0 mg. cholesterol; 21 g. carbohydrates; 1563 mg. sodium; 7 g. fiber

Meat and Vegetable Soup

8 cups water
1½ pounds beef bones with meat for soup
1 can (16 ounces) tomatoes
2 ribs celery, chopped
1 medium onion, chopped
½ medium green pepper, seeded and chopped
½ cup dry lima beans
3 tablespoons large pearl barley
½ small bunch parsley, chopped
2 medium carrots, peeled and diced
1 medium sweet potato, peeled and cubed
1 can (16 ounces) drained green beans, or 1 package (10 ounces) frozen green beans
1 can (16 ounces) drained peas, or 1 package (10 ounces) frozen peas
1 can (8 ounces) creamed-style corn
1 can (8 ounces) tomato sauce
Salt and pepper to taste

In large saucepot or Dutch oven, place 4 cups water, bones, undrained tomatoes, celery, onions, green peppers, lima beans, barley and parsley. Bring to boil. Reduce heat to medium-low; cover and cook 2 hours.

Add remaining ingredients and remaining 4 cups water. Cook 45 to 55 minutes more, or until vegetables and meat are tender. Remove bones. Season with salt and pepper. Makes 12 servings.

Per serving: 157 calories; 10 g. protein; 3 g. fat; 19% calories from fat; 20 mg. cholesterol; 22 g. carbohydrates; 285 mg. sodium; 6 g. fiber

Sweet-and-Sour Cabbage Soup

8 cups water
2 pounds short ribs or beef chuck, fat removed
1 large onion, sliced
1 head (about 2 pounds) cabbage, shredded
2 cans (16 ounces) stewed tomatoes
½ cup sugar
3 tablespoons lemon juice
1 teaspoon salt
½ teaspoon ground ginger
¼ teaspoon pepper

In large saucepot over high heat, place water, chuck or short ribs and onions. Bring to boil. Reduce heat to low; cover and simmer 1½ hours, skimming fat as necessary.

Add remaining ingredients. Cover and cook 30 to 45 minutes more, or until meat is tender. Remove meat; cut into bite-size pieces. Add to soup. Makes 12 servings.

Per serving: 206 calories; 17 g. protein; 7 g. fat; 32% calories from fat; 50 mg. cholesterol; 19 g. carbohydrates; 354 mg. sodium; 3 g. fiber

Green Split Pea Soup

10 cups water
1 package (16 ounces) green split peas, rinsed and drained
1 ham hock
12 green onions, sliced with ½ tops also sliced
1 cup diced carrots
1 cup diced celery
1 slice lemon
1 bay leaf
½ teaspoon white or black pepper
Salt to taste

In large saucepot or Dutch oven over high heat, combine all ingredients. Bring to boil. Reduce heat to low; simmer, uncovered, for 2 hours, or until peas are tender. Stir frequently. Add more water as needed.

Remove and discard lemon and bay leaf. Remove ham hock; chop edible ham coarsely. Return to soup. Makes 8 servings.

Per serving: 328 calories; 24 g. protein; 1 g. fat; 5% calories from fat; 7 mg. cholesterol; 55 g. carbohydrates; 223 mg. sodium; 13 g. fiber

Mushroom-Barley Soup

3 cups (about ½ pound) sliced mushrooms
½ cup chopped onions
½ cup chopped green peppers
⅓ cup butter or margarine
⅓ cup all-purpose flour
3 cups water
2 cups skim milk
½ cup quick-cooking barley
2 teaspoons Worcestershire sauce
1½ teaspoons salt
1 teaspoon dried parsley flakes
Pepper to taste

Heat butter or margarine in large saucepot over medium heat. Sauté mushrooms, onions and green peppers. Blend in flour; cook, stirring, until flour is browned. Gradually stir in water and milk. Add remaining ingredients. Bring to boil. Reduce heat to low; cover and simmer 10 to 12 minutes, or until barley is tender. Makes 12 servings.

Note: Thin with additional milk or water if soup becomes too thick upon standing.

Per serving: 96 calories; 2 g. protein; 5 g. fat; 49% calories from fat; 14 mg. cholesterol; 10 g. carbohydrates; 334 mg. sodium; 1 g. fiber

Vegetarian Chowder

- 1 package (16 ounces) dried white beans (large or baby limas, navy beans or Great Northerns), rinsed and picked over
- 8 cups hot water
- 1½ teaspoons salt
- 1½ cups chopped celery
- 1 cup chopped onions
- ¼ cup butter or margarine
- ¼ cup all-purpose flour
- ⅛ teaspoon pepper
- 3 cups skim milk
- 1 can (16 ounces) tomatoes
- 1 can (12 ounces) vacuum-packed whole-kernel corn
- 1 cup (4 ounces) shredded Monterey Jack or sharp Cheddar cheese

In large saucepot or Dutch oven over high heat, place beans, water and salt. Bring to boil. Reduce heat to low; cover and cook until tender (about 1 hour for limas, about 2 to 2½ hours for navy and Great Northerns). Don't drain.

Heat butter or margarine in medium saucepan over medium heat. Sauté celery and onions. Stir in flour and pepper. Gradually stir in milk; bring to boil, stirring. Add to beans with remaining ingredients. Heat through. Makes 12 servings.

Note: For extra zip, add a few dashes of hot pepper sauce.

Per serving: 278 calories; 14 g. protein; 8 g. fat; 26% calories from fat; 21 mg. cholesterol; 39 g. carbohydrates; 286 mg. sodium; 12 g. fiber

Winter Spinach Soup

5 cups water
1 medium carrot, shredded
¼ cup medium barley
¼ cup dried lentils
¼ cup dried green split peas
¼ cup chopped onions
1 tablespoon dried parsley
2 teaspoons salt
Pepper to taste
2 cups skim milk
1 package (10 ounces) frozen chopped spinach, thawed
2 tablespoons butter or margarine
¼ teaspoon ground nutmeg
1 hard cooked egg, chopped (optional)

In large saucepot or Dutch oven over high heat, place water, carrots, barley, lentils, peas, onions, parsley, salt and pepper. Bring to boil. Reduce heat to low; cover and simmer, stirring occasionally, 1 hour, or until beans are tender.

Add milk, spinach, butter or margarine and nutmeg. Heat through (do not boil). Top with chopped egg, if desired. Makes 8 servings.

Per serving: 110 calories; 6 g. protein; 3 g. fat; 25% calories from fat; 627 mg. cholesterol; 15 g. carbohydrates; 627 mg. sodium; 3 g. fiber

Lentil Soup

- 8 cups vegetable stock or water
- 1 package (16 ounces) lentils, rinsed
- 2 bay leaves
- ¼ cup canola, peanut, soybean or sunflower oil
- 1 medium onion, finely chopped
- 1 large rib celery with leaves, chopped
- 1 large carrot, coarsely shredded
- 1 small zucchini, coarsely shredded
- 2 cloves garlic, minced
- 2 tablespoons minced fresh parsley, or 2 teaspoons dried parsley
- 1 teaspoon dried thyme
- 1½ cups tomato juice
- ¼ cup red wine vinegar
- 1 teaspoon salt or to taste
- Shredded reduced-fat Cheddar cheese (optional)

In large saucepot or Dutch oven over high heat, place stock or water, lentils and bay leaves. Bring to boil. Reduce heat to low; cover and simmer for 1 to 1½ hours, or until lentils are almost tender.

Heat oil in small skillet over medium heat. Sauté onions until tender. Add celery, carrots, zucchini, garlic, parsley and thyme. Cook 5 minutes. Add to lentils with tomato juice, vinegar and salt. Cover and simmer 30 minutes. Top with cheese, if desired. Makes 6 servings.

Per serving: 332 calories; 19 g. protein; 9 g. fat; 26% calories from fat; 0 mg. cholesterol; 45 g. carbohydrates; 606 mg. sodium; 10 g. fiber

Chicken-Spinach Soup

- 1 broiler-fryer chicken (about 3 pounds), cut into quarters and skinned
- 6 quarts water
- 2 cups diced carrots
- 2 cups diced celery
- 1 cup diced onions
- ¼ cup chopped fresh parsley
- 3 packages (10 ounces each) frozen chopped spinach, thawed
- 1 package (10 ounces) frozen peas
- 4 eggs, lightly beaten
- Salt and pepper to taste
- Grated Parmesan cheese (optional)

In large saucepot or Dutch oven over high heat, place chicken and water. Bring to boil, skimming top as necessary. Reduce heat to low; cover and simmer 40 to 45 minutes, or until chicken is tender. Remove chicken from broth; cool slightly and remove from bones. Cut into bite-size pieces; set aside.

To broth, add carrots, celery, onions and parsley; cook 20 minutes. Add spinach and peas; cook 15 minutes. Add reserved chicken. Heat through. Remove from heat. Stirring constantly, gradually add eggs. Season with salt and pepper. Top with cheese, if desired. Makes 20 servings.

Per serving: 146 calories; 18 g. protein; 5 g. fat; 31% calories from fat; 100 mg. cholesterol; 6 g. carbohydrates; 124 mg. sodium; 2 g. fiber

Cauliflower Soup

2 cups chicken broth or stock
1 medium cauliflower (about 1¼ pounds), cut into small florets
2 cups skim milk
¼ cup butter or margarine, melted
2 tablespoons all-purpose flour
Grated nutmeg to taste
Salt to taste

In large saucepan over high heat, bring broth or stock to boil. Reduce heat to low; add cauliflower florets. Cook gently for 7 minutes. With slotted spoon, remove florets from liquid; set aside.

Add milk to liquid. Bring to boil. Reduce heat to low; whisk in butter or margarine and flour. Simmer 5 minutes. Season with nutmeg and salt. Add reserved florets. Makes 4 servings.

Per serving: 198 calories; 9 g. protein; 12 g. fat; 55% calories from fat; 33 mg. cholesterol; 13 g. carbohydrates; 568 mg. sodium; 3 g. fiber

SUPER SALADS

Florida Chicken Salad

¼ cup light mayonnaise
2 tablespoons lime juice
¼ teaspoon salt
⅛ teaspoon pepper
1 can (16 ounces) grapefruit sections, well drained
2 cups diced cooked chicken
1 cup diced celery
6 cups assorted salad greens
Additional grapefruit sections for garnish (optional)

In large bowl, mix mayonnaise, lime juice, salt and pepper. Add grapefruit, chicken and celery. Toss gently to evenly coat. To serve, line bowl with greens and top with chicken salad and extra grapefruit sections, if desired. Makes 6 servings.

Per serving: 172 calories; 14 g. protein; 7 g. fat; 36% calories from fat; 45 mg. cholesterol; 12 g. carbohydrates; 229 mg. sodium; 2 g. fiber

Tuna-Rice Salad

1 cup uncooked rice
1 can (7 ounces) solid white tuna, drained
1½ cups finely chopped carrots
1 cup finely chopped celery
3 green onions, finely sliced
1 medium green pepper, finely chopped
1 pimiento, diced (optional)
¼ cup sweet pickle relish
¾ cup light mayonnaise
½ cup fresh parsley, chopped
¼ cup canola, corn, cottonseed, soybean or safflower oil
¼ cup cider vinegar
¼ teaspoon pepper
Sliced tomatoes for garnish (optional)

Cook rice according to package directions; cool. In large bowl, place rice, tuna, carrots, celery, onions, green peppers, pimientos, if desired, and relish. Mix well. In small bowl, mix mayonnaise, ⅓ cup parsley, oil, vinegar and pepper. Pour over tuna mixture; toss gently to evenly coat.

Into 2-quart bowl, sprinkle remaining parsley. Spoon tuna-rice mixture into prepared bowl, pressing down. Chill thoroughly. To serve, run a knife around edge and turn out onto serving platter. Place sliced tomatoes around edge, if desired. Makes 8 servings.

Per serving: 289 calories; 8 g. protein; 16 g. fat; 51% calories from fat; 11 mg. cholesterol; 26 g. carbohydrates; 326 mg. sodium; 2 g. fiber

Oriental Salad

- 2 pounds skinless, boneless chicken breasts, cut into 1-inch-wide strips
- 4 tablespoons soy sauce
- ⅔ cup canola, corn, cottonseed, soybean or safflower oil
- 1 clove garlic, scored
- 1 teaspoon shredded lemon peel
- ¼ cup lemon juice
- 1 bag (10 ounces) fresh spinach, washed and well drained
- ½ head iceberg lettuce, torn into bite-size pieces
- 3 cups fresh or canned bean sprouts, rinsed and well drained
- ¼ cup toasted sesame seeds
- Salt to taste

In small bowl or plastic bag, place chicken, 1 tablespoon soy sauce, 2 tablespoons oil, garlic and ½ teaspoon lemon peel; chill for several hours.

Divide chicken mixture into 3 batches. Heat 2 tablespoons oil in large skillet or wok over high heat. Place ⅓ chicken mixture in hot oil. Cook, stirring, 3 to 5 minutes until chicken is firm; remove to bowl. Repeat with next 2 batches of chicken. Discard garlic.

To chicken, add remaining soy sauce, oil, lemon peel and lemon juice. Toss gently until evenly coated. Chill. In large salad bowl, toss chicken mixture with spinach, lettuce, bean sprouts, sesame seeds and salt. Serve immediately. Makes 8 servings.

Per serving: 201 calories; 30 g. protein; 6 g. fat; 28% calories from fat; 71 mg. cholesterol; 6 g. carbohydrates; 613 mg. sodium; 3 g. fiber

Curried Chicken Salad

- 3 tablespoons instant minced onions
- 3 tablespoons water
- 2 tablespoons butter or margarine
- 1¼ teaspoons curry powder
- ¾ cup light mayonnaise
- 1 tablespoon lemon juice
- ½ teaspoon salt
- Dash cayenne pepper
- 3 cups diced cooked chicken
- 1 can (20 ounces) pineapple chunks, drained
- 1 red apple, cored and diced
- 2 tablespoons coarsely chopped nuts
- ⅓ cup golden raisins
- 4-6 lettuce leaves
- 2 tablespoons shredded or flaked coconut

In small bowl, mix onions and water; let stand 10 minutes. Melt butter or margarine in small skillet over medium heat. Add onions and curry powder; cook, stirring, 3 to 5 minutes. Set aside to cool.

In large bowl, stir curry mixture, mayonnaise, lemon juice, salt and pepper until well combined. Add chicken, pineapple, apples, nuts and raisins; toss gently to evenly coat. To serve, line salad bowl with lettuce; fill with chicken salad. Sprinkle with coconut. Makes 6 servings.

Note: Cooked turkey may be substituted for chicken.

Per serving: 368 calories; 21 g. protein; 21 g. fat; 52% calories from fat; 82 mg. cholesterol; 23 g. carbohydrates; 507 mg. sodium; 2 g. fiber

Potato-Brussels Salad

1 cup Brussels sprouts
1 tablespoon nonfat plain yogurt
1 tablespoon light mayonnaise
1 tablespoon orange juice
¼ cup chopped fresh parsley
Salt and pepper to taste
1 large orange, peeled and sectioned
1 pound potatoes, peeled, cooked and diced

In small saucepan over medium heat, cook Brussels sprouts in salted water 5 minutes, or until tender. Drain. Cool and slice.

In large bowl, stir yogurt, mayonnaise, orange juice, parsley, salt and pepper until well blended. Reserve a few orange sections for garnish. Add remaining orange sections, Brussels sprouts and potatoes; toss gently to evenly coat. Cover and chill several hours. To serve, top with reserved orange sections. Makes 6 servings.

Per serving: 91 calories; 2 g. protein; 1 g. fat; 10% calories from fat; 0 mg. cholesterol; 19 g. carbohydrates; 27 mg. sodium; 3 g. fiber

Wintery Turkey Salad

2 cups coarsely chopped cooked turkey
½ cup light mayonnaise
¼ cup thinly sliced celery
2 tablespoons finely chopped pimientos
2 tablespoons drained capers
1 tablespoon finely chopped green onions
1 tablespoon finely chopped parsley
1 tablespoon lemon juice or to taste
1 teaspoon Dijon mustard
Salt to taste
Few drops hot-pepper sauce
Bibb lettuce for garnish (optional)

In large bowl, place all ingredients except lettuce; toss gently to evenly coat. Serve on bed of lettuce, if desired. Makes 4 servings.

Per serving: 223 calories; 20 g. protein; 13 g. fat; 56% calories from fat; 63 mg. cholesterol; 3 g. carbohydrates; 835 mg. sodium; 0 g. fiber

Molded Vegetable Salad

1 package (4-serving size) lemon, lime or orange gelatin
¾ teaspoon salt
1 cup boiling water
¾ cup cold water
¼ cup finely chopped green peppers
2 tablespoons cider vinegar
2 teaspoons grated onions
Ground pepper to taste
¾ cup finely chopped cabbage
¾ cup finely chopped celery
2 tablespoons diced pimientos

In medium bowl, place gelatin and salt. Pour in boiling water; stir until dissolved. Stir in cold water, green peppers, vinegar, onions and pepper. Chill until slightly thickened, about 1½ hours. Fold in cabbage, celery and pimiento; pour into 1-quart mold. Chill until firm, about 4 hours. Makes 6 servings.

Note: Equal quantities of diced tomatoes, cucumbers, shredded carrots, stuffed olives and/or thin onion rings may be substituted for the vegetables.

Per serving: 60 calories; 1 g. protein; 0 g. fat; 1% calories from fat; 0 mg. cholesterol; 14 g. carbohydrates; 317 mg. sodium; 0 g. fiber

Health Salad

1 head Boston lettuce, rinsed
1 small cucumber, thinly sliced
2 small tomatoes, peeled and sliced
1 medium green pepper, sliced
½ large avocado, peeled and sliced
5 radishes, sliced
1 medium peach, peeled and cubed
6 thin slices pineapple
½ can (11 ounces) mandarin orange segments
1 pint strawberries, hulled
Fat-free dressing (optional)

On large serving platter or in salad bowl, tear lettuce into bite-size pieces. Top with arrangement of remaining ingredients. Serve with dressing, if desired. Makes 6 servings.

Per serving: 73 calories; 2 g. protein; 3 g. fat; 33% calories from fat; 0 mg. cholesterol; 12 g. carbohydrates; 9 mg. sodium; 5 g. fiber

Spinach Salad Veronique

4 cups torn fresh spinach leaves
½ small red onion, thinly sliced
½ cup thinly sliced seedless green grapes
4 tablespoons fat-free Italian dressing
1 tablespoon chopped fresh mint leaves for garnish (optional)

In each of 2 salad bowls, place 2 cups spinach; top with onions and grapes. Top each with 2 tablespoons dressing. Garnish with mint, if desired. Makes 2 servings.

Per serving: 71 calories; 4 g. protein; 0 g. fat; 8% calories from fat; 0 mg. cholesterol; 15 g. carbohydrates; 235 mg. sodium; 5 g. fiber

Red Cabbage and Apple Salad

½ small red cabbage, finely shredded
3 Delicious or Golden Delicious apples, cored and coarsely shredded
¼-⅓ cup fat-free French dressing

In large bowl, place cabbage and apples. Add dressing; toss to evenly coat. Makes 4 servings.

Per serving: 118 calories; 1 g. protein; 0 g. fat; 5% calories from fat; 0 mg. cholesterol; 29 g. carbohydrates; 154 mg. sodium; 5 g. fiber

Fruit Slaw

¼ cup light mayonnaise
1 tablespoon pineapple juice
¼ teaspoon salt
4 cups shredded cabbage
3 medium oranges, peeled and cut into sections
⅓ cup drained crushed pineapple
½ cup chopped green peppers

In large bowl, mix mayonnaise, pineapple juice and salt until well blended. Add cabbage, orange sections, pineapple and green peppers; toss gently until evenly coated. Makes 6 servings.

Per serving: 80 calories; 1 g. protein; 3 g. fat; 37% calories from fat; 3 mg. cholesterol; 12 g. carbohydrates; 174 mg. sodium; 3 g. fiber

Zucchini Salad

6 medium zucchini, thinly sliced
1 large onion, sliced
1 clove garlic, sliced
Fat-free French dressing
3 large tomatoes, thinly sliced
Lettuce leaves
Parmesan cheese for garnish (optional)

In large saucepan over medium heat, cook zucchini in salted water 2 to 3 minutes; drain well. In large bowl, place zucchini, onions and garlic; cover with French dressing. Cover and chill overnight.

To serve, drain zucchini; discard onions and garlic. On large platter, arrange tomato slices over bed of lettuce; top with zucchini. Garnish with cheese, if desired. Makes 6 servings.

Per serving: 48 calories; 2 g. protein; 0 g. fat; 7% calories from fat; 0 mg. cholesterol; 10 g. carbohydrates; 154 mg. sodium; 3 g. fiber

Lima Bean Salad

2 cans (17 ounces each) lima beans
¾ cup wine vinegar
1 clove garlic, minced
¼ cup finely minced onions
¼ cup chopped fresh parsley
2 tablespoons sugar
½ teaspoon salt
¼ teaspoon pepper

Drain lima beans, reserving ⅔ cup bean liquid. In large bowl, mix reserved bean liquid, vinegar, garlic, onions, parsley, sugar, salt and pepper until well blended. Add lima beans; toss gently to evenly coat. Cover and chill several hours. Makes 4 servings.

Per serving: 214 calories; 11 g. protein; 0 g. fat; 2% calories from fat; 0 mg. cholesterol; 43 g. carbohydrates; 1030 mg. sodium; 16 g. fiber

Layered Vegetable Salad

1 package (10 ounces) frozen baby lima beans
2 cups fresh cauliflower florets, cut into bite-size pieces
1 small red onion, thinly sliced
1 cup alfalfa sprouts
1 cup fresh broccoli or broccoflower florets, cut into bite-size pieces
1 cup (4 ounces) shredded reduced-fat Cheddar cheese
2 tablespoons chopped walnuts
Fat-free Italian dressing (optional)

In small saucepan over medium heat, cook lima beans in salted water 5 minutes; drain. In medium glass salad bowl, place ½ each lima beans and cauliflower, onions, sprouts, and broccoli or broccoflower. Repeat layers using remaining vegetables. Top with cheese and walnuts. To serve, toss gently and, if desired, top with dressing. Makes 6 servings.

Per serving: 130 calories; 10 g. protein; 4 g. fat; 31% calories from fat; 6 mg. cholesterol; 14 g. carbohydrates; 156 mg. sodium; 6 g. fiber

Dilled Cucumber and Yogurt Salad

1 cup water
¼ cup cider or white vinegar
1 slice onion
1 teaspoon dried dill
2 cucumbers, thinly sliced
1 cup nonfat plain yogurt
½ teaspoon salt
⅛ teaspoon turmeric
Dash pepper
¼ cup diced cooked potatoes
4 cups torn leafy lettuce or mixed greens

In large bowl, place water, vinegar, onion and dill. Add cucumber slices; let stand at least 30 minutes. Discard onion and drain well.

In serving bowl, mix yogurt, salt, turmeric and pepper. Add cucumbers and potatoes; toss gently to evenly coat. On serving platter, arrange lettuce or greens; top with cucumber mixture. Makes 4 servings.

Per serving: 60 calories; 5 g. protein; 0 g. fat; 6% calories from fat; 1 mg. cholesterol; 10 g. carbohydrates; 316 mg. sodium; 2 g. fiber

Carrot Salad

2 cans (16 ounces each) sliced carrots, drained
1 small onion, finely chopped
1 medium pepper, finely chopped
3 ribs celery, finely chopped
1 cup undiluted condensed tomato soup
1 cup sugar
¾ cup cider vinegar
¼ cup canola, corn, cottonseed, safflower or soybean oil
1 tablespoon dry mustard
1 tablespoon Worcestershire sauce
Lettuce leaves for garnish (optional)

In large bowl, place carrots, onions, peppers and celery; set aside. In small saucepan over high heat, mix tomato soup, sugar, vinegar, oil, mustard and Worcestershire sauce. Bring to boil, stirring until smooth. Pour over carrot mixture. Cool slightly. Cover and chill overnight. Serve over lettuce, if desired. Makes 10 servings.

Per serving: 179 calories; 1 g. protein; 6 g. fat; 30% calories from fat; 0 mg. cholesterol; 31 g. carbohydrates; 482 mg. sodium; 1 g. fiber

Spicy Lentil Salad

2 cups dry lentils, rinsed and picked over
3 cloves garlic, peeled
2 hot red or green chili peppers, seeded and chopped
4 tablespoons olive oil
1 teaspoon salt
3-6 tablespoons cider vinegar
½ cup finely chopped onions
Pepper to taste

In large saucepot over high heat, place lentils and enough water to cover. Bring to boil. Reduce heat to low; add garlic and chili peppers. Cover and simmer 20 to 30 minutes, or until lentils are tender. Discard garlic; drain well.

In large bowl, mix cooked lentils, oil and salt; cover and chill 2 hours. Just before serving, stir in vinegar, onions and peppers until well blended. Makes 6 servings.

Per serving: 306 calories; 18 g. protein; 9 g. fat; 27% calories from fat; 0 mg. cholesterol; 39 g. carbohydrates; 363 mg. sodium; 8 g. fiber

Garbanzo Bean Salad

1 can (15 to 19 ounces) garbanzo beans (chickpeas), drained
3 green onions, chopped
¾ cup chopped celery
½ cup sliced pitted green olives
¼ cup chopped pimientos
2 tablespoons olive oil
2 tablespoons tarragon vinegar
½ teaspoon salt
¼ teaspoon garlic powder
Dash of pepper
Lettuce for garnish (optional)

In medium bowl, place all ingredients except lettuce; toss gently to evenly coat. Cover and chill 24 hours. Serve in lettuce cups, if desired. Makes 4 servings.

Per serving: 225 calories; 8 g. protein; 11 g. fat; 44% calories from fat; 0 mg. cholesterol; 25 g. carbohydrates; 675 mg. sodium; 7 g. fiber

Garden Pea Salad

1 package (10 ounces) frozen peas
¼ cup canola, corn, cottonseed, safflower or soybean oil
2½ tablespoons cider vinegar
¾ teaspoon salt
¼ teaspoon dried thyme
⅛ teaspoon pepper
1 cup alfalfa sprouts
½ cup (2 ounces) cubed reduced-fat Cheddar cheese
¼ cup chopped celery
¼ cup coarsely chopped unsalted cashews
2 tablespoons nonfat plain yogurt
1 tablespoon light mayonnaise

In small saucepan over medium heat, place ½ cup water and peas. Bring to boil. Remove from heat; let stand 1 or 2 minutes, or just until peas are heated through. Drain; place in medium bowl.

In small bowl, mix oil, vinegar, salt, thyme and pepper; pour over peas. Cover and chill several hours. Just before serving, drain off marinade; add remaining ingredients. Toss gently to evenly coat. Makes 6 servings.

Per serving: 128 calories; 6 g. protein; 7 g. fat; 52% calories from fat; 4 mg. cholesterol; 9 g. carbohydrates; 179 mg. sodium; 3 g. fiber

Confetti Salad

2 cups cooked mixed vegetables
½ cup shredded carrots
½ cup chopped celery
¼ cup chopped green peppers
1 tablespoon minced onions
¼ cup fat-free French dressing
¼ cup crumbled Roquefort or blue cheese
Lettuce for garnish (optional)

In medium bowl, place mixed vegetables, carrots, celery, peppers and onions. Add dressing; stir until well mixed. Add cheese; toss gently to evenly coat. Cover and chill several hours. To serve, toss again and place in lettuce cups, if desired. Makes 4 servings.

Per serving: 93 calories; 4 g. protein; 2 g. fat; 20% calories from fat; 5 mg. cholesterol; 15 g. carbohydrates; 294 mg. sodium; 4 g. fiber

Grapefruit Salad

2 large firm grapefruits
2 tablespoons light mayonnaise
1 tablespoon nonfat sour cream
2 teaspoons lemon juice
1 teaspoon thawed frozen orange juice concentrate
⅛ teaspoon paprika
1 cup diced cooked potatoes
½ cup diced unpeeled cucumbers
Parsley for garnish (optional)

With sharp knife, slice top off grapefruit. Remove grapefruit sections, keeping them intact; drain sections and set aside. Cut design in edge of grapefruit shell with kitchen shears as desired. If necessary, slice small amount off bottom of grapefruit to keep in upright position.

In medium bowl, stir mayonnaise, sour cream, lemon juice, orange juice concentrate and paprika. Add reserved grapefruit sections, potatoes and cucumbers. Toss gently to evenly coat. Cover and chill several hours. To serve, spoon into grapefruit shells. Top with parsley, if desired. Makes 2 servings.

Per serving: 260 calories; 4 g. protein; 5 g. fat; 18% calories from fat; 6 mg. cholesterol; 50 g. carbohydrates; 132 mg. sodium; 5 g. fiber

Tabbouleh Salad

1 cup bulgur (cracked wheat)
1½ cups boiling water
1 bunch parsley, finely chopped
2 medium tomatoes, peeled and finely chopped
1 large cucumber, finely chopped
¼ cup lemon juice
¼ cup olive oil
12 chopped fresh mint leaves, or 2 tablespoons dried mint leaves
½ teaspoon garlic salt
Salt and pepper to taste

In large bowl, place bulgur and boiling water; let stand 2 hours. Drain well.

In large bowl, place soaked bulgur and remaining ingredients. Toss until well blended. Cover and chill several hours. Makes 8 servings.

Note: May be made a day ahead.

Per serving: 149 calories; 3 g. protein; 7 g. fat; 42% calories from fat; 0 mg. cholesterol; 19 g. carbohydrates; 37 mg. sodium; 5 g. fiber

BOUNTIFUL BREADS

Basic Muffins

2 cups all-purpose flour
⅓ cup sugar
1 tablespoon baking powder
1 teaspoon salt
1 egg
1 cup skim milk
⅓ cup canola, corn, safflower or soybean oil

Preheat oven to 400°F. Grease 12 (2½-inch) muffin cups well or line with paper baking cups. In large bowl, mix flour, sugar, baking powder and salt. In separate bowl, blend egg, milk and oil. Add to flour mixture all at once, stirring just until dry ingredients are moistened. Spoon into prepared muffin cups, filling each about halfway. Bake 20 to 25 minutes, or until muffins are lightly browned. Makes 12 muffins.

Per muffin: 158 calories; 3 g. protein; 6 g. fat; 35% calories from fat; 23 mg. cholesterol; 22 g. carbohydrates; 277 mg. sodium; trace g. fiber

VARIATIONS

Blueberry Muffins: Increase sugar to ½ cup. Lightly blend in ¾ cup fresh or drained canned blueberries when combining liquid and dry ingredients. Do not crush berries.

Per muffin: 176 calories; 3 g. protein; 6 g. fat; 32% calories from fat; 23 mg. cholesterol; 26 g. carbohydrates; 277 mg. sodium; 1 g. fiber

Oatmeal-Raisin Muffins: Reduce flour to 1¼ cups. Mix 1 cup quick-cooking rolled oats and 1½ cup raisins with dry ingredients before adding liquid.

Per muffin: 217 calories; 4 g. protein; 6 g. fat; 26% calories from fat; 23 mg. cholesterol; 37 g. carbohydrates; 279 mg. sodium; 2 g. fiber

Honey Corn Muffins

- ¾ cup sifted all-purpose flour
- ⅓ cup cornmeal
- 1¼ teaspoon baking powder
- ½ teaspoon salt
- 1 egg, well beaten
- ⅓ cup skim milk
- ¼ cup honey
- 3 tablespoons canola, corn, safflower or soybean oil
- ¼ cup peeled diced apple

Preheat oven to 400°F. Grease 8 (2-inch) muffin cups well or line with paper baking cups. In large bowl, mix flour, cornmeal, baking powder and salt. In separate bowl, blend egg, milk, honey and oil. Add to flour mixture all at once, stirring just until dry ingredients are moistened. Gently stir in apple. Spoon into prepared muffin cups. Bake 15 to 20 minutes, or until muffins are well browned. Makes 8 muffins.

Per muffin: 148 calories; 2 g. protein; 5 g. fat; 34% calories from fat; 34 mg. cholesterol; 22 g. carbohydrates; 220 mg. sodium; trace g. fiber

Nutty Carrot Muffins

- 1 cup whole-wheat pastry flour
- ¾ cup all-purpose flour
- ¼ cup firmly packed brown sugar
- ¼ cup nonfat dry milk powder
- 2½ teaspoons baking powder
- 1 teaspoon salt
- ⅔ cup water
- ⅓ cup canola, corn, safflower or soybean oil
- 1 egg
- 1 large carrot, cut into ½-inch slices
- ½ cup unsalted peanuts

Preheat oven to 400°F. Grease 12 (2½-inch) muffin cups well or line with paper baking cups. In large bowl, mix flours, sugar, dry milk, baking powder and salt. In blender, place remaining ingredients; blend until smooth. Add carrot-peanut mixture to flour mixture all at once, stirring just until dry ingredients are moistened. Spoon into prepared muffin cups. Bake 20 to 25 minutes, or until muffins are firm to touch. Serve warm. Makes 12 muffins.

Per muffin: 177 calories; 4 g. protein; 9 g. fat; 45% calories from fat; 23 mg. cholesterol; 20 g. carbohydrates; 265 mg. sodium; 2 g. fiber

Oatmeal Muffins

1 cup whole-wheat flour
¾ cup rolled oats
½ cup raisins or chopped prunes, figs, apricots or dates
¼ cup firmly packed light brown sugar
1 tablespoon baking powder
¾ teaspoon salt
½ teaspoon baking soda
¼ teaspoon nutmeg
1 egg, lightly beaten
1 cup skim milk
¼ cup canola, corn, safflower or soybean oil

Preheat oven to 400°F. Grease 12 (2½-inch) muffin cups well or line with paper baking cups. In large bowl, mix flour, oats, raisins or prunes, figs, apricots or dates, sugar, baking powder, salt, baking soda, and nutmeg. In separate bowl, blend egg, milk and oil. Add to flour mixture all at once, stirring just until dry ingredients are moistened. Spoon into prepared muffin cups, filling each about halfway. Bake 20 to 25 minutes, or until muffins are well browned. Makes 12 muffins.

Per muffin: 146 calories; 3 g. protein; 5 g. fat; 33% calories from fat; 23 mg. cholesterol; 21 g. carbohydrates; 136 mg. sodium; 2 g. fiber

Prune-Nugget Muffins

½ cup all-purpose flour
½ cup whole-wheat pastry flour
¼ cup wheat germ
2 teaspoons baking powder
1 teaspoon grated lemon peel
½ teaspoon salt
1 egg, lightly beaten
⅔ cup skim milk
¼ cup honey
¼ cup canola, corn, safflower or soybean oil
1 cup coarsely chopped prunes
⅓ cup chopped walnuts or pecans

Preheat oven to 400°F. Grease 12 (2½-inch) muffin cups well or line with paper baking cups. In large bowl, mix flours, wheat germ, baking powder, lemon peel and salt. In separate bowl, blend egg, milk, honey and oil. Add to flour mixture all at once, stirring just until dry ingredients are moistened. Gently stir in prunes and nuts. Spoon into prepared muffin cups. Bake 18 to 20 minutes, or until muffins are lightly browned. Makes 12 muffins.

Per muffin: 185 calories; 3 g. protein; 7 g. fat; 34% calories from fat; 23 mg. cholesterol; 28 g. carbohydrates; 158 mg. sodium; 3 g. fiber

Ginger Muffins

- 2 cups sifted all-purpose flour
- ⅔ cup sugar
- 1½ teaspoons baking soda
- 1½ teaspoons ground ginger
- 1½ teaspoons ground cinnamon
- ¼ teaspoon ground nutmeg
- ⅔ cup dark molasses
- ⅔ cup buttermilk
- ⅓ cup canola, corn, safflower or soybean oil
- 1 egg, slightly beaten

Preheat oven to 425°F. Grease 12 (2½-inch) muffin cups well or line with paper baking cups. In large bowl, mix flour, sugar, baking soda, ginger, cinnamon and nutmeg. In separate bowl, blend molasses, buttermilk, oil and egg. Add to flour mixture all at once, stirring just until dry ingredients are moistened. Spoon into prepared muffin cups. Bake 15 to 20 minutes, or until muffins are done. Makes 12 muffins.

Per muffin: 213 calories; 3 g. protein; 5 g. fat; 25% calories from fat; 23 mg. cholesterol; 37 g. carbohydrates; 140 mg. sodium; trace g. fiber

Applesauce-Banana Muffins

1 cup whole-wheat flour
⅔ cup all-purpose flour
2½ teaspoons baking powder
½ teaspoon salt
¾ cup unsweetened applesauce
1 very ripe small banana, mashed
1 egg
¼ cup canola, corn, safflower or soybean oil
½ cup raisins (optional)

Preheat oven to 375°F. Grease 12 (2½-inch) muffin cups well or line with paper baking cups. In large bowl, mix flours, baking powder and salt. In separate bowl, blend applesauce, banana, egg and oil. Add to flour mixture all at once, with raisins, if desired, stirring just until dry ingredients are moistened. Spoon into prepared muffin cups. Bake 20 to 25 minutes, or until muffins are golden brown. Serve warm. Makes 12 muffins.

Per muffin: 122 calories; 2 g. protein; 5 g. fat; 38% calories from fat; 22 mg. cholesterol; 16 g. carbohydrates; 164 mg. sodium; 2 g. fiber

Honey Rye Bread

- 2 envelopes dry active yeast
- ½ cup lukewarm (105-111°F) water
- 1½ cups lukewarm (105-111°F) milk
- ¼ cup honey
- 2 tablespoons butter, softened
- 3 teaspoons salt
- 3¼ cups medium rye flour
- 2½ cups all-purpose flour

Grease two 9 x 5-inch loaf pans; set aside. In large bowl, dissolve yeast in water. With wooden spoon, stir in milk, honey, butter, salt and 1¼ cups rye flour. Beat in more rye flour, 1 cup at a time, until mixture is smooth. Work in any remaining rye flour and all-purpose flour until dough leaves sides of bowl. Turn out on well-floured surface; knead 10 minutes until elastic. Place in greased bowl; turn dough to grease top. Cover; let rise in warm, draft-free place until doubled in bulk, 1 to 1½ hours. Punch down; turn out on well-floured surface.

Divide into two equal portions. Shape each portion into loaf, and place each into prepared loaf pans. Cover; let rise 1 to 1¼ hours until doubled. Bake in preheated 375°F oven 30 to 35 minutes. Turn out on wire racks to cool. Makes 2 loaves (15 slices each).

Per slice: 101 calories; 3 g. protein; 1 g. fat; 10% calories from fat; 2 mg. cholesterol; 20 g. carbohydrates; 227 mg. sodium; 2 g. fiber

Whole-Wheat Date Biscuits

2 cups whole-wheat flour
2 teaspoons baking powder
½ teaspoon salt
½ teaspoon ground cloves
4 tablespoons shortening or margarine
¾ cup finely chopped dates
½ cup finely chopped nuts (optional)
¾ cup skim milk

Preheat oven to 450°F. Grease large baking sheet; set aside. In large bowl, mix flour, baking powder, salt and cloves. With pastry blender or 2 knives used scissor fashion, cut in shortening or margarine until mixture resembles coarse cornmeal. Add dates; stir in nuts, if desired. Add milk, stirring just until ingredients are moistened. Turn out on lightly floured surface and knead briefly. Roll ¾ inch thick; with small biscuit cutter or glass, cut into rounds. Place on prepared baking sheet. Bake 15 minutes until golden brown. Makes 22 biscuits.

Per biscuit: 95 calories; 2 g. protein; 4 g. fat; 39% calories from fat; 0 mg. cholesterol; 13 g. carbohydrates; 83 mg. sodium; 2 g. fiber

Orange-Nut Bread

- 2 cups sifted all-purpose flour
- ¾ cup sifted whole-wheat flour
- ⅓ cup wheat germ
- ½ cup sugar
- 1 tablespoon baking powder
- ½ teaspoon baking soda
- 1 cup orange juice
- ⅓ cup canola, corn, safflower or soybean oil
- 1 egg, lightly beaten
- ⅓ cup walnuts, chopped
- 2 tablespoons shredded orange peel

Preheat oven to 350°F. Grease 9 x 5-inch loaf pan. In large bowl, mix flours, wheat germ, sugar, baking powder and baking soda. In separate bowl, blend orange juice, oil and egg. Add to flour mixture all at once with nuts and orange peel until well blended. Spoon into prepared pan. Bake 55 to 60 minutes, or until pick inserted into center comes out clean. Remove from pan to wire rack; cool completely. Makes 1 loaf (16 slices).

Per slice: 167 calories; 3 g. protein; 6 g. fat; 33% calories from fat; 17 mg. cholesterol; 24 g. carbohydrates; 92 mg. sodium; 1 g. fiber

Spoonbread

2 cups boiling water
1 cup yellow cornmeal
3 tablespoons butter
1 teaspoon salt
Cholesterol-free, fat-free egg substitute, equivalent to 3 eggs
1 cup skim milk

Preheat oven to 375°F. Grease 2-quart ovenproof casserole; set aside. In large bowl, place boiling water; slowly add cornmeal, stirring constantly until thick and smooth. Add butter and salt; cool to lukewarm. Add egg substitute and milk. Beat for 2 minutes; pour into prepared casserole. Bake 35 minutes, or until golden brown. Spoon out while piping hot. Serves 8.

Per serving: 123 calories; 4 g. protein; 4 g. fat; 34% calories from fat; 12 mg. cholesterol; 15 g. carbohydrates; 356 mg. sodium; 1 g. fiber

Steamed Brown Bread

1 cup medium rye flour
1 cup whole-wheat flour
1 cup cornmeal
2 teaspoons baking soda
1 teaspoon salt
2 cups buttermilk or sour 1% low-fat milk
¾ cup molasses
1 cup raisins

Grease two 1-pound coffee cans; set aside. In large bowl, mix flours, cornmeal, baking soda and salt. In separate bowl, blend milk and molasses. Add to flour mixture, stirring until well blended. Stir in raisins. Spoon evenly into prepared cans. Tightly cover cans with waxed paper.

In large saucepot, place wire rack and enough water to just cover rack. Place cans on rack; cover saucepot tightly. Steam over low heat 3 hours. Makes 2 loaves (12 slices each).

Per slice: 104 calories; 2 g. protein; 0 g. fat; 4% calories from fat; 0 mg. cholesterol; 23 g. carbohydrates; 189 mg. sodium; 2 g. fiber

Molasses Brown Bread

- 2 tablespoons lemon juice
- 2 cups skim milk
- 1 cup all-purpose flour
- 1 cup whole-wheat flour
- 1 cup cornmeal
- 2 teaspoons baking soda
- 1 teaspoon salt
- ¾ cup unsulfured molasses
- ¾ cup diced candied fruit, raisins or nuts (optional)

Preheat oven to 350°F. Grease four 16-ounce cans or three 20-ounce cans; set aside. Add lemon juice to milk; set aside at least 5 minutes.

In large bowl, mix flours, cornmeal, baking soda and salt. In another bowl, blend milk mixture and molasses. Add to flour mixture, stirring just until dry ingredients are moistened. Stir in candied fruit, raisins or nuts, if desired. Spoon mixture evenly into prepared cans. Bake 45 to 50 minutes, or until pick inserted near center comes out clean. Cool in cans 10 minutes; turn out onto wire rack. Serve warm, if desired. Makes 3 or 4 loaves (24 servings).

Per serving: 108 calories; 2 g. protein; 0 g. fat; 2% calories from fat; 0 mg. cholesterol; 24 g. carbohydrates; 190 mg. sodium; 1 g. fiber

Corn Bread

1 cup cornmeal
1 cup all-purpose flour
4 teaspoons baking powder
1 tablespoon sugar
½ teaspoon salt
1½ cups skim milk
1 egg
¼ cup canola, corn, safflower or soybean oil

Preheat oven to 450°F. Grease 8 x 8-inch baking pan. In large bowl, mix cornmeal, flour, baking powder, sugar and salt. In separate bowl, blend milk, egg and oil. Add to flour mixture all at once, stirring until well blended. Spoon into prepared baking pan. Bake 25 to 30 minutes, or until golden brown. Makes 12 servings.

Per serving: 139 calories; 3 g. protein; 5 g. fat; 35% calories from fat; 23 mg. cholesterol; 18 g. carbohydrates; 220 mg. sodium; 1 g. fiber

Zucchini Bread

- 2 cups whole-wheat flour
- ¼ cup wheat germ
- ¼ cup unprocessed bran
- 3½ teaspoons ground cinnamon
- 1 teaspoon baking soda
- ¼ teaspoon baking powder
- Cholesterol-free, fat-free egg substitute, equivalent to 3 eggs
- 1 cup honey
- 1 cup canola, corn, safflower or soybean oil
- 2 teaspoons vanilla extract
- 2 cups shredded, unpeeled zucchini
- ¾ cup chopped walnuts or pecans
- ½ cup raisins (optional)

Preheat oven to 325°F. Grease two 8½ x 4½-inch loaf pans. In large bowl, mix flour, wheat germ, bran, cinnamon, baking soda and baking powder. In separate bowl, blend egg substitute, honey, oil and vanilla. Add with zucchini and nuts to flour mixture all at once, stirring until blended. Stir in raisins, if desired. Spoon into prepared loaf pans. Bake 60 to 70 minutes, or until pick inserted into center comes out clean. Makes 2 loaves (12 slices each).

Per slice: 201 calories; 3 g. protein; 11 g. fat; 50% calories from fat; 0 mg. cholesterol; 23 g. carbohydrates; 52 mg. sodium; 2 g. fiber

Nutty Brown Bread

1 cup all-purpose flour
1 cup whole-wheat flour
½ cup firmly packed light brown sugar
½ cup walnuts, finely grated (makes about ¾ cup)
2 teaspoons baking powder
¾ teaspoon salt
¼ teaspoon baking soda
1 egg
1¼ cups skim milk

Preheat oven to 350°F. Grease 8½ x 4½-inch loaf pan. In large bowl, mix flours, sugar, walnuts, baking powder, salt and baking soda. In separate bowl, blend egg and milk. Add to flour mixture all at once, stirring just until dry ingredients are moistened. Spoon into prepared loaf pan. Bake 50 minutes, or until pick inserted into center comes out clean. (Top will have crack.) Turn out on wire rack; cool completely right side up. Makes 1 loaf (12 slices).

Note: Inexpensive rotary-type, hand-operated grater works well for grating nuts.

Per slice: 154 calories; 4 g. protein; 4 g. fat; 22% calories from fat; 23 mg. cholesterol; 26 g. carbohydrates; 229 mg. sodium; 2 g. fiber

Easy Whole-Wheat Bread

1	envelope dry active yeast
1	teaspoon salt
1	teaspoon honey
3	cups fairly hot (120-130°F) water
4	cups whole-wheat flour
½-1	cup wheat flakes, rye flakes, rolled oats or wheat germ

Preheat oven to 400°F. Grease 9 x 5-inch loaf pan; set aside. In large bowl, place yeast, salt and honey. Pour in water; let stand until surface is bubbly. Stir in flour and enough flakes, oats or wheat germ to make thick yet softer, more liquid bread dough. Place dough in loaf pan; let stand in warm, draft-free place 10 minutes. Bake 45 minutes, or until loaf sounds hollow when lightly tapped. Makes 1 loaf (12 slices).

Per slice: 164 calories; 6 g. protein; 1 g. fat; 9% calories from fat; 0 mg. cholesterol; 33 g. carbohydrates; 190 mg. sodium; 5 g. fiber

Whole-Wheat Irish Soda Bread

4 cups whole-wheat flour
1 tablespoon baking powder
2 teaspoons salt
½ teaspoon baking soda
2 cups buttermilk

Preheat oven to 350°F. Grease large baking sheet; set side. In large bowl, mix flour, baking powder, salt and baking soda. Add buttermilk, stirring to form soft dough. Turn out on floured surface; knead lightly for 1 minute. Shape into two flat, round patties, about 8 inches in diameter. Slash large cross in each top. Place on prepared baking sheet. Bake 40 minutes, or until bread sounds hollow when lightly tapped. Cool 5 minutes on wire rack before cutting. Makes 2 loaves (12 slices each).

Per slice: 75 calories; 3 g. protein; 0 g. fat; 7% calories from fat; 0 mg. cholesterol; 15 g. carbohydrates; 258 mg. sodium; 2 g. fiber

Banana Bread

- ¾ cup sugar
- ½ cup shortening
- Cholesterol-free, fat-free egg substitute, equivalent to 2 eggs
- 1 cup mashed banana
- 1¾ cups all-purpose flour
- 2 teaspoons baking powder
- ½ teaspoon baking soda
- ½ teaspoon salt

Preheat oven to 350°F. Grease 9 x 5-inch loaf pan; set aside. In large bowl with mixer, beat sugar, shortening and egg substitute until light and well combined. Stir in banana. Stir in flour, baking powder, baking soda and salt just until smooth. Spoon into prepared pan. Bake 50 to 60 minutes, or until firm when lightly touched on top. Cool in pan on wire rack 10 minutes. Remove and cool completely. Makes 1 loaf (16 slices).

Per slice: 160 calories; 2 g. protein; 6 g. fat; 37% calories from fat; 0 mg. cholesterol; 23 g. carbohydrates; 147 mg. sodium; trace g. fiber

VARIATION

Orange-Banana Bread: Add 1 tablespoon grated orange peel to sugar-egg mixture.

Per slice: 160 calories; 2 g. protein; 6 g. fat; 37% calories from fat; 0 mg. cholesterol; 23 g. carbohydrates; 147 mg. sodium; trace g. fiber

Apricot Bran Loaf

- 1 cup dried apricots, cut into small pieces
- ½ cup plus 2 tablespoons sugar
- 1½ cups sifted all-purpose flour
- 4 teaspoons baking powder
- ½ teaspoon salt
- 1½ cups whole-bran cereal
- 1 cup skim milk
- Cholesterol-free, fat-free egg substitute equivalent to 2 eggs
- ⅓ cup canola, corn, safflower or soybean oil

Preheat oven to 350°F. Grease 9 x 5-inch loaf pan; set aside. In medium bowl, place apricots in enough boiling water to cover; let stand 10 minutes. Drain; stir in 2 tablespoons sugar and set aside.

In large bowl, mix remaining ½ cup sugar, flour, baking powder and salt. In separate bowl, blend cereal, milk, egg substitute and oil. Add to flour mixture all at once, stirring just until dry ingredients are moistened. Stir in apricot mixture. Spoon into prepared loaf pan. Bake 60 minutes, or until pick inserted into center comes out clean. Remove from pan; cool completely on wire rack. Makes 1 loaf (16 slices).

Note: Dried pears, prunes or apples may be substituted for apricots.

Per slice: 156 calories; 4 g. protein; 5 g. fat; 28% calories from fat; 34 mg. cholesterol; 26 g. carbohydrates; 257 mg. sodium; 3 g. fiber

Vegetable-Stuffed Green Peppers

4 medium green peppers
1 cup drained canned corn or thawed frozen whole-kernel corn
¾ cup diced tomatoes
½ cup soft bread crumbs
¼ cup finely chopped celery
Cholesterol-free, fat-free egg substitute, equivalent to 2 eggs
2 tablespoons butter or margarine, melted
1 tablespoon finely chopped onion
Salt and pepper to taste

Preheat oven to 325°F. Grease baking dish or casserole large enough to hold peppers standing up; set aside. Cut tops from peppers and remove seeds. In large saucepan or Dutch oven over medium heat, place peppers and ½ cup water. Cover and cook 5 minutes. Drain well upside down.

In medium bowl, combine remaining ingredients until thoroughly blended. Place peppers cut end up; fill evenly with corn mixture. Add 3 tablespoons water to dish. Bake about 1 hour, or until stuffing is set. Makes 4 servings.

Per serving: 143 calories; 6 g. protein; 6 g. fat; 38% calories from fat; 15 mg. cholesterol; 18 g. carbohydrates; 211 mg. sodium; 3 g. fiber

Spinach, Mushroom and Cheese Squares

2 pounds fresh spinach, trimmed
3 tablespoons butter or margarine
12 ounces fresh mushrooms, sliced
Cholesterol-free, fat-free egg substitute, equivalent to 8 eggs
1½ cups soft whole-wheat bread crumbs
1¾ teaspoons salt
2 tablespoons Worcestershire sauce
2 cups low-fat cottage cheese

Preheat oven to 350°F. Grease 11 x 7-inch baking pan. Rinse spinach; drain or spin until almost dry. In large saucepot over medium heat, place damp spinach. Cover tightly and cook 2 to 3 minutes, or until just limp. Drain well and squeeze dry.

Heat butter or margarine in large skillet over medium heat. Sauté mushrooms 3 minutes, or until tender. In large bowl, combine spinach, ⅔ cooked mushrooms, egg substitute equivalent to 6 eggs, bread crumbs, 1 teaspoon salt and 1 tablespoon Worcestershire sauce until well blended. In medium bowl, combine remaining egg substitute, remaining 1 tablespoon Worcestershire sauce, remaining ¾ teaspoon salt and cottage cheese until well blended.

Into prepared baking pan, spoon ½ spinach mixture; top with all of cheese mixture, then remaining spinach mixture. Bake, uncovered, 30 minutes, or until firm. Let stand 10 minutes. Top with heated reserved mushrooms. Makes 6 servings.

Per serving: 225 calories; 25 g. protein; 8 g. fat; 30% calories from fat; 25 mg. cholesterol; 17 g. carbohydrates; 1345 mg. sodium; 8 g. fiber

Italian Stuffed Mushrooms

3 pounds large fresh mushrooms
2 medium onions, chopped
1-2 cloves garlic, minced
2 tablespoons dry sherry or white wine
1 tablespoon olive or other vegetable oil
1 package (10 ounces) frozen chopped spinach, thawed and squeezed dry
3 tablespoons Italian-seasoned dry bread crumbs
Pinch dried oregano
Pinch dried nutmeg
Salt and pepper to taste
2 tablespoons grated sharp Romano or Parmesan cheese

Preheat oven to 375°F. Spray jelly-roll pan with nonstick cooking spray; set aside. Remove and finely chop stems from mushrooms. Reserve caps.

Spray large nonstick skillet with nonstick cooking spray; place over high heat. Add chopped mushrooms, onions, garlic, sherry or wine and oil; cook until liquid evaporates and mixture begins to lightly brown. Add spinach; cook until heated through. Remove from heat; stir in bread crumbs, oregano, nutmeg, salt and pepper until well mixed. On prepared pan, place mushroom caps top-side down; fill evenly with spinach mixture. Sprinkle with cheese. Bake 12 to 15 minutes, or until heated through. Makes 8 servings.

Per serving: 95 calories; 6 g. protein; 3 g. fat; 25% calories from fat; 1 mg. cholesterol; 14 g. carbohydrates; 78 mg. sodium; 5 g. fiber

Southern Pickled Shrimp

½ cup chopped celery leaves
¼ cup whole mixed pickling spice
1½ pounds frozen raw, peeled, deveined shrimp, thawed
2 cups sliced onions
5 bay leaves
1½ cups salad oil
1½ cups white vinegar
¼ cup chopped pimientos
2 tablespoons capers, undrained
1½ teaspoons celery seed
1½ teaspoons salt
¼ teaspoon hot-pepper sauce
Salad greens for garnish (optional)

In small piece of cheesecloth, place celery and pickling spice; tie securely. In large saucepot or Dutch oven over high heat, bring to boil 2 quarts water and spice bag; boil 10 minutes. Add shrimp. Reduce heat to low; cover and simmer 3 to 5 minutes, or until shrimp are cooked. Drain.

In large bowl, arrange in layers onions and shrimp. Add bay leaves. In medium bowl, combine oil, vinegar, pimientos, capers, celery seed, salt and hot-pepper sauce until well mixed; pour over shrimp mixture. Cover and chill 6 hours, stirring occasionally. Drain well. To serve, place on bed of greens, if desired. Makes 6 servings.

Per serving: 193 calories; 24 g. protein; 8 g. fat; 39% calories from fat; 221 mg. cholesterol; 4 g. carbohydrates; 975 mg. sodium; 1 g. fiber

Broccoli Casserole

1 package (10 ounces) frozen chopped broccoli
1¼ cups lukewarm skim milk
Cholesterol-free, fat-free egg substitute, equivalent to 3 eggs
½ cup grated Parmesan or Romano cheese
½ teaspoon salt
½ teaspoon ground nutmeg

Preheat oven to 350°F. Grease 1½- to 2-quart casserole; set aside. Cook broccoli according to package directions; drain.

In small bowl, combine remaining ingredients; beat until well blended. Pour into prepared casserole. Add broccoli. Bake 25 to 30 minutes, or until knife inserted into center comes out clean. Serve immediately. Makes 4 servings.

Per serving: 115 calories; 13 g. protein; 3 g. fat; 25% calories from fat; 9 mg. cholesterol; 8 g. carbohydrates; 586 mg. sodium; 2 g. fiber

Spinach-Stuffed Tomatoes

6 medium firm, ripe tomatoes
Salt
1 pound fresh, trimmed, chopped spinach, or 2 packages (10 ounces each) frozen chopped spinach, thawed
1 hard-cooked egg, finely chopped
1 tablespoon vinegar
½ teaspoon dried basil or tarragon (or ¼ teaspoon each)
¼ teaspoon dried oregano
⅛ teaspoon dried mustard
⅛ teaspoon garlic powder
¼ cup buttered bread crumbs*

Preheat oven to 350°F. Grease shallow casserole large enough to hold tomatoes; set aside. Cut tops off tomatoes; scoop out and reserve pulp, leaving ½-inch shells. Sprinkle shells with salt; invert to drain. Chop pulp. In small saucepan over low heat, place chopped tomato pulp, spinach and ¼ cup water; cook 5 minutes, stirring occasionally. Drain.

In medium bowl, combine tomato-spinach mixture, egg, vinegar, basil or tarragon, oregano, mustard and garlic powder until well blended. Place tomatoes cut end up in prepared casserole; fill with tomato-spinach mixture. Sprinkle tops with bread crumbs. Bake 20 minutes, or until tomato pierces easily with fork. Makes 3 servings.

* *Recipe for buttered bread crumbs is on page 154.*

Per serving: 171 calories; 11 g. protein; 4 g. fat; 21% calories from fat; 95 mg. cholesterol; 27 g. carbohydrates; 277 mg. sodium; 9 g. fiber

Eggplant Italiano

- 2 medium eggplants (about 1 pound each), peeled and cut into 1-inch cubes
- 3 tablespoons olive or other vegetable oil
- 1 medium onion, finely chopped
- 2 cloves garlic, minced
- ⅓ cup finely chopped fresh parsley
- 2 medium green peppers, finely chopped
- 1 can (28 ounces) Italian-style tomatoes, broken up
- 3 tablespoons tomato paste
- 1½ teaspoons salt
- 1 teaspoon dried basil
- ½-1 teaspoon dried oregano
- ¼ teaspoon ground coriander
- ½ teaspoon pepper
- 3 tablespoons catsup
- 3 tablespoons chili sauce
- Salad greens, lemon slices, carrot curls, cherry tomatoes, black olives for garnish (optional)

Preheat oven to 350°F. Grease large baking pan; add eggplant cubes. Bake 45 minutes, or until soft, stirring frequently.

Heat oil in large heavy saucepan over medium heat. Sauté onions, garlic and parsley 5 to 7 minutes, or until soft. Add peppers; cook 3 minutes. Add tomatoes, tomato paste, salt, basil, oregano, coriander and pepper, mixing well. Reduce heat to low; cover and cook 20 to 30 minutes, stirring frequently.

In food processor or by hand, finely chop eggplant; add to tomato mixture. Cover and cook 20 minutes. Stir in catsup and chili sauce until well blended. Cover and chill several hours.

Serve on bed of greens with lemon slices and vegetable garnish, if desired. Makes 4 servings.

Per serving: 248 calories; 6 g. protein; 11 g. fat; 37% calories from fat; 0 mg. cholesterol; 36 g. carbohydrates; 1447 mg. sodium; 12 g. fiber

Ratatouille (Mixed Vegetables)

4 tablespoons canola, corn, cottonseed, safflower or soybean oil
3 large onions, finely chopped
3 large green peppers, coarsely chopped
6 small zucchini, thinly sliced
1 medium eggplant, unpeeled and cut into 1-inch cubes
6 large tomatoes, peeled, seeded and coarsely chopped
1 cup chopped fresh parsley
3 cloves garlic, minced
Salt and pepper to taste
Grated Parmesan cheese (optional)

Heat oil in large heavy skillet over medium heat. Sauté onions 5 minutes, or until light golden brown. Add peppers; cook 2 minutes. Stir in zucchini and eggplant; cook 5 minutes. Add tomatoes, parsley, garlic, salt and pepper, stirring until well mixed. Reduce heat to low; cook, covered, 15 to 20 minutes. Serve sprinkled with cheese, if desired.

Per serving: 258 calories; 5 g. protein; 15 g. fat; 49% calories from fat; 0 mg. cholesterol; 30 g. carbohydrates; 32 mg. sodium; 9 g. fiber

Eggplant Creole

1 medium eggplant, peeled and cut into 1-inch cubes
1¼ teaspoons salt
4 tablespoons butter or margarine
3 tablespoons all-purpose flour
3 large tomatoes, peeled and chopped
1 small green pepper, chopped
1 small onion, chopped
1 tablespoon brown sugar
2 whole cloves
1 small bay leaf
¼ cup dry bread crumbs

Preheat oven to 350°F. Grease 1½-quart casserole; set aside. In medium saucepan over medium heat, cook eggplant, ¾ teaspoon salt and ½ cup water, uncovered, 10 minutes, or until eggplant is tender. Drain well; place in prepared casserole.

Melt 3 tablespoons butter or margarine in large skillet over medium heat. Stir in flour until blended. Add remaining ½ teaspoon salt, tomatoes, peppers, onions, brown sugar, cloves and bay leaf. Cook, uncovered, 5 minutes, stirring occasionally. Remove bay leaf; pour mixture over eggplant. Sprinkle with bread crumbs; dot with remaining tablespoon butter or margarine. Bake 30 minutes. Makes 4 servings.

Per serving: 199 calories; 3 g. protein; 12 g. fat; 51% calories from fat; 31 mg. cholesterol; 22 g. carbohydrates; 780 mg. sodium; 6 g. fiber

Stuffed Squash

- 2 acorn squash
- 2 cups chopped mushrooms
- 1 cup chopped onions
- 2 cloves garlic, crushed
- 2 tablespoons dry white wine
- ¼ cup chopped parsley
- 1 teaspoon tamari or lite soy sauce
- ½ teaspoon dried basil or thyme
- Pepper to taste
- 1 cup low-fat cottage cheese
- ¾ cup cooked brown rice or bread crumbs

Preheat oven to 350°F. Pierce squash with fork; bake in oven or microwave until tender. Cut in half and remove seeds; set aside. In large skillet over medium heat, cook mushrooms, onions, garlic and wine 3 minutes, or until onions are tender. Add parsley, tamari or soy sauce, basil or thyme and pepper; cook 1 minute. Remove from heat; stir in cottage cheese and rice or bread crumbs until well blended. Let stand 2 minutes; drain, reserving liquid for sauce.

In large casserole, place acorn squash; fill with vegetable-cheese mixture. Bake for 30 minutes, or until heated through. In small saucepan, cook drained liquid until of desired sauce consistency, stirring occasionally. Serve over squash. Makes 4 servings.

Per serving: 235 calories; 11 g. protein; 1 g. fat; 5% calories from fat; 7 mg. cholesterol; 49 g. carbohydrates; 289 mg. sodium; 8 g. fiber

Spicy Yellow Squash

2 tablespoons butter or margarine
8 medium yellow summer squash, sliced 1-inch thick
1 medium onion, finely chopped
2 hot chili peppers, stems and seeds removed
2 medium tomatoes, peeled and chopped
½ cup diced ham
Salt and pepper to taste
¼ cup shredded reduced-fat Cheddar cheese

Preheat oven to 350°F. Grease 2- to 2½-quart casserole; set aside. Melt butter or margarine in large skillet over medium heat. Sauté squash, onions and chili peppers 3 minutes, or until onions are tender. Add tomatoes, ham, salt and pepper. Cook, stirring, 1 minute; pour into prepared casserole. Sprinkle with cheese. Bake 10 to 15 minutes, or until cheese melts and browns slightly. Makes 4 servings.

Note: If desired, ½ large green pepper, chopped, may be substituted for chili peppers.

Per serving: 170 calories; 10 g. protein; 8 g. fat; 42% calories from fat; 27 mg. cholesterol; 16 g. carbohydrates; 343 mg. sodium; 5 g. fiber

Vegetable Casserole

- 4 medium potatoes (about 1¼ pounds), peeled and thinly sliced
- Salt and pepper to taste
- 4 tablespoons butter or margarine, cut into pieces
- 2 medium onions, thinly sliced and separated into rings
- 4 small yellow summer squash (about 1¼ pounds), thinly sliced
- 1 cup nonfat sour cream
- ½ cup grated Parmesan cheese

Preheat oven to 350°F. Grease 2½-quart ovenproof and broilerproof casserole; layer ½ potatoes, salt, pepper and ½ tablespoon butter or margarine; ½ onions, salt, pepper and ½ tablespoon butter or margarine; and ½ squash, salt, pepper and 1 tablespoon butter. Repeat layers.

Cover tightly; bake 1 to 1¼ hours, or until potatoes are fork-tender. In small bowl, stir sour cream and cheese until well blended; spoon over casserole. Broil until lightly browned. To serve, spoon down through all layers. Makes 6 servings.

Per serving: 260 calories; 7 g. protein; 10 g. fat; 35% calories from fat; 32 mg. cholesterol; 34 g. carbohydrates; 252 mg. sodium; 3 g. fiber

Baked Zucchini and Rice Soufflé

3 medium zucchini (about 1 pound), thickly sliced
½ cup cooked rice
6 ounces nonfat sour cream
1 cup (4 ounces) shredded Swiss cheese
Cholesterol-free, fat-free egg substitute, equivalent to 2 eggs
Salt and pepper to taste

Preheat oven to 350°F. Grease 1-quart casserole; set aside. In medium saucepan over medium heat, cook zucchini in lightly salted water 7 to 10 minutes, or until tender. Drain well; place into prepared casserole. Top with rice. In small bowl, stir sour cream, cheese, egg substitute, salt and pepper until well blended; pour over rice. Bake for 40 minutes, or until brown. Makes 4 servings.

Per serving: 202 calories; 14 g. protein; 8 g. fat; 37% calories from fat; 32 mg. cholesterol; 16 g. carbohydrates; 181 mg. sodium; 1 g. fiber

Potato and Spinach Casserole

- 3 medium potatoes (about 1 pound), peeled and cut into eighths
- 2 eggs, at room temperature, separated
- 4 tablespoons butter or margarine
- ½ teaspoon white pepper or to taste
- ¼ teaspoon ground nutmeg or to taste
- 1½ bags (10 ounces each) fresh spinach, trimmed
- 3 tablespoons grated Parmesan cheese
- Parsley sprigs for garnish (optional)

Preheat oven to 400°F. Grease 2-quart casserole; set aside. In medium saucepan over medium-high heat, place potatoes and ½ cup lightly salted water. Cover and cook 20 minutes, or until fork-tender; drain. Mash or put through potato ricer. Add egg yolks, 1½ tablespoons butter or margarine, pepper and nutmeg, stirring until almost smooth. In small bowl with mixer, beat egg whites until stiff peaks form; fold into potato mixture and set aside.

Rinse spinach; drain or spin almost dry. In large saucepot over medium heat, place damp spinach. Cover tightly and cook 2 to 3 minutes, or until just limp. Drain well; add 1½ tablespoons butter or margarine; toss until well coated.

Spoon ½ potato mixture into prepared casserole; top with spinach mixture, then remaining potato mixture. Sprinkle with cheese and dot with remaining 1 tablespoon butter or margarine. Bake 30 minutes, or until heated through. Garnish with parsley, if desired. Makes 4 servings.

Per serving: 263 calories; 8 g. protein; 14 g. fat; 49% calories from fat; 168 mg. cholesterol; 27 g. carbohydrates; 226 mg. sodium; 5 g. fiber

Spinach Pie

- 2 packages (10 ounces each) frozen chopped spinach, cooked and drained
- Cholesterol-free, fat-free egg substitute, equivalent to 2 eggs
- 1 cup (4 ounces) shredded Swiss cheese
- 1 unbaked 9-inch pie crust
- 1 cup nonfat sour cream
- 1 tablespoon butter or margarine
- 4 tablespoons Italian-seasoned dry bread crumbs

Preheat oven to 350°F. In medium bowl, combine spinach, egg substitute and cheese; spoon into pie crust. Cover top completely with layer of sour cream. Melt butter or margarine in small skillet. Cook bread crumbs, stirring, until lightly browned; sprinkle over top. Bake 45 minutes, or until knife comes out clean. Makes 8 servings.

Per serving: 195 calories; 6 g. protein; 9 g. fat; 43% calories from fat; 9 mg. cholesterol; 21 g. carbohydrates; 298 mg. sodium; 2 g. fiber

Broccoli-Mushroom Stir-Fry

- 2 tablespoons corn oil
- ¾ pound broccoli, trimmed and cut into florets, with stems sliced
- 1¼ cups sliced mushrooms
- 1 large carrot, cut into 2-inch strips
- 1 clove garlic, minced
- 1 teaspoon shredded lemon peel
- ½ teaspoon salt
- ¼ teaspoon dried thyme

Heat oil in large skillet or wok over medium-high heat. Add remaining ingredients. Cook, stirring constantly, 5 to 8 minutes, or until vegetables are tender. Makes 4 servings.

Per serving: 97 calories; 3 g. protein; 7 g. fat; 61% calories from fat; 0 mg. cholesterol; 7 g. carbohydrates; 297 mg. sodium; 3 g. fiber

Cauliflower-Pasta Toss

3 cups uncooked penne, rigatoni or ziti
2 tablespoons butter or margarine
2 tablespoons olive oil
1 clove garlic, minced
1 package (10 ounces) frozen cauliflower, cooked
¼ teaspoon dried oregano
½ tablespoon dehydrated parsley flakes
Salt and pepper to taste
Grated Parmesan cheese (optional)

Prepare pasta according to package directions. Heat butter or margarine and oil in large skillet over medium heat. Sauté garlic 2 minutes. Add cauliflower; sauté 5 minutes, or until lightly browned. Drain pasta; add to cauliflower with oregano, parsley, salt and pepper. Heat through. Serve sprinkled with cheese, if desired. Makes 4 servings.

Per serving: 517 calories; 14 g. protein; 14 g. fat; 24% calories from fat; 15 mg. cholesterol; 82 g. carbohydrates; 63 mg. sodium; 6 g. fiber

Asparagus-Tomato Stir-Fry

1 tablespoon cold water
2 teaspoons soy sauce
1 teaspoon cornstarch
¼ teaspoon salt
1 tablespoon corn or blended vegetable oil
1 pound fresh asparagus, diagonally sliced into 1-inch pieces
4 green onions with tops, diagonally sliced into 1-inch pieces
½ cup sliced fresh mushrooms
2 small tomatoes, cut into thin wedges

In small bowl or custard cup, stir water, soy sauce, cornstarch and salt until thoroughly blended; set aside. Heat oil in large skillet or wok over medium-high heat. Add asparagus and onions. Cook, stirring constantly, 4 minutes. Add mushrooms; cook, stirring constantly, 2 minutes more. Push vegetables to side; stir cornstarch mixture and add to skillet or wok. Cook, stirring into vegetables, until sauce thickens and bubbles. Add tomatoes. Toss gently to combine. Serve immediately. Makes 6 servings.

Per serving: 49 calories; 3 g. protein; 2 g. fat; 40% calories from fat; 0 mg. cholesterol; 5 g. carbohydrates; 208 mg. sodium; 2 g. fiber

Bulgur-Cheese Stuffed Peppers

6 large green peppers
3 tablespoons olive oil
1 small onion, finely chopped
1 large carrot, shredded
½ teaspoon dried basil
½ teaspoon dried oregano
2 cloves garlic, minced
2½ cups cooked bulgur (cracked wheat)
1½ cups (6 ounces) shredded part-skim milk mozzarella cheese
2 eggs, beaten
Salt and pepper to taste
1 cup tomato juice

Preheat oven to 350°F. Grease baking dish or casserole large enough to hold peppers standing up; set aside. Cut tops from peppers and remove seeds. In large saucepan or Dutch oven over medium heat, place peppers and ½ cup water. Cover and cook 5 minutes. Drain well upside down.

Heat oil in small skillet over medium heat. Sauté onions and carrots 3 minutes, or until tender. Add basil, oregano and garlic. In large bowl, stir onion-carrot mixture, bulgur, cheese, eggs, salt and pepper. In prepared dish, place peppers cut end up; fill evenly with bulgur mixture. Add tomato juice to dish. Cover and bake 20 to 25 minutes, or until stuffing is set. Makes 6 servings.

Per serving: 306 calories; 15 g. protein; 14 g. fat; 43% calories from fat; 43 mg. cholesterol; 28 g. carbohydrates; 328 mg. sodium; 6 g. fiber

Green and Yellow Pasta

8 ounces spinach pasta
8 ounces regular pasta
2 tablespoons butter or margarine
3 cups cubed zucchini
2 cloves garlic, minced
2 cups nonfat plain yogurt
3 tablespoons chopped fresh basil or parsley
Grated Parmesan cheese (optional)

Cook pasta al dente according to package directions. Melt butter or margarine in large skillet over medium heat. Sauté zucchini and garlic until golden. Turn off heat; stir in yogurt and basil or parsley. Drain pasta; toss immediately with yogurt mixture. Serve with cheese, if desired. Makes 4 servings.

Note: For slightly thicker, richer sauce, 1 cup each nonfat plain yogurt and nonfat sour cream may be used instead of all yogurt.

Per serving: 294 calories; 13 g. protein; 6 g. fat; 20% calories from fat; 17 mg. cholesterol; 45 g. carbohydrates; 138 mg. sodium; 3 g. fiber

All Green and White Sandwich

4 large (7- to 8-inch) pita breads (Middle Eastern pocket bread)
1 small zucchini, thinly sliced
1 small green pepper, chopped
4 green onions, chopped
1 cup bean sprouts or alfalfa sprouts
1 cup coarsely chopped spinach leaves
4 ounces feta cheese, crumbled
4 ounces nonfat plain yogurt

Slice off top inch of pita breads. Holding bread open, drop cut-off portion into bottom. In small bowl, combine zucchini, peppers, green onions, sprouts, spinach, and cheese. Place ¼ vegetable mixture in each pita. Stir yogurt until thinned down; pour ¼ over vegetable mixture in each pita. Makes 4 servings.

Per serving: 278 calories; 14 g. protein; 7 g. fat; 23% calories from fat; 25 mg. cholesterol; 40 g. carbohydrates; 690 mg. sodium; 3 g. fiber

Kidney Bean and Corn Chili

- 2 tablespoons canola, corn, cottonseed, safflower or soybean oil
- 1 small onion, chopped
- 1 clove garlic, minced
- ½ cup chopped green peppers
- 2 cups thawed frozen or drained canned whole-kernel corn
- 1 cup water
- 1½ tablespoons tomato paste
- 3 cups cooked or drained canned kidney beans
- 1 teaspoon dried oregano
- ½-1 teaspoon chili powder
- ¼ teaspoon ground cumin

Heat oil in large skillet over medium heat. Sauté onions and garlic 3 minutes. Add peppers; cook 3 minutes. Add corn, water and tomato paste. In small bowl with fork, mash 1 cup beans. Add mashed beans, remaining 2 cups whole beans, oregano, chili powder and cumin to skillet mixture. Bring to boil. Reduce heat to low; simmer 30 minutes, or until thickened. Makes 4 servings.

Per serving: 311 calories; 14 g. protein; 7 g. fat; 21% calories from fat; 0 mg. cholesterol; 50 g. carbohydrates; 12 mg. sodium; 15 g. fiber

Vegetable Loaf

- 1 large carrot
- 1 rib celery
- ½ cup chopped broccoli
- 2 ounces green beans, cooked
- 1 tablespoon safflower oil
- 1 small onion, chopped
- 1 cup soft bread crumbs
- 1 egg
- Salt and pepper to taste
- ¼ teaspoon nutmeg or ground ginger

Preheat oven to 350°F. Grease shallow baking dish; set aside. Through grinder or in food processor, coarsely grind or chop carrot, celery, broccoli and green beans. Heat oil in large skillet over medium heat. Sauté onions 3 minutes or until tender. Add to chopped vegetables with remaining ingredients; shape into loaf. Place in prepared dish. Bake 45 minutes, or until firm. Makes 4 servings.

Per serving: 107 calories; 4 g. protein; 5 g. fat; 44% calories from fat; 68 mg. cholesterol; 11 g. carbohydrates; 92 mg. sodium; 2 g. fiber

Vegetable Stew

2 potatoes, peeled and cubed
2 carrots, peeled and sliced
2 ribs celery, cut into slices
2 medium onions, sliced
1 large red pepper, cut into strips
1 clove garlic, minced
½ head broccoflower, cut into florets
½ pound mushrooms, sliced
1 can (13¾ ounces) ready-to-use chicken broth
2 tablespoons chopped fresh dill, or 2 teaspoons dried dill
2 teaspoons salt
⅛ teaspoon pepper

Preheat oven to 350°F. Place all ingredients in 3-quart casserole. Cover and bake 45 to 60 minutes, or until vegetables are of desired doneness. Makes 8 servings.

Per serving: 88 calories; 4 g. protein; 0 g. fat; 7% calories from fat; 0 mg. cholesterol, 18 g. carbohydrates; 723 mg. sodium; 4 g. fiber

Lentil Burgers

2 cups cooked lentils*
2 eggs, lightly beaten
1 cup soft whole-wheat bread crumbs
½ cup wheat germ
½ cup finely chopped onions
1¼ teaspoons salt
Dash hot-pepper sauce
2 tablespoons canola, corn, cottonseed, safflower or soybean oil
Whole-wheat hamburger rolls or pita breads (optional)

In medium bowl, mash lentils slightly. Add eggs, bread crumbs, wheat germ, onions, salt and hot-pepper sauce. Shape ½-cup portions lentil mixture into six 3 ½-inch patties. Heat oil in large skillet over medium heat. Fry patties, turning once, 5 minutes, or until golden brown. Serve in rolls or pitas, if desired. Makes 6 servings.

* *About ¾ cup uncooked lentils equals 2 cups cooked.*

Per serving: 204 calories; 11 g. protein; 10 g. fat; 34% calories from fat; 91 mg. cholesterol; 22 g. carbohydrates; 508 mg. sodium; 5 g. fiber

Chicken à la King

- ⅓ cup water
- 1 cup frozen green peas
- ¼ cup chopped green peppers
- 2 tablespoons finely chopped onions
- ⅔ cup all-purpose flour
- 1 cup cold skim milk
- 2 cups chicken broth or bouillon
- 2 teaspoons salt
- ½ teaspoon poultry seasoning
- Pepper to taste
- 2 cups diced cooked chicken or turkey
- 1 can (4 ounces) mushroom stems and pieces, drained and coarsely chopped
- 1 tablespoon chopped pimientos
- Toast, biscuits or cooked rice (optional)

In medium saucepan over medium heat, place water, peas, peppers and onions. Cover and cook 5 minutes, or until peas are tender. Drain, saving liquid.

In same saucepan, blend flour and milk until well blended; stir in reserved cooking liquid, broth or bouillon, salt, poultry seasoning and pepper. Bring to boil, stirring constantly. Cook 1 minute. Add cooked vegetables, chicken or turkey, mushrooms and pimientos. Heat through. Serve over rice, toast or biscuits, if desired. Makes 6 servings.

Per serving: 178 calories; 17 g. protein; 3 g. fat; 18% calories from fat; 39 mg. cholesterol; 18 g. carbohydrates; 1113 mg. sodium; 2 g. fiber

Mushroom and Chicken Kabobs

1 can (8 ounces) pineapple chunks in juice
2 tablespoons canola, corn, cottonseed, safflower or soybean oil
¾ teaspoon garlic powder
¾ teaspoon ground ginger
¼ teaspoon salt
1½ pounds boneless, skinless chicken breasts, cut into 1½-inch chunks
1 pound fresh mushrooms, cut in half
1 large green pepper, cut into chunks
Hot cooked rice (optional)

Drain pineapple, reserving juice; set chunks aside. In small bowl, combine reserved juice, oil, garlic powder, ginger and salt until well mixed. In large bowl, place chicken; pour in oil mixture and toss to coat evenly. Cover and chill for 2 hours, stirring occasionally.

Preheat broiler. Assemble 12 7-inch skewers. Drain chicken, reserving marinade. Thread each skewer with mushroom half, pepper chunk and chicken chunk; repeat. Place pineapple chunk on end. Place any remaining pineapple chunks on skewers. Brush skewers with reserved marinade. Broil 6 inches from heat source, turning frequently, 5 minutes, or until chicken is tender. Serve over rice, if desired. Makes 6 servings.

Per serving: 209 calories; 28 g. protein; 6 g. fat; 27% calories from fat; 65 mg. cholesterol; 10 g. carbohydrates; 166 mg. sodium; 2 g. fiber

Curried Chicken with Rice

- 2½ pounds whole chicken breasts, split
- 1 teaspoon salt
- 3 tablespoons canola, corn, cottonseed, safflower or soybean oil
- 1 cup green pepper strips
- ¼ pound fresh mushrooms, sliced
- ½ cup chopped onions
- 1 clove garlic, minced
- 2 cans (10½ ounces each) condensed chicken broth
- 1½ cups uncooked long-grain rice
- 1 teaspoon curry powder
- 1 package (6 ounces) frozen snow pea pods, thawed
- 1 medium tomato, chopped

Sprinkle chicken with ¾ teaspoon salt. Heat oil in large skillet over medium-high heat. Add chicken; cook 7 minutes, or until brown on both sides. Push to one side of skillet. Add peppers, mushrooms, onions and garlic; sauté 5 minutes or until onions are tender.

In 4-cup measure, add enough water to chicken broth to make 3¼ cups. To chicken-vegetable mixture, add diluted broth, remaining ¼ teaspoon salt, rice and curry powder. Rearrange chicken breasts on top of rice mixture. Bring to boil. Reduce heat to low; cover and simmer, stirring occasionally, for 15 minutes, or until chicken is tender. Add pea pods and tomatoes. Cover and cook for 2 minutes, or until rice is tender and liquid is absorbed. Serve immediately. Makes 6 servings.

Per serving: 426 calories; 39 g. protein; 9 g. fat; 20% calories from fat; 82 mg. cholesterol; 43 g. carbohydrates; 944 mg. sodium; 3 g. fiber

Chicken Cacciatore

- ¼ cup all-purpose flour
- 1 teaspoon salt
- ¼ teaspoon pepper
- 1 broiler-fryer chicken (about 2½ pounds), cut into pieces and skinned
- 3 tablespoons olive or other vegetable oil
- ½ cup drained canned small white pearl onions, or thawed frozen small white pearl onions
- 1 medium green pepper, cut into strips
- 1 can (4 ounces) mushrooms, drained
- 1 clove garlic, minced
- ½ cup water
- 1 can (10½ ounces) condensed tomato soup
- 2 tablespoons vinegar or lemon juice
- 1 tablespoon Worcestershire sauce
- ½ teaspoon dried oregano
- Hot cooked spaghetti (optional)

On wax paper, mix flour, salt and pepper. Roll chicken into flour mixture until well coated. Heat oil in large skillet over medium heat. Cook chicken 7 minutes, or until brown on both sides; remove and keep warm. To same skillet, add onions, peppers, mushrooms and garlic; sauté 5 minutes, or until tender.

In small bowl, combine water, undiluted tomato soup, vinegar or lemon juice, Worcestershire sauce and oregano until well blended; pour into skillet. Add chicken; cover and simmer, stirring occasionally, about 30 minutes, or until chicken is fork-tender. Serve over spaghetti, if desired. Makes 4 servings.

Per serving: 412 calories; 40 g. protein; 16 g. fat; 36% calories from fat; 119 mg. cholesterol; 26 g. carbohydrates; 1577 mg. sodium; 2 g. fiber

Tomatoes Stuffed with Chicken

1 cup nonfat plain yogurt
½ teaspoon salt
¼ teaspoon tarragon
1½ cups diced cooked chicken
1 can (8 ounces) crushed pineapple, drained
3 tablespoons toasted slivered almonds
1 rib celery, finely chopped
6 large tomatoes

In small bowl, combine yogurt, salt and tarragon; set aside. In large bowl, combine chicken, pineapple, almonds and celery. Add yogurt mixture; toss gently to evenly coat. To serve, cut tomatoes into wedges almost to bottom; gently spread out. Fill each with ⅙ chicken mixture. Makes 6 servings.

Per serving: 151 calories; 14 g. protein; 5 g. fat; 30% calories from fat; 32 mg. cholesterol; 13 g. carbohydrates; 253 mg. sodium; 3 g. fiber

Poule au Pot

1 stewing or roasting chicken (about 5 pounds)
16 cups water
12 small pearl onions, peeled
6 ribs celery, cut into 2-inch lengths
4 small turnips, peeled and quartered (2 cups)
3 medium carrots, cut into 2-inch lengths
2 green peppers, cored, seeded and cut into quarters
1½ cups chopped leeks
2 bay leaves
2 cloves garlic, peeled and left whole
12 peppercorns
1½ teaspoons dried thyme
Salt and pepper to taste
3 small zucchini, cut into 1-inch lengths
2 medium parsnips, peeled and cut into quarters
⅔ cup uncooked rice

In large Dutch oven over high heat, place chicken, water, onions, celery, turnips, carrots, green peppers, leeks, bay leaves, garlic, peppercorns, thyme, salt and pepper. Bring to boil. Reduce heat to low; cover and cook 45 to 75 minutes, or until chicken is almost tender. Add remaining ingredients; cook 15 minutes, or until rice is tender. Remove bay leaves; skin chicken. Makes 8 servings.

Per serving: 511 calories; 58 g. protein; 14 g. fat; 25% calories from fat; 164 mg. cholesterol; 35 g. carbohydrates; 207 mg. sodium; 7 g. fiber

Moo Goo Gai Pan (Chicken with Pea Pods)

1 pound boneless, skinless chicken, cut into strips
3 tablespoons soy sauce
4 ribs celery, cut into 1-inch strips
2 medium onions, sliced
1 can (16 ounces) mixed Chinese vegetables, drained
1 can (4 ounces) mushrooms, drained
¾ cup hot water
2 chicken bouillon cubes
2 tablespoons cornstarch
1 package (6 ounces) frozen snow pea pods
Hot cooked rice (optional)

In large skillet over medium heat, place chicken and 2 tablespoons soy sauce. Cook, stirring, 5 minutes, or until chicken is no longer pink; remove. To skillet, add celery, onions, Chinese vegetables and mushrooms. In 1-cup measure, combine water, remaining tablespoon soy sauce and bouillon cubes, stirring until bouillon is dissolved. Add to vegetables; cook 15 minutes. Add chicken; cook 5 minutes. In small bowl, blend 2 tablespoons cold water and cornstarch until well mixed. Add to skillet with pea pods; cook, stirring occasionally, 3 minutes, or until thickened. Makes 4 servings.

Per serving: 254 calories; 33 g. protein; 2 g. fat; 8% calories from fat; 65 mg. cholesterol; 26 g. carbohydrates; 1392 mg. sodium; 7 g. fiber

Braised Chicken and Vegetables

- 5 tablespoons all-purpose flour
- Salt and pepper to taste
- 1 broiler-fryer chicken (about 2½ pounds), cut up
- 2 tablespoons corn oil
- 3 medium carrots, cut up
- ½ pound mushrooms, sliced
- 4 ribs celery, chopped
- ½ large onion, chopped
- ½ large green pepper, chopped
- 1½ cups water

On wax paper, mix well 3 tablespoons flour, salt and pepper. Roll chicken into flour mixture until well coated. Heat oil in large saucepot or Dutch oven over medium heat. Cook chicken 7 minutes, or until brown on both sides; remove and keep warm. To same saucepot, add remaining flour and remaining ingredients. Bring to boil. Add reserved chicken. Reduce heat to low; cover and cook 45 minutes, or until chicken is tender. Makes 4 servings.

Per serving: 375 calories; 45 g. protein; 12 g. fat; 30% calories from fat; 139 mg. cholesterol; 18 g. carbohydrates; 206 mg. sodium; 4 g. fiber

Hawaiian Chicken

- 1 broiler-fryer chicken (about 2½ pounds), cut up
- Salt and pepper to taste
- 1¼ cups orange juice
- ½ cup prepared chutney
- ½ cup raisins
- ½ teaspoon ground cinnamon
- ½ teaspoon curry powder
- ½ teaspoon dried thyme
- ¼ cup blanched slivered almonds

Preheat oven to 425°F. Grease baking dish or roasting pan large enough to hold chicken in single layer; add chicken. Season with salt and pepper. Bake 15 minutes.

In medium saucepan over high heat, combine orange juice, chutney, raisins, cinnamon, curry powder and thyme; bring to boil. Pour over chicken. Bake 45 to 50 minutes more, or until chicken is fork-tender. Sprinkle with almonds last 5 minutes. Makes 4 servings.

Per serving: 383 calories; 45 g. protein; 9 g. fat; 23% calories from fat; 139 mg. cholesterol; 29 g. carbohydrates; 154 mg. sodium; 3 g. fiber

Turkey-Leek Rotini

1 package (16 ounces) rotini or other short pasta
3 tablespoons butter or margarine
1 pound leeks, white part and 2 inches of green stem quartered lengthwise and sliced
¼ cup all-purpose flour
Salt and pepper to taste
1 pound boneless turkey breast fillets, cut into 1x1¼-inch slivers
2 tablespoons canola, corn, cottonseed, safflower or soybean oil
¼ cup white port, other dry white wine or chicken broth
¾ cup skim milk
½ cup (2 ounces) shredded Muenster cheese
¼ cup (1 ounce) blue cheese, crumbled
¼ cup chopped fresh Italian parsley

Cook pasta according to package directions. Meanwhile, melt 1 tablespoon butter or margarine in large skillet over medium-high heat. Sauté leeks, stirring often, 5 minutes, or until leeks are wilted. Remove leeks; keep warm.

On wax paper, combine flour, salt and pepper. Dip turkey into flour mixture to coat well. To same skillet, add remaining butter or margarine and oil. Add coated turkey in batches; cook, stirring, 5 minutes, or until golden. Remove; keep warm.

Add wine or broth to skillet over medium-high heat, scraping skillet bottom to remove browned bits. Cook 1 minute. Add reserved leeks, browned turkey, milk, cheeses and parsley. Drain pasta. On large platter, place pasta; top with sauce. Toss gently to evenly coat. Serve immediately. Makes 6 servings.

Per serving: 303 calories; 22 g. protein; 16 g. fat; 50% calories from fat; 67 mg. cholesterol; 13 g. carbohydrates; 238 mg. sodium; 1 g. fiber

Turkey and Rice Stuffed Peppers

- 4 large green peppers
- 2 cups ½-inch cubes cooked turkey
- 1 cup hot, cooked rice
- ¼ pound fresh mushrooms, chopped
- 1 jar (2 ounces) chopped pimientos, undrained
- ½ cup light mayonnaise
- ¼ cup nonfat sour cream
- 2 tablespoons instant chicken bouillon granules
- 1 tablespoon dried parsley
- ½ teaspoon celery salt
- ½ teaspoon hot pepper sauce
- ¼ teaspoon ground thyme

Preheat oven to 375°F. Grease baking dish or casserole large enough to hold peppers standing up. Cut tops from peppers and remove seeds. Place cut end up in prepared dish; set aside. In large bowl, combine remaining ingredients until well blended; fill peppers. Add 1 cup water to dish; cover tightly with lid or foil. Bake 45 to 50 minutes, or until peppers are tender-crisp. Makes 4 servings.

Per serving: 322 calories; 23 g. protein; 14 g. fat; 41% calories from fat; 66 mg. cholesterol; 23 g. carbohydrates; 587 mg. sodium; 2 g. fiber

Turkey Parmigiana

- 2 egg whites or cholesterol-free, fat-free egg substitute, equivalent to 2 eggs
- 2 tablespoons canola, cottonseed, corn, safflower or soybean oil
- ⅓ cup Italian-seasoned dry bread crumbs
- ½ teaspoon salt
- Dash pepper
- 1 pound raw turkey breast slices
- ¾ cup defatted turkey or chicken broth
- 3 tablespoons tomato paste
- 1 clove garlic, minced
- 1 teaspoon dried oregano
- 1 cup (4 ounces) part-skim milk mozzarella cheese

Preheat oven to 450°F. Spray jelly-roll pan with nonstick cooking spray; set aside. In shallow dish, beat eggs and oil until well blended. On wax paper, mix bread crumbs, salt and pepper. Dip each turkey slice into egg mixture, then into bread crumbs to lightly coat both sides. Arrange in single layer on prepared pan. Bake 8 to 10 minutes, or until golden and crisp. Place in single layer in ovenproof and broilerproof casserole or platter; keep warm.

Preheat broiler. In small saucepan over medium heat, combine broth, tomato paste, garlic and oregano. Cook, uncovered, until thickened to desired consistency. Spoon over turkey; top with cheese. Broil until cheese lightly browns. Makes 4 servings.

Per serving: 324 calories; 36 g. protein; 14 g. fat; 42% calories from fat; 75 mg. cholesterol; 10 g. carbohydrates; 825 mg. sodium; 1 g. fiber

Vegetable-Burger Potpourri

8 ounces ground chicken, turkey or beef
2 cups water
1 can (16 ounces) stewed tomatoes, cut up
1 can (8 ounces) tomato sauce
1 package (10 ounces) frozen mixed vegetables
½ envelope (¼ cup) dry onion soup mix
1 teaspoon sugar
Dash Worcestershire sauce
Dash garlic salt

In large heavy saucepan or Dutch oven over medium heat, cook chicken, turkey or beef, stirring occasionally, 5 minutes, or until browned; drain off excess fat. Stir in remaining ingredients. Bring to boil. Reduce heat to low; cover and simmer 20 minutes, or until vegetables are cooked. Makes 6 servings.

Per serving: 121 calories; 9 g. protein; 4 g. fat; 28% calories from fat; 35 mg. cholesterol; 13 g. carbohydrates; 450 mg. sodium; 3 g. fiber

Noodles Milanese

2 tablespoons canola, corn, cottonseed, safflower or soybean oil
2 medium onions, chopped
1 clove garlic, minced
1 pound lean ground beef
1 can (8 ounces) tomato sauce
1 can (6 ounces) tomato paste
1 teaspoon dried oregano
Salt to taste
8 ounces uncooked noodles
2 eggs
¾ pound fresh spinach, trimmed, cooked, and chopped, or 1 package (10 ounces) frozen chopped spinach, thawed
1 cup low-fat cottage cheese
½ cup chopped fresh parsley
½ cup grated Parmesan cheese
1 teaspoon dried basil

Preheat oven to 350°F. Grease 12 x 8-inch baking dish; set aside. Heat oil in large skillet over medium heat. Sauté onions and garlic 3 minutes, or until tender. Add beef; cook, stirring, 5 minutes, or until brown. Add tomato sauce, tomato paste, oregano and salt. Reduce heat to low; simmer 15 minutes.

Cook noodles according to package directions; drain. In large bowl, stir drained noodles and 1 egg; set aside. In another bowl, stir remaining egg, spinach, cottage cheese, parsley, ¼ cup Parmesan cheese and basil until well blended. In prepared pan, layer ½ noodle mixture, ⅓ tomato-beef mixture, and ½ spinach mixture; repeat layers. Top with remaining tomato-beef mixture and ¼ cup Parmesan cheese. Bake 45 minutes, or until heated through. Let stand 5 minutes. Makes 6 servings.

Per serving: 526 calories; 35 g. protein; 27 g. fat; 46% calories from fat; 201 mg. cholesterol; 36 g. carbohydrates; 608 mg. sodium; 5 g. fiber

Carrot Meat Loaf

1 pound lean ground beef
2 large carrots, shredded (about 1½ cups)
1 medium onion, chopped
½ cup cornflake crumbs
½ cup skim milk
1 egg
1 teaspoon Worcestershire sauce
1 teaspoon salt
½ teaspoon pepper

Preheat oven to 350°F. In large bowl, combine all ingredients until well blended. Place in 8 x 4-inch loaf pan; bake 50 to 60 minutes, or until done. Drain off fat; let stand 10 minutes. Remove from pan and slice. Makes 6 servings.

Per serving: 261 calories; 21 g. protein; 15 g. fat; 53% calories from fat; 112 mg. cholesterol; 9 g. carbohydrates; 505 mg. sodium; 1 g. fiber

Little Joes

¾ pound fresh spinach, trimmed, or 1 bag (10 ounces) fresh spinach, trimmed
1 tablespoon canola, corn, cottonseed, safflower or soybean oil
1 cup finely chopped onions
1 pound lean ground beef
Salt and pepper to taste
Cholesterol-free, fat-free egg substitute, equivalent to 4 eggs
Hot-pepper sauce to taste
¼ cup grated Parmesan cheese

Rinse spinach; drain or spin dry. In large saucepot over medium heat, place damp spinach. Cover and cook 1 to 2 minutes, or until wilted. Cool and squeeze dry; chop and set aside. Heat oil in medium heavy skillet over medium heat. Sauté onions 3 minutes, or until tender. Add beef; cook, stirring, to brown and break up lumps. Add spinach, salt and pepper, stirring until blended. Pour eggs and hot-pepper sauce over meat-spinach mixture. Cook, gently stirring, until eggs are set. Top with cheese. Makes 6 servings.

Per serving: 284 calories; 26 g. protein; 17 g. fat; 56% calories from fat; 68 mg. cholesterol; 5 g. carbohydrates; 240 mg. sodium; 2 g. fiber

Fish Fillets on Spinach

1½ pounds boneless, skinless fish fillets (cod, turbot, flounder, orange roughy)
2 tablespoons lemon juice
1½ pounds fresh spinach, trimmed and chopped, or 2 bags (10 ounces each) frozen chopped spinach
1 tablespoon canola, cottonseed, corn, safflower or soybean oil
1 medium onion, chopped
½ teaspoon salt
½ teaspoon ground nutmeg
⅛ teaspoon white pepper
2 medium tomatoes, sliced
¼ cup (1 ounce) shredded part-skim milk mozzarella cheese

Preheat oven to 350°F. Grease shallow 2½-quart casserole; set aside. Sprinkle fish with lemon juice; let stand 10 minutes. Rinse spinach; drain or spin dry. Heat oil in large skillet over medium heat. Sauté onions in hot oil 3 minutes, or until tender. Add fish; cook, turning once, until fish is golden brown. Remove and set aside.

In same skillet, sauté spinach 1 minute, or until wilted. Spoon into prepared pan; top with reserved fillets and onions. Sprinkle with salt, nutmeg and pepper. Top with layer of tomatoes, then cheese. Bake 15 minutes, or until heated through and cheese melts. Makes 6 servings.

Per serving: 162 calories; 24 g. protein; 4 g. fat; 23% calories from fat; 51 mg. cholesterol; 7 g. carbohydrates; 331 mg. sodium; 3 g. fiber

Sole with Sweet-Sour Vegetables

- 1 pound boneless, skinless sole or flounder fillets, loosely rolled
- 1 tablespoon lemon juice
- 1 tablespoon canola, corn, cottonseed, safflower or soybean oil
- 2 cups julienne-cut carrots (cut 2¼ x ¼-inch)
- ½ cup thinly sliced onions
- 2 tablespoons water
- 2 cups sliced celery
- ½ cup sliced water chestnuts
- 1 can (8¼ ounces) pineapple chunks in juice
- 3 tablespoons cider vinegar
- 1½ tablespoons brown sugar
- 1½ tablespoons soy sauce
- 1½ teaspoons cornstarch

In large skillet over medium-low heat, place fish rolls with enough boiling water to barely cover; add lemon juice. Cover and simmer 8 to 10 minutes, or until fish flakes easily with fork. Keep warm.

Heat oil in another skillet over medium-high heat. Add carrots and onions; cook, stirring constantly, 5 minutes. Reduce heat to medium; add water. Cover and steam 4 minutes. Uncover; add celery and water chestnuts. Cook, stirring constantly, 2 minutes. Add undrained pineapple.

In small bowl, combine remaining ingredients. Add to skillet mixture; cook, stirring, 2 minutes, or until sauce coats vegetables and pineapple. Remove fish rolls from liquid; drain well. Serve fish topped with sweet-sour sauce. Makes 4 servings.

Note: Sauce is also good over broiled or baked fish or poultry.

Per serving: 262 calories; 23 g. protein; 5 g. fat; 17% calories from fat; 54 mg. cholesterol; 31 g. carbohydrates; 588 mg. sodium; 5 g. fiber

Halibut Hawaiian

2 halibut steaks (1 pound each), fresh or thawed frozen
1¾ teaspoons salt
1 cup soft bread cubes
1 cup drained crushed pineapple
1 cup cooked rice
2 tablespoons lemon juice
½ teaspoon curry powder
2 tablespoons butter or margarine, melted

Preheat oven to 350°F. Grease 12 x 8-inch baking dish or pan; set aside. Sprinkle steaks with 1 teaspoon salt. Place 1 steak in prepared dish; set aside. In medium bowl, stir bread cubes, pineapple, rice, lemon juice, remaining ¾ teaspoon salt and curry powder; place over steak. Top with remaining steak. Secure with toothpicks or skewers. Brush top steak with butter or margarine. Bake 30 to 40 minutes, or until fish flakes easily when tested with fork. Makes 6 servings.

Per serving: 271 calories; 32 g. protein; 7 g. fat; 26% calories from fat; 58 mg. cholesterol; 15 g. carbohydrates; 776 mg. sodium; 0 g. fiber

Mediterranean Baked Fish

- 1 pound boneless, skinless fish fillets (sole, flounder, sea perch, turbot)
- 1 tablespoon corn oil
- 1 large onion, diced
- 3 large tomatoes, chopped, or 1 can (16 ounces) tomatoes, drained
- 1 clove garlic, minced
- 1 cup bottled clam juice
- ½ cup dry white wine
- 1 bay leaf
- 1 tablespoon shredded orange rind
- 1 teaspoon fennel seeds, crushed
- ½ teaspoon dried oregano
- ¼ teaspoon dried thyme
- ¼ teaspoon dried basil
- Salt and pepper to taste

Preheat oven to 375°F. Grease 11 x 7-inch baking dish; place fish in single layer and set aside. Heat oil in large skillet over medium heat. Sauté onions 3 minutes, or until tender. Add remaining ingredients. Reduce heat to low; simmer, stirring occasionally, in uncovered skillet 30 minutes. Remove bay leaf. Pour sauce over fish. Bake 15 to 20 minutes, or until fish flakes easily with fork. Makes 4 servings.

Per serving: 193 calories; 23 g. protein; 5 g. fat; 24% calories from fat; 54 mg. cholesterol; 8 g. carbohydrates; 231 mg. sodium; 2 g. fiber

Fish in Green Tomato Sauce

- 2 tablespoons canola, corn, cottonseed, safflower or soybean oil
- 1 large onion, thinly sliced
- 2 cans Mexican green tomatoes (tomatillos), drained
- ⅓ cup chopped fresh cilantro
- 1-2 small hot green chili peppers, seeded
- 2 pounds boneless fish fillets (red snapper, cod, turbot), cut into 2-inch pieces
- 2 cups thinly sliced zucchini
- Hot cooked rice (optional)
- Nonfat sour cream (optional)

Heat oil in a large skillet over medium heat. Sauté onions 3 minutes, or until tender; remove from pan with slotted spoon and set aside. In blender or food processor, combine green tomatoes, cilantro and peppers until of desired consistency. Place fish in same skillet; top with reserved onions, then green tomato sauce. Cook over medium heat 5 minutes. Add zucchini; cook 5 minutes more, or until fish flakes easily when tested with fork. Serve over rice with dollop of sour cream, if desired. Makes 8 servings.

Per serving: 147 calories; 20 g. protein; 4 g. fat; 27% calories from fat; 46 mg. cholesterol; 6 g. carbohydrates; 74 mg. sodium; 2 g. fiber

West African Tuna Casserole

- 2 cups cooked black-eyed peas
- 2 tablespoons canola, corn, cottonseed, safflower or soybean oil
- ½ cup finely chopped onions
- 1 large tomato, chopped
- 1½-2 teaspoons chopped, seeded hot red pepper
- 2 cans (6½ ounces) chunk light tuna, drained and flaked
- 2 tablespoons tomato paste
- ½ teaspoon salt
- ½ cup dry bread crumbs
- 1 tablespoon butter or margarine, melted

Preheat oven to 350°F. Place peas in 9- or 10-inch baking dish. Heat oil in large skillet over medium heat. Sauté onions 3 minutes, or until tender. Spoon over peas with tomatoes and peppers. Cover and bake 15 minutes. Remove from oven; top with tuna, tomato paste and salt. Cover and bake 15 minutes. In small bowl, combine bread crumbs and butter or margarine until well blended; sprinkle over casserole. Uncover and bake 5 minutes more, or until lightly browned. Makes 6 servings.

Per serving: 242 calories; 22 g. protein; 7 g. fat; 28% calories from fat; 36 mg. cholesterol; 21 g. carbohydrates; 459 mg. sodium; 8 g. fiber

Hot Baked Po-Tunas

- 4 large baking potatoes, baked
- 2 cans (7 ounces each) solid white tuna, drained and flaked
- ¾ cup light mayonnaise
- ½ cup plus 2 tablespoons (2½ ounces) shredded reduced-fat Cheddar cheese
- ¼ cup chopped green peppers
- ¼ cup chopped pimientos
- ¼ cup chopped green onions
- 1 egg white, stiffly beaten

Preheat oven to 400°F. Scoop potatoes from skins, leaving ½-inch shell. In medium bowl, mash scooped potatoes; add tuna, ½ cup mayonnaise, ½ cup cheese, peppers, pimientos and green onions, stirring until well combined. Spoon back into shells; bake 10 minutes.

In small bowl with mixer, beat egg white until stiff peaks form; fold in remaining ¼ cup mayonnaise and 2 tablespoons cheese. Spoon evenly over stuffed potatoes. Bake 10 minutes more. Makes 4 servings.

Per serving: 531 calories; 35 g. protein; 18 g. fat; 31% calories from fat; 67 mg. cholesterol; 55 g. carbohydrates; 795 mg. sodium; 5 g. fiber

Vegetable-Topped Fish Fillets

¼ cup canola, corn, cottonseed, safflower or soybean oil
6 carp, pike or whitefish fillets (4 ounces each)
1 teaspoon salt
¾ teaspoon pepper
2 large tomatoes, diced
1 package (10 ounces) frozen mixed vegetables, thawed
3 medium potatoes (about 1 pound), peeled and diced
2 medium onions, sliced
¼ teaspoon garlic powder

Preheat oven to 425°F. Place oil in 13 x 9-inch baking dish. Place dish in oven until oil is hot. Sprinkle fish with half salt and pepper; place in dish with hot oil. Bake 10 minutes. Add tomatoes, mixed vegetables, potatoes, onions, garlic powder and remaining salt and pepper. Cover. Reduce heat to 350°F. Bake 40 minutes more; remove cover for last 15 minutes. Makes 6 servings.

Per serving: 273 calories; 24 g. protein; 7 g. fat; 24% calories from fat; 65 mg. cholesterol; 27 g. carbohydrates; 463 mg. sodium; 4 g. fiber

Italian Tuna and Peppers for Two

- 1 can (7 ounces) solid white tuna packed in water
- 1 large Spanish or other sweet onion, cut in half and thinly sliced
- 2 medium green peppers, thinly sliced
- 1 cup tomato juice
- ¼ teaspoon dried oregano

Drain tuna; reserve liquid and flake tuna. In large nonstick skillet over medium heat, combine tuna liquid and remaining ingredients. Cover and simmer 5 minutes. Uncover and cook 5 minutes, or until tomato juice evaporates into thick sauce. Add flaked tuna; toss gently to evenly mix. Heat through. Makes 2 servings.

Per serving: 149 calories; 26 g. protein; 0 g. fat; 5% calories from fat; 46 mg. cholesterol; 9 g. carbohydrates; 737 mg. sodium; 2 g. fiber

DELECTABLE SIDE DISHES

Cucumbers in Dill

- 4 medium cucumbers, peeled and thinly sliced
- 1 cup boiling water
- ¾ cup nonfat sour cream
- ¼ cup lemon juice
- 3 tablespoons minced fresh dill, or 3 teaspoons dried dill
- 1½ teaspoons salt
- 1 teaspoon sugar
- ⅛ teaspoon pepper

Place cucumbers in medium bowl; pour on boiling water. Let stand 5 minutes; drain. Plunge cucumbers into ice water; drain and place back in bowl. In small bowl, mix remaining ingredients until well blended. Add to cucumbers; toss gently to evenly coat. Cover and chill 30 minutes. Makes 6 servings.

Per serving: 61 calories; 2 g. protein; 0 g. fat; 4% calories from fat; 5 mg. cholesterol; 12 g. carbohydrates; 577 mg. sodium; 2 g. fiber

Marinated Vegetables

- 1 pound baby carrots, cooked and drained
- ½ pound green beans, cooked and drained
- 1 package (10 ounces) frozen asparagus spears, cooked and drained
- 1 pint cherry tomatoes, cut into halves
- 1½ cups tomato juice
- 1 tablespoon lemon juice
- 1 teaspoon white vinegar
- ¼ cup thinly sliced green onions
- ¼ cup finely chopped fresh parsley, or 1 tablespoon dried parsley
- 1 clove garlic, minced
- 1 teaspoon salt
- Dash pepper
- Dash hot-pepper sauce

In large, shallow glass baking dish, casserole or plastic container, arrange carrots, green beans, asparagus and tomatoes in separate groups. In medium bowl, stir tomato juice and remaining ingredients until well blended; pour over vegetables. Cover and chill 3 to 4 hours. Makes 8 servings.

Per serving: 48 calories; 3 g. protein; 0 g. fat; 6% calories from fat; 0 mg. cholesterol; 10 g. carbohydrates; 575 mg. sodium; 3 g. fiber

Red Cabbage

2 tablespoons canola, corn, cottonseed, safflower or soybean oil
2 small onions, sliced
1 large head red cabbage (about 2 pounds), shredded
2 tablespoons cider vinegar
1 large tart apple, peeled, cored and finely chopped
1 piece (2 ounces) salt pork
½ cup red wine or water
½ cup hot beef broth
1 teaspoon sugar
Salt to taste

Heat oil in large saucepan or Dutch oven over medium heat. Sauté onions 3 minutes, or until tender. Add cabbage; immediately pour vinegar over cabbage and toss well. Add remaining ingredients, stirring until well blended. Bring to boil. Reduce heat to low; cover and simmer 45 to 60 minutes, or until cabbage is tender-crisp. Makes 8 servings.

Per serving: 120 calories; 3 g. protein; 6 g. fat; 46% calories from fat; 7 mg. cholesterol; 12 g. carbohydrates; 68 mg. sodium; 3 g. fiber

Quick Zucchini—Genoa Style

3 tablespoons canola, corn, cottonseed, safflower or soybean oil
4 medium zucchini, cut into thin strips
1 clove garlic, minced
1 tablespoon fresh chopped parsley, or 1 teaspoon dried parsley
1 teaspoon dried oregano
1 teaspoon lemon juice
½ teaspoon salt
½ teaspoon pepper

Heat oil in large skillet over medium heat. Sauté zucchini and garlic for 5 minutes, stirring frequently. Add remaining ingredients. Reduce heat to low; cook 5 minutes longer. Makes 4 servings.

Per serving: 107 calories; 1 g. protein; 10 g. fat; 83% calories from fat; 0 mg. cholesterol; 3 g. carbohydrates; 269 mg. sodium; 1 g. fiber

Sautéed Squash and Potatoes

4 tablespoons olive oil
3 large zucchini, sliced
3 large yellow summer squash, sliced
1 large onion, cut into wedges
3 potatoes, peeled if desired and cut into 1-inch cubes
3 medium tomatoes, coarsely chopped (optional)
Salt to taste
¼ teaspoon Italian seasoning
⅛ teaspoon pepper

Heat oil in large skillet over medium heat. Sauté zucchini, yellow squash, onions and potatoes, stirring frequently, 10 minutes, or until tender. Add tomatoes, if desired. Season with salt, Italian seasoning and pepper. Makes 8 servings.

Per serving: 139 calories; 3 g. protein; 7 g. fat; 44% calories from fat; 0 mg. cholesterol; 17 g. carbohydrates; 9 mg. sodium; 3 g. fiber

Zucchini and Tomato Casserole

4 tablespoons canola, corn, cottonseed, safflower or soybean oil
1 small onion, chopped
½ clove garlic, minced
2 medium zucchini, sliced
2 medium tomatoes, peeled and coarsely chopped, or 1 cup canned tomatoes, coarsely chopped
½ teaspoon salt
¼ teaspoon dried basil
¼ teaspoon pepper
2 tablespoons grated Parmesan cheese

Heat oil in large ovenproof skillet over medium heat. Sauté onions and garlic 3 minutes, or until tender. Add zucchini. Reduce heat to low; cover and cook 5 minutes, or until tender-crisp. Add tomatoes, salt, basil and pepper. Cook, uncovered, 10 minutes, or until of desired doneness. Preheat broiler. Sprinkle with cheese. Broil until top is lightly browned. Makes 4 servings.

Per serving: 159 calories; 2 g. protein; 14 g. fat; 80% calories from fat; 2 mg. cholesterol; 5 g. carbohydrates; 320 mg. sodium; 2 g. fiber

Spanish Carrots

2 tablespoons butter or margarine
1 small clove garlic, minced
1 pound young carrots (about 7 or 8), cut diagonally ¼-inch thick
¼ teaspoon salt
¼ large green pepper, cut into strips
1 tablespoon catsup
Chili powder to taste

Melt butter or margarine in large skillet over medium heat. Sauté garlic for 1 minute. Add carrots and salt; cook, tightly covered, 10 minutes, shaking pan occasionally. Add peppers, catsup and chili powder; cook 5 minutes more, or until carrots are tender-crisp. Makes 4 servings.

Per serving: 105 calories; 1 g. protein; 6 g. fat; 49% calories from fat; 15 mg. cholesterol; 12 g. carbohydrates; 266 mg. sodium; 3 g. fiber

Zucchini with Dill Sauce

4 cups sliced zucchini
1 teaspoon dried dill
1 package (1.25 ounces) sour cream sauce mix
½ cup cold skim milk
2 teaspoons lemon juice

In medium saucepan over medium heat, cook zucchini and ½ teaspoon dill in ½ cup lightly salted water for 3 minutes, or until tender-crisp; drain well. Return to saucepan; keep warm.

In small bowl, place sour cream sauce mix and milk; with spoon, beat 1 to 1½ minutes, or until well blended. Let stand 10 minutes. Stir in lemon juice and remaining ½ teaspoon dill; pour over zucchini. Cook 3 to 4 minutes, or until heated through. Makes 4 servings.

Per serving: 104 calories; 5 g. protein; 3 g. fat; 25% calories from fat; 12 mg. cholesterol; 13 g. carbohydrates; 146 mg. sodium; 2 g. fiber

Hot Brussels Sprouts in Dilled "Hollandaise" Sauce

1 package (10 ounces) fresh or frozen Brussels sprouts
Onion salt to taste
Pepper to taste
½ cup water
2 tablespoons light mayonnaise
¼ teaspoon dried dill

In medium saucepan over medium heat, cook Brussels sprouts, onion salt, pepper and water 7 to 10 minutes, or until sprouts are tender-crisp. With slotted spoon, remove Brussels sprouts to serving bowl; keep warm.

Add mayonnaise and dill to seasoned water, stirring until well blended. Cook, uncovered, until of desired sauce consistency; pour over warm sprouts. Makes 3 servings.

Per serving: 73 calories; 3 g. protein; 3 g. fat; 41% calories from fat; 3 mg. cholesterol; 8 g. carbohydrates; 98 mg. sodium; 4 g. fiber

Zucchini and Cheese Bake

8 ounces low-fat cottage cheese
½ teaspoon dried basil
2 tablespoons canola, corn, cottonseed, safflower or soybean oil
2 medium zucchini, sliced
1 small onion, chopped
2 tablespoons grated Parmesan cheese

Preheat oven to 350°F. Grease 1½-quart casserole; set aside. In food processor or blender, puree cottage cheese and basil until smooth; set aside. Heat oil in large skillet over medium heat. Sauté zucchini and onions 3 minutes, or until crisp-tender; drain. In prepared casserole, place layer of ½ zucchini, then ½ cheese mixture; repeat. Top with Parmesan cheese. Bake 20 to 25 minutes, or until heated through. Makes 4 servings.

Per serving: 90 calories; 2 g. protein; 7 g. fat; 73% calories from fat; 2 mg. cholesterol; 4 g. carbohydrates; 49 mg. sodium; 1 g. fiber

Brown Rice Cheese Strata

1 cup uncooked brown rice
1 cup low-fat cottage cheese
2 tablespoons chopped pimientos
1 egg, beaten
¼ teaspoon salt
2 tablespoons butter or margarine
½ cup sliced celery
½ cup sliced onions
2 cups shredded reduced-fat Cheddar cheese
Paprika to taste
Tomato slices or green pepper rings for garnish (optional)

Preheat oven to 375°F. Cook rice according to package directions. In large bowl, stir cooked rice, cottage cheese, pimientos, egg and salt until well blended. Melt butter or margarine in small skillet over medium heat. Sauté celery and onions for 3 minutes, or until onions are tender. Stir into rice mixture.

In 2-quart casserole, spoon ½ rice mixture; sprinkle with 1 cup Cheddar cheese. Repeat layers. Cover and bake 25 to 30 minutes, or until heated through. Sprinkle with paprika. Top with tomato slices or pepper rings, if desired. Makes 6 servings.

Per serving: 284 calories; 18 g. protein; 11 g. fat; 36% calories from fat; 74 mg. cholesterol; 28 g. carbohydrates; 538 mg. sodium; 1 g. fiber

Orange Rice

2 tablespoons butter or margarine
½ cup thinly sliced celery
3 tablespoons finely chopped onions
1½ cups water
1 cup orange juice
2 tablespoons shredded orange peel
½ teaspoon salt
Pepper to taste
1 cup uncooked long-grain rice

Melt butter or margarine in medium saucepan over medium heat. Sauté celery and onions 3 minutes, or until tender. Add water, orange juice, orange peel, salt and pepper. Bring to boil. Add rice. Reduce heat to low; cover and cook 20 minutes, or until rice is tender. Makes 6 servings.

Per serving: 170 calories; 2 g. protein; 4 g. fat; 22% calories from fat; 20 mg. cholesterol; 30 g. carbohydrates; 222 mg. sodium; 1 g. fiber

Arroz Verde

- 1 small bunch parsley
- 3 sprigs cilantro
- 2 large romaine lettuce leaves, torn into pieces
- 2 canned green chilies
- ¼ small onion, chopped
- ½ cup water
- ⅓ cup canola, corn, cottonseed, safflower or soybean oil
- 1½ cups uncooked long-grain rice
- 3 cups defatted chicken broth or bouillon

In blender or food processor, puree parsley, cilantro, lettuce, chilies, onions and water until smooth; set aside.

Heat oil in large skillet over medium heat. Add rice and cook, stirring, until golden. Drain off excess oil. Add pureed parsley mixture; cook, stirring, until rice is almost dry. Add broth or bouillon; cook, uncovered, 15 minutes, or until all liquid is absorbed. Cover and let stand 5 minutes, or until ready to serve. Makes 8 servings.

Per serving: 220 calories; 4 g. protein; 8 g. fat; 37% calories from fat; 0 mg. cholesterol; 29 g. carbohydrates; 298 mg. sodium; 1 g. fiber

Spanish Rice

- 2 tablespoons canola, corn, cottonseed, safflower or soybean oil
- 2 tablespoons diced onions
- 2 tablespoons diced green peppers
- 1 can (16 ounces) tomatoes
- 1 can (8 ounces) tomato sauce
- 2 beef bouillon cubes
- 2 teaspoons chili powder
- Salt and pepper to taste
- Worcestershire sauce to taste
- 1 cup uncooked long-grain rice

Heat oil in large skillet over medium heat. Sauté onions and peppers 5 minutes, or until slightly brown. Add tomatoes, tomato sauce, bouillon, chili powder, salt, pepper and Worcestershire sauce. Bring to boil. Add rice. Reduce heat to low; cover and simmer, stirring occasionally, 20 to 30 minutes, or until rice is done. Makes 6 servings.

Per serving: 186 calories; 3 g. protein; 5 g. fat; 25% calories from fat; 0 mg. cholesterol; 31 g. carbohydrates; 694 mg. sodium; 2 g. fiber

Parsley Rice

- 1 cup uncooked rice
- 2 cups water
- 2 chicken bouillon cubes
- 1 teaspoon salt
- 2 teaspoons butter or margarine
- ⅓ cup minced green peppers
- ¼ cup sliced green onions
- ¼ cup chopped slivered almonds
- ½ cup chopped parsley

In medium saucepan over medium heat, cook rice in water, bouillon and salt for 15 minutes, or until rice is tender. Melt butter or margarine in small saucepan over medium heat. Sauté peppers, green onions and almonds for 3 minutes. Stir into rice with parsley. Makes 6 servings.

Per serving: 167 calories; 3 g. protein; 4 g. fat; 24% calories from fat; 3 mg. cholesterol; 27 g. carbohydrates; 636 mg. sodium; 2 g. fiber

Curried Rice with Peas

- 2 cans (13¾ ounces each) ready-to-use chicken broth
- 1¾ cups uncooked long-grain rice
- 1 package (10 ounces) frozen peas
- 2 tablespoons canola, corn, cottonseed, safflower or soybean oil
- 1 tablespoon curry powder
- 2 teaspoons salt

Preheat oven to 350°F. Grease 3-quart casserole. Place all ingredients in casserole; stir until well mixed. Cover and bake 1 hour, or until rice is tender. Fluff mixture with fork before serving. Makes 10 servings.

Per serving: 203 calories; 5 g. protein; 6 g. fat; 28% calories from fat; 0 mg. cholesterol; 30 g. carbohydrates; 705 mg. sodium; 2 g. fiber

Black-Eyed Peas Supreme

2 cans (16 ounces each) black-eyed peas, drained
1 onion, thinly sliced into rings
¼ cup olive oil
¼ cup wine vinegar
1 clove garlic, minced
1 tablespoon Worcestershire sauce
1 teaspoon salt
Pepper to taste

Place peas and onions in medium bowl; set aside. In small saucepan over high heat, bring to boil remaining ingredients; pour immediately over peas and onions. Cover and chill several hours or overnight. Makes 8 servings.

Per serving: 134 calories; 4 g. protein; 7 g. fat; 48% calories from fat; 0 mg. cholesterol; 13 g. carbohydrates; 551 mg. sodium; 6 g. fiber

Tomato Sauced Green Beans and Potatoes

1 tablespoon canola oil
1 clove garlic, minced
1 package (10 ounces) frozen cut green beans, or
  1 can (16 ounces) cut green beans, drained
2 medium potatoes, cut into 1-inch cubes
1 can (8 ounces) tomato sauce
  Salt and pepper to taste
  French or Italian bread (optional)

Heat oil in large skillet over medium heat. Sauté garlic for 3 minutes, or until brown. Add green beans, potatoes, tomato sauce, salt and pepper. Bring to boil. Reduce heat to low; cover and simmer 20 to 25 minutes, or until vegetables are fork-tender. Serve with bread, if desired. Makes 4 servings.

Per serving: 124 calories; 2 g. protein; 3 g. fat; 25% calories from fat; 0 mg. cholesterol; 21 g. carbohydrates; 355 mg. sodium; 4 g. fiber

Make-Believe "Sweet Potatoes"

2 packages (10 ounces each) frozen sliced yellow squash
Sugar or artificial sweetener to taste
½ teaspoon ground cinnamon
½ teaspoon ground ginger
⅛ teaspoon salt
1 tablespoon butter or margarine (optional)

In large saucepan over medium heat, bring to boil squash and ½ cup water; cook 10 minutes, or until tender. Drain. In serving bowl, place hot cooked squash, enough sugar or artificial sweetener to sweeten, cinnamon, ginger and salt; toss gently to evenly coat. If desired, top with butter or margarine. Makes 6 servings.

Per serving: 20 calories; 1 g. protein; 0 g. fat; 8% calories from fat; 0 mg. cholesterol; 4 g. carbohydrates; 44 mg. sodium; 1 g. fiber

Oven French Fries

1 tablespoon oil
1 tablespoon water
3 medium potatoes, peeled and cut into thin strips

Preheat oven to 475°F. In medium bowl, mix oil and water; add potatoes, turning until well coated. On large baking sheet lined with foil, place potatoes in single layer. Bake 25 to 30 minutes, or until potatoes are cooked. Makes 4 servings.

Per serving: 154 calories; 2 g. protein; 3 g. fat; 20% calories from fat; 0 mg. cholesterol; 28 g. carbohydrates; 8 mg. sodium; 2 g. fiber

Broccoli with Tart Sauce

- 1 head broccoli or broccoflower (about 1 pound), separated into florets
- 2 tablespoons butter or margarine, melted
- 1½ teaspoons prepared white horseradish
- 1½ teaspoons sugar
- ½ teaspoon salt
- ½ teaspoon paprika

In large saucepan over medium heat, bring to boil broccoli or broccoflower and ½ cup water. Reduce heat to medium; cook 10 minutes, or until tender. Drain. In serving bowl, stir remaining ingredients until well blended. Add broccoli or broccoflower; toss gently to evenly coat. Makes 4 servings.

Per serving: 91 calories; 3 g. protein; 6 g. fat; 54% calories from fat; 15 mg. cholesterol; 8 g. carbohydrates; 329 mg. sodium; 3 g. fiber

Italian-Style Broccoli Pasta

1 cup uncooked elbow macaroni or other small pasta
2 cups coarsely chopped cooked broccoli or broccoflower
2 tablespoons olive oil
1 small clove garlic, minced
Salt to taste

Cook macaroni or other pasta according to package directions; drain and place into large serving bowl. Immediately toss with remaining ingredients. Serve immediately. Makes 4 servings.

Per serving: 86 calories; 2 g. protein; 6 g. fat; 66% calories from fat; 0 mg. cholesterol; 5 g. carbohydrates; 22 mg. sodium; 2 g. fiber

Stuffed Celery

½ cup low-fat cottage cheese
⅓ cup chopped sweet gherkins (about 2)
1 tablespoon chopped celery leaves
¼ teaspoon Worcestershire sauce
¼ teaspoon salt
6 ribs celery, cut into 8-inch pieces

In small bowl, stir cottage cheese, gherkins, celery leaves, Worcestershire sauce and salt until well mixed. Spread cheese mixture evenly on celery pieces. Makes 6 servings.

Per serving: 36 calories; 2 g. protein; 0 g. fat; 9% calories from fat; 2 mg. cholesterol; 6 g. carbohydrates; 277 mg. sodium; 0 g. fiber

Beans and Sprouts

1 pound green beans, trimmed and cut diagonally into ½-inch pieces
¼ cup boiling water
2 tablespoons canola, corn, cottonseed, safflower or soybean oil
2 tablespoons sesame oil
1 pound fresh mung-bean sprouts
½ cup loosely packed thinly sliced Spanish or other sweet onions
2 tablespoons minced fresh ginger
1 clove garlic, minced
3 tablespoons soy sauce mixed with 2 teaspoons sugar

In wok or large heavy skillet over high heat, bring to boil green beans, water and oils. Reduce heat; partially cover and simmer 5 to 8 minutes, or until beans are tender-crisp and water has evaporated. Add bean sprouts, onions, ginger, garlic and soy sauce mixture; cook, stirring constantly, 1 minute, or until onions are tender-crisp. Makes 8 servings.

Per serving: 105 calories; 3 g. protein; 7 g. fat; 55% calories from fat; 0 mg. cholesterol; 9 g. carbohydrates; 392 mg. sodium; 3 g. fiber

Tomatoes Stuffed with Spinach

5 medium tomatoes
½ teaspoon salt
2 packages (10 ounces each) frozen chopped spinach
2 tablespoons butter or margarine
1 small onion, grated
½ cup nonfat sour cream
¼ cup grated Parmesan cheese
Pepper to taste
Dash cayenne pepper to taste
⅓ cup Italian-seasoned dry bread crumbs

Preheat oven to 350°F. Grease baking dish large enough to hold tomatoes; set aside. Cut tops off tomatoes; scoop out pulp, reserving for another use, leaving ½-inch shell. Sprinkle with ¼ teaspoon salt; invert to drain.

Meanwhile, cook spinach according to package directions. Drain; cool, then squeeze dry. Melt 1 tablespoon butter or margarine in medium skillet over medium heat. Sauté onions 3 minutes, or until tender. Stir in spinach, sour cream, cheese, remaining ¼ teaspoon salt and peppers. Spoon into tomato shells. Place in prepared pan. Sprinkle top with bread crumbs; dot with remaining tablespoon butter or margarine. Bake 20 to 25 minutes, or until heated through. Makes 5 servings.

Per serving: 137 calories; 8 g. protein; 3 g. fat; 20% calories from fat; 9 mg. cholesterol; 21 g. carbohydrates; 379 mg. sodium; 5 g. fiber

Spiced Garbanzo Beans

3 tablespoons canola, corn, cottonseed, safflower or soybean oil
1 medium onion, finely chopped
1 clove garlic, finely chopped
1 tomato, peeled and chopped
2 jalapeño peppers, seeded and chopped
2 teaspoons chili powder
¼ teaspoon dried oregano
1 can (15 to 19 ounces) garbanzo beans (chickpeas), drained
Salt to taste

Heat oil in large skillet over medium heat. Cook onions and garlic for 3 minutes. Add tomatoes, peppers, chili powder and oregano. Cook over low heat, stirring frequently, 10 minutes, or until most liquid has evaporated. Add garbanzo beans and salt; cover and simmer 20 minutes more. Makes 6 servings.

Per serving: 172 calories; 5 g. protein; 8 g. fat; 43% calories from fat; 0 mg. cholesterol; 19 g. carbohydrates; 7 mg. sodium; 4 g. fiber

Hungarian Asparagus

1 pound fresh trimmed asparagus, cooked, or 2 packages (10 ounces each) frozen asparagus spears, cooked
¼ cup nonfat sour cream
1 cup buttered bread crumbs*

Preheat oven to 350°F. Grease 11 x 7-inch baking dish or 2½-quart shallow casserole; arrange asparagus in single layer. Cover with sour cream, then bread crumbs. Bake about 15 minutes, or until bread crumbs are golden brown. Serves 6.

* *To make buttered crumbs:* Heat 3 tablespoons butter, margarine or oil until hot in small saucepan over medium heat. Add 1 cup bread crumbs. Cook, stirring, until crumbs are lightly browned.

Per serving: 143 calories; 5 g. protein; 3 g. fat; 41% calories from fat; 18 mg. cholesterol; 16 g. carbohydrates; 186 mg. sodium; 1 g. fiber

Stuffed Mushrooms

1½ pounds large fresh mushrooms (about 24)
2 tablespoons butter or margarine
1 large onion, finely chopped
½ cup Italian-seasoned dry bread crumbs

Preheat oven to 350°F. Remove mushroom stems; finely chop and set aside. Melt butter or margarine in small saucepan over medium heat. Sauté onions 3 minutes, or until tender. Add chopped mushrooms. Cook 3 minutes, or until tender. Add bread crumbs, stirring until well combined. On large baking or jelly-roll pan, place mushroom caps top-side down; fill with bread crumb mixture. Add enough water to cover bottom of pan. Bake 20 minutes, or until mushrooms are tender. Makes 6 servings.

Per serving: 93 calories; 3 g. protein; 4 g. fat; 41% calories from fat; 10 mg. cholesterol; 11 g. carbohydrates; 74 mg. sodium; 3 g. fiber

Stewed Okra and Tomatoes

2 tablespoons canola, corn, cottonseed, safflower or soybean oil
1 small onion, chopped
1 package (10 ounces) frozen okra
1 can (16 ounces) tomatoes, undrained
½ teaspoon salt
¼ teaspoon pepper

Heat oil in large saucepan over medium heat. Sauté onions 5 minutes, or until lightly browned. Add remaining ingredients. Cook, stirring occasionally, 10 to 15 minutes, or until okra is tender. Makes 6 servings.

Per serving: 76 calories; 2 g. protein; 5 g. fat; 53% calories from fat; 0 mg. cholesterol; 8 g. carbohydrates; 302 mg. sodium; 2 g. fiber

Italian Peppers

2 cups chopped red and/or green peppers
1 can (8 ounces) tomatoes, broken up
3 tablespoons chopped onions
Pinch dried oregano or pizza herbs
Grated Parmesan or Romano cheese (optional)

In large saucepan over medium heat, combine peppers, tomatoes, onions and oregano or herbs; cover and simmer 5 minutes. Uncover; cook until thickened to desired sauce consistency. Top with cheese, if desired. Makes 4 servings.

Note: To bake in oven, if desired: Preheat oven to 425°F. In 1½-quart casserole, combine all ingredients except cheese. Cover and bake 20 to 25 minutes. Top with cheese.

Per serving: 25 calories; 1 g. protein; 0 g. fat; 12% calories from fat; 0 mg. cholesterol; 5 g. carbohydrates; 94 mg. sodium; 1 g. fiber

Green Bean–Mushroom Casserole

- 2 packages (10 ounces each) frozen cut green beans
- ¼ cup finely chopped onions
- 1 teaspoon salt
- 1 can (10½ ounces) condensed cream of mushroom soup
- 1 can (4 ounces) mushroom stems and pieces, drained and chopped
- ½ cup canned French-fried onion rings

Preheat oven to 350°F. Grease 1½-quart casserole; set aside. In large saucepan over medium heat, bring to boil ¼ cup water, green beans and onions. Cook 12 minutes, or until tender. Drain; return to saucepan. Stir in undiluted soup and mushrooms; pour into prepared casserole. Top with onion rings. Cover and bake 30 minutes, or until mixture is heated through. Uncover last 5 minutes to brown top. Makes 6 servings.

Per serving: 123 calories; 3 g. protein; 6 g. fat; 47% calories from fat; 1 mg. cholesterol; 13 g. carbohydrates; 1051 mg. sodium; 4 g. fiber

Tossed Rice Bowl

1 clove garlic, cut in half
1 can (16 ounces) bean sprouts, drained and rinsed
1 cup thinly sliced radishes
1 cup diced unpeeled cucumbers
1 cup thinly sliced celery
1 cup chopped watercress or lettuce
2 small Spanish or other sweet onions, chopped
¼ cup chopped green peppers
1½ cups cold cooked rice
1 cup light mayonnaise
Soy sauce to taste (optional)

Rub garlic on sides of large salad bowl. Layer vegetables and rice in order given. Top with mayonnaise. Just before serving, toss gently to blend well. Serve with soy sauce, if desired. Makes 6 servings.

Per serving: 206 calories; 2 g. protein; 13 g. fat; 60% calories from fat; 13 mg. cholesterol; 18 g. carbohydrates; 342 mg. sodium; 3 g. fiber

Mexican-Style Beans

- 1 package (16 ounces) pinto beans, rinsed and picked over
- 2 cups chopped tomatoes
- 1 medium onion, diced
- 1 can or jar (12 ounces) prepared taco sauce
- 1 can (4 ounces) green chilies, chopped
- 2 cloves garlic, minced
- 1½ teaspoons salt
- ½ teaspoon ground cumin
- ½ teaspoon pepper

In large saucepot or Dutch oven, place beans and enough water to cover by 2 inches. Let stand overnight, or boil 2 minutes, then let stand 1 hour. Stir in remaining ingredients. Bring to boil. Reduce heat to low; cover and simmer 1½ to 3 hours, or until beans are tender, adding boiling water if needed. Makes 12 servings.

Per serving: 128 calories; 7 g. protein; 0 g. fat; 4% calories from fat; 0 mg. cholesterol; 24 g. carbohydrates; 430 mg. sodium; 9 g. fiber

Tomatoes Provençales

1½ cups soft bread crumbs
¾ cup finely minced onions
¾ cup chopped parsley
2 tablespoons olive oil
3 cloves garlic, minced
1 teaspoon salt
¾ teaspoon dried thyme, crumbled
⅛ teaspoon pepper
2 pints cherry tomatoes

Preheat oven to 425°F. Grease shallow baking dish large enough to hold tomatoes in single layer; set aside. In medium bowl, combine bread crumbs, onions, parsley, oil, garlic, salt, thyme and pepper until well blended. Place tomatoes in prepared pan. Sprinkle bread crumb mixture over tomatoes; bake for 8 to 10 minutes, or until tomatoes are fork-tender. Makes 6 servings.

Per serving: 123 calories; 2 g. protein; 7 g. fat; 53% calories from fat; 0 mg. cholesterol; 12 g. carbohydrates; 426 mg. sodium; 3 g. fiber

Vegetable Medley

- ¼ cup butter or margarine, melted
- ½ cup cornflake crumbs
- ¼ cup grated Parmesan cheese
- 1 cup French-cut green beans
- 1 cup cauliflower florets, cooked
- 1 cup sliced carrots, cooked
- 2 teaspoons instant minced onions
- 1 cup (4 ounces) shredded reduced-fat Cheddar cheese
- 1 can (10½ ounces) condensed cream of mushroom soup
- 1 cup sliced potatoes, cooked

Preheat oven to 350°F. Grease 11 x 7-inch (1½-quart) baking dish; set aside. In small bowl, combine butter or margarine, cornflake crumbs and Parmesan cheese until well mixed; set aside. In prepared baking dish, place green beans, cauliflower, carrots and onions. Add Cheddar cheese and soup; stir until well mixed. Arrange potatoes in layer over vegetable mixture. Evenly top with crumb mixture. Bake 30 minutes, or until thoroughly heated. Makes 8 servings.

Per serving: 186 calories; 7 g. protein; 12 g. fat; 60% calories from fat; 23 mg. cholesterol; 11 g. carbohydrates; 739 mg. sodium; 2 g. fiber

Braised Leeks

3 bunches leeks, cut in half lengthwise and well rinsed
2 tablespoons butter or margarine
1 medium Bermuda onion, thinly sliced
2 cups beef broth or bouillon
2 whole cloves
1 bay leaf
½ teaspoon salt
⅛ teaspoon pepper

Cut off tops of leeks within 1½ inches of white part; save tops for another use. Melt butter or margarine in large skillet over medium heat. Sauté onions 5 minutes, or until lightly browned. Add leeks and remaining ingredients. Partially cover and simmer 30 minutes, or until leeks are tender and broth has almost evaporated. Remove cloves and bay leaf. Makes 6 servings.

Per serving: 136 calories; 2 g. protein; 4 g. fat; 27% calories from fat; 10 mg. cholesterol; 23 g. carbohydrates; 274 mg. sodium; 4 g. fiber

Orange-Buttered Acorn Squash

2 medium acorn squash, cut in half and seeded
½ teaspoon salt
2 tablespoons firmly packed brown sugar
2 tablespoons butter or margarine
¼ cup orange juice

Preheat oven to 350°F. In 13 x 9-inch baking dish, place squash cut-side down. Bake 40 minutes; turn cut-side up. Sprinkle with salt; into each cavity, place ½ tablespoon brown sugar, ½ tablespoon butter or margarine and 1 tablespoon orange juice. Return to oven; bake 15 to 20 minutes more, or until squash is fork-tender. Makes 4 servings.

Per serving: 152 calories, 1 g. protein; 4 g. fat; 33% calories from fat; 15 mg. cholesterol; 26 g. carbohydrates; 324 mg. sodium; 3 g. fiber

Cranberry Ice

1 can (8 ounces) jellied cranberry sauce
1-2 drops red food coloring
½ cup lemon-lime carbonated beverage

In small bowl with mixer, beat cranberry sauce and food coloring until smooth. Slowly beat in lemon-lime beverage. Pour into small refrigerator tray. Cover and freeze until firm. In chilled small mixer bowl, break up cranberry mixture into chunks; beat until fluffy. Return to tray. Cover and refreeze. To serve, scoop into dessert glasses. Makes 2 servings.

Per serving: 196 calories; 0 g. protein; 0 g. fat; 1% calories from fat; 0 mg. cholesterol; 50 g. carbohydrates; 39 mg. sodium; 2 g. fiber

Three-Fruit Salad

1 apple (Red Delicious, Gala), cored, unpeeled and cut into small pieces
1 banana, peeled and sliced
¼ cup pineapple chunks, drained
¼ cup nonfat plain yogurt
1 tablespoon pineapple juice
1 teaspoon sugar
⅛ teaspoon nutmeg
Lettuce for garnish (optional)

In small bowl, mix apples, bananas and pineapple. For dressing, in another small bowl, mix yogurt, pineapple juice, sugar and nutmeg until well blended. Pour over fruit; toss gently to coat. Serve on bed of lettuce, if desired. Makes 4 servings.

Per serving: 76 calories; 1 g. protein; 0 g. fat; 4% calories from fat; 0 mg. cholesterol; 18 g. carbohydrates; 11 mg. sodium; 2 g. fiber

Melon Cooler

- 1 package (4-serving size) lemon gelatin
- 1 cup hot water
- 1 cup cold water
- 1 tablespoon lemon juice
- 1½ cups melon balls (cantaloupe, honeydew)
- Additional melon balls and lettuce for garnish (optional)

In medium bowl, stir gelatin and hot water until gelatin is dissolved. Add cold water and lemon juice. Chill until slightly thickened; fold in melon balls. Turn into 1-quart mold or bowl; chill until firm. To serve, unmold onto serving platter. Place melon balls and lettuce around mold, if desired. Makes 6 servings.

Per serving: 68 calories; 1 g. protein; 0 g. fat; 1% calories from fat; 0 mg. cholesterol; 16 g. carbohydrates; 39 mg. sodium; trace g. fiber

Jellied Blueberries and Peaches

1 envelope unflavored gelatin
½ cup cold water
1 cup boiling water
⅓ cup sugar
¼ cup fresh lime juice
¼ teaspoon grated lime peel
1 cup fresh blueberries
1 cup ¼-inch cubes peeled peaches

In medium bowl, sprinkle gelatin over cold water; let stand 5 minutes, or until softened. Stir in boiling water, sugar, lime juice and lime peel until gelatin and sugar dissolve. Chill until slightly thickened. In small bowl, gently stir blueberries and peaches; fold into gelatin mixture. Spoon into 6 individual ½-cup dessert dishes or glasses. Chill until firm. Makes 6 servings.

Per serving: 75 calories; 1 g. protein; 0 g. fat; 2% calories from fat; 0 mg. cholesterol; 18 g. carbohydrates; 2 mg. sodium; 1 g. fiber

Red, White and Blue Mold

2 packages (4-serving size) strawberry gelatin
3 cups boiling water
1 package (10 ounces) frozen strawberries in syrup, thawed
2 packages (4-serving size) lemon gelatin
1 can (15¼ ounces) crushed pineapple in juice
4 cups nonfat sour cream
2 packages (4-serving size) black cherry gelatin
3 cups fresh or canned blueberries

For red layer: In medium bowl, stir strawberry gelatin and 1 cup boiling water until gelatin is dissolved. In 4-cup measure, place strawberries and syrup; add enough water to make 4 cups. Stir into dissolved gelatin. Pour into 16-cup mold or bowl. Chill until firm, about 4 hours.

For white layer: In medium bowl, stir lemon gelatin and 1 cup boiling water until gelatin is dissolved. In 4-cup measure, place pineapple and juice; add enough water to make 3 cups. Stir into dissolved gelatin with 2 cups sour cream. Pour into mold over strawberry layer. Chill until firm, about 4 hours.

For blue layer: In medium bowl, stir black cherry gelatin and 1 cup boiling water until gelatin is dissolved. In 4-cup measure, place blueberries; add enough water to make 3 cups. Stir into dissolved gelatin with remaining 2 cups sour cream. Pour into mold over pineapple layer. Chill until firm, about 4 hours. To serve, unmold onto serving platter. Makes 24 servings.

Per serving: 154 calories; 3 g. protein; 0 g. fat; 1% calories from fat; 6 mg. cholesterol; 34 g. carbohydrates; 109 mg. sodium; 1 g. fiber

Sparkling Dainties

1 package (4-serving size) sugar-free imitation flavor gelatin dessert
½ cup boiling water
2 tablespoons nonfat dry milk powder

In 8-inch baking dish or pan, stir gelatin and boiling water until gelatin is dissolved. Chill until firm. Cut into 1-inch squares; roll in milk powder to coat. Makes 64 dainties.

Per serving: 0 calories; 0 g. protein; 0 g. fat; 0% calories from fat; 0 mg. cholesterol; 0 g. carbohydrates; 0 mg. sodium; 0 g. fiber

Cantaloupe Frappé

1 medium ripe cantaloupe, peeled, seeded and cubed
¼ cup dry sherry (optional)
2 tablespoons honey
2 tablespoons lemon juice
Fresh mint leaves for garnish (optional)

In blender or food processor, puree cantaloupe cubes in batches until smooth. In medium bowl, stir cantaloupe puree, sherry, if desired, honey and lemon juice. Chill well and serve soft or freeze to thicker frappé stage. To serve, spoon into dessert dishes or glasses. Top with mint sprigs, if desired. Makes 8 servings.

Per serving: 40 calories; 0 g. protein; 0 g. fat; 4% calories from fat; 0 mg. cholesterol; 10 g. carbohydrates; 6 mg. sodium; trace g. fiber

Raspberry Lime Float

½ cup fresh or frozen unsweetened raspberries
¾ cup prepared lemonade
¼ cup (1 scoop) lime sherbet

In tall glass, place raspberries; pour in lemonade. Top with sherbet. Serve with long spoon. Makes 1 serving.

Note: Other fruit, such as blueberries, banana slices, or strawberries may be substituted.

Per serving: 172 calories; 1 g. protein; 1 g. fat; 7% calories from fat; 3 mg. cholesterol; 41 g. carbohydrates; 23 mg. sodium; 4 g. fiber

Ambrosia

1 can (8 ounces) mandarin orange segments, drained
1 can (8 ounces) pineapple tidbits, drained
1½ cups (about 8 ounces) green seedless grapes
2¼ cups (about 8 ounces) miniature marshmallows
1 container (8 ounces) nonfat sour cream
1⅓ cups shredded or flaked coconut
Maraschino cherries for garnish (optional)

Place oranges, pineapple, grapes, marshmallows, sour cream and coconut in large serving bowl; toss gently to coat. Garnish with cherries, if desired. Chill at least 4 hours. Makes 6 servings.

Per serving: 231 calories; 2 g. protein; 5 g. fat; 18% calories from fat; 4 mg. cholesterol; 46 g. carbohydrates; 99 mg. sodium; 3 g. fiber

Upside-Down Cake

½ cup firmly packed brown sugar
1 can (8 ounces) pineapple slices, drained
4 eggs, at room temperature, separated
1 cup sugar
1 cup all-purpose flour
1 teaspoon vanilla extract

Preheat oven to 350°F. Grease 9 x 9-inch or 9-inch round baking pan. Evenly sprinkle with brown sugar; top with pineapple slices and set aside.

In small bowl with mixer, beat egg whites, gradually adding ½ cup sugar until stiff peaks form; set aside.

In large bowl with mixer, beat egg yolks with remaining ½ cup sugar until thick and lemony-looking. Stir in flour until well blended. Fold in egg whites and vanilla until well blended. Spoon into prepared pan. Bake 30 minutes, or until toothpick inserted into center comes out clean. Immediately invert onto serving platter. Makes 8 servings.

Note: If desired, fresh sliced apples or canned or fresh sliced peaches can be substituted for the pineapple.

Per serving: 259 calories; 4 g. protein; 3 g. fat; 10% calories from fat; 137 mg. cholesterol; 54 g. carbohydrates; 41 mg. sodium; trace g. fiber

Carrot Kugel

2 eggs, at room temperature, separated
1 cup cooked or canned diced carrots
⅔ cup sifted cake flour
4 tablespoons sugar
2 tablespoons orange juice
½ teaspoon cinnamon
½ teaspoon salt

Preheat oven to 350°F. Spray 11 x 7-inch baking pan with nonstick cooking spray; set aside. In blender or food processor, place egg yolks and remaining ingredients; blend until smooth. In small bowl with mixer, beat egg whites until stiff peaks form. Fold into carrot mixture. Spoon into prepared pan. Bake 50 to 60 minutes, or until cake pulls away from sides of pan. Cut into squares. Makes 8 servings.

Per serving: 80 calories; 2 g. protein; 1 g. fat; 17% calories from fat; 68 mg. cholesterol; 14 g. carbohydrates; 86 mg. sodium; trace g. fiber

Fresh Harvest Pie

- 3 large apples peeled, cored and sliced (3 cups)
- 2 large pears peeled, cored and sliced (2 cups)
- 1½ cups seedless grapes
- ½ cup sugar
- 2 tablespoons all-purpose flour
- 1 tablespoon lemon juice
- ½ teaspoon grated lemon peel
- ½ teaspoon ground cinnamon
- ¼ teaspoon ground nutmeg
- Pastry for 2-crust pie

Preheat oven to 350°F. In large bowl, place apples, pears, grapes, sugar, flour, lemon juice, lemon peel, cinnamon and nutmeg; mix well.

Divide pastry in half. On lightly floured surface, roll out half of pastry into 12-inch circle. Fit pastry into 9-inch pie plate; trim, leaving 1-inch overhang. Spoon in fruit mixture. Roll remaining pastry into 10-inch circle. Cut pastry into ½-inch strips; weave strips over fruit to form lattice top. Press strips onto bottom crust. Fold crust over strips, forming rim, then flute. Bake for 50 to 60 minutes, or until fruit is tender. Makes 8 servings.

Per serving: 377 calories; 3 g. protein; 14 g. fat; 33% calories from fat; 0 mg. cholesterol; 49 g. carbohydrates; 277 mg. sodium; 3 g. fiber

Pumpkin Pie

⅔ cup sugar
½ teaspoon ground cinnamon
½ teaspoon ground ginger
½ teaspoon ground nutmeg
⅛ teaspoon salt
Pinch ground cloves
1½ cups canned pumpkin
1½ cups evaporated skim milk
3 egg whites, slightly beaten
1 teaspoon vanilla extract
½ teaspoon grated orange peel
1 unbaked 9-inch pie crust
Lite nondairy whipped topping for garnish (optional)

Preheat oven to 450°F. In small bowl, mix sugar, cinnamon, ginger, nutmeg, salt and cloves. In large bowl with mixer, beat pumpkin, milk, egg whites, vanilla and orange peel until smooth. Beat in sugar mixture. Pour into pie crust. Bake 10 minutes. Reduce heat to 325°F; bake 45 minutes more, or until knife inserted into center comes out clean. Serve in wedges topped with whipped topping, if desired. Makes 8 servings.

Per serving: 229 calories; 6 g. protein; 7 g. fat; 30% calories from fat; 2 mg. cholesterol; 34 g. carbohydrates; 246 mg. sodium; 1 g. fiber

Bean Bars

1 cup whole-wheat pastry flour
⅓ cup nonfat dry milk powder
½ cup firmly packed brown sugar
1 teaspoon baking soda
1 teaspoon ground cinnamon
½ teaspoon ground nutmeg
½ teaspoon ground cloves
½ teaspoon salt
2 cups cooked or drained canned green beans
1 egg
½ cup canola, cottonseed, safflower or soybean oil
½ cup unsweetened applesauce
¾ cup chopped walnuts
½ cup currants
2 tablespoons confectioners' sugar

Preheat oven to 350°F. Grease 11 x 7-inch baking pan. In large bowl, place flour, milk powder, sugar, baking soda, cinnamon, nutmeg, cloves and salt. In blender or food processor, place green beans, egg, oil and applesauce; process until smooth. Add to flour mixture, stirring until well blended. Stir in walnuts and currants. Pour into prepared pan. Bake 25 to 30 minutes, or until pick inserted into center comes out clean. Sprinkle with confectioners' sugar while warm. Cut into bars. Makes 24 bars.

Per bar: 120 calories; 2 g. protein; 7 g. fat; 52% calories from fat; 11 mg. cholesterol; 13 g. carbohydrates; 90 mg. sodium; 1 g. fiber

Carrot-Date Bars

1 cup whole-wheat pastry flour
1 teaspoon baking powder
½ teaspoon salt
Cholesterol-free, fat-free egg substitute, equivalent to 2 eggs
½ cup honey
1 teaspoon vanilla extract
1 cup chopped dates
1 cup shredded carrots
½ cup chopped walnuts

Preheat oven to 350°F. Grease 8 x 8-inch baking pan. In large bowl, mix flour, baking powder and salt. In small bowl, beat egg substitute, honey and vanilla until creamy. Add to flour mixture, stirring until well blended. Stir in dates, carrots and walnuts. Spoon into prepared baking pan; spread evenly. Bake 30 minutes. Cool completely on wire rack; cut into bars. Makes 16 bars.

Per bar: 125 calories; 2 g. protein; 3 g. fat; 22% calories from fat; 34 mg. cholesterol; 23 g. carbohydrates; 99 mg. sodium; 2 g. fiber

Broiled Fruit Cups

6 medium oranges
2 apples, cored, unpeeled and coarsely chopped
1 cup seedless grapes
6 tablespoons sugar

Preheat broiler. With sharp knife, slice tops off oranges. Remove insides of oranges, keeping sections intact. Cut design in edge of shell with kitchen shears, if desired. If necessary, slice small amount off bottom of orange to keep in upright position.

In small bowl, mix orange sections, apples and grapes. Sprinkle with sugar. Fill orange shells with sweetened fruit mixture. Place on broiler pan; broil 6 inches from heat source, or until warm through. Makes 6 servings.

Per serving: 154 calories; 1 g. protein; 0 g. fat; 3% calories from fat; 0 mg. cholesterol; 39 g. carbohydrates; 1 mg. sodium; 4 g. fiber

No-Bake Bran Fruit Squares

- 3 cups bran flakes cereal
- 1½ cups chopped raisins
- 1 cup chopped walnuts
- ¾ cup chopped dried figs
- ¾ cup chopped dates
- ¾ cup sweetened condensed milk
- 1 tablespoon lemon juice
- 1 tablespoon honey

In large bowl, mix all ingredients until well blended. Press firmly into 9 x 9-inch baking pan; cut into squares. Remove to platter; let stand 2 hours to dry. Store tightly covered. Makes 36 squares.

Per serving: 93 calories; 1 g. protein; 2 g. fat; 25% calories from fat; 2 mg. cholesterol; 17 g. carbohydrates; 40 mg. sodium; 1 g. fiber

Plum Brulee

4 large plums, cut in half and pitted
¾ cup nonfat sour cream
1 tablespoon granulated sugar
1 teaspoon orange liqueur or ¼ teaspoon grated orange peel
¼ teaspoon vanilla extract
⅛ teaspoon ground nutmeg
¼ cup firmly packed brown sugar

Preheat broiler. In small broiler-proof baking dish, place plums cut side up. In small bowl, mix sour cream, sugar, orange liqueur or orange peel, vanilla and nutmeg. Spoon over plum halves. Sprinkle with brown sugar. Broil 6 inches from heat source 5 minutes, or until sugar has melted and plums are heated through. Serve warm or chilled. Makes 4 servings.

Per serving: 158 calories; 2 g. protein; 0 g. fat; 3% calories from fat; 7 mg. cholesterol; 35 g. carbohydrates; 66 mg. sodium; 1 g. fiber

Peachy Yogurt Pie

1 envelope unflavored gelatin
¼ cup cold water
2 tablespoons peach brandy or peach nectar
6 tablespoons sugar
½ cup peach or apricot nectar
1 cup nonfat plain yogurt
1 ready-to-fill graham cracker pie crust
3 cups peeled peach or nectarine slices

In small saucepan, sprinkle gelatin over water; let stand 1 minute to soften. Cook over medium-low heat, stirring, until gelatin dissolves. Stir in brandy or nectar and sugar. In small bowl, stir ½ gelatin-brandy mixture with nectar. Chill 10 to 15 minutes, or until slightly thickened; set aside.

In small bowl, stir remaining gelatin-brandy mixture with yogurt; spoon into pie crust. Freeze to set slightly. Remove from freezer; arrange peach or nectarine slices in overlapping concentric circles on top of yogurt filling. Spoon thickened gelatin mixture over fruit to form glaze. Chill until firm and set. Makes 8 servings.

Per serving: 259 calories; 4 g. protein; 11 g. fat; 37% calories from fat; 0 mg. cholesterol; 37 g. carbohydrates; 262 mg. sodium; 2 g. fiber

Orange Sherbet

1 cup skim milk
2 tablespoons thawed frozen orange juice concentrate
2 tablespoons sugar
4-5 ice cubes

In blender or food processor, process all ingredients until smooth yet still icy. Pour into 2 dessert dishes; freeze about 1 hour, or until of desired consistency. Makes 2 servings.

Note: If desired, sherbet may be put in tall glasses and sipped. Other frozen fruit juice concentrates may be substituted.

Per serving: 119 calories; 4 g. protein; 0 g. fat; 2% calories from fat; 2 mg. cholesterol; 25 g. carbohydrates; 63 mg. sodium; 0 g. fiber

Pineapple Ice

½ cup water
⅓ cup pineapple juice
1 tablespoon lemon juice
1 egg white, at room temperature

In small freezer tray, stir water, pineapple juice and lemon juice; freeze, stirring often, until almost firm. In chilled small mixer bowl, break up fruit mixture into chunks; beat until fluffy. In another small bowl, beat egg white until stiff; fold into pineapple ice. Serve immediately or refreeze. Makes 1 serving.

Per serving: 60 calories; 3 g. protein; 0 g. fat; 1% calories from fat; 0 mg. cholesterol; 12 g. carbohydrates; 50 mg. sodium; trace g. fiber

Fruited Yogurt Parfait

1 can (16 ounces) sliced peaches, drained
2 containers (8 ounces each) nonfat vanilla yogurt
1 cup quartered seedless grapes
2 medium pears, peeled and sliced
1 can (8 ounces) pineapple chunks, drained
Lite nondairy whipped topping (optional)
4 maraschino cherries (optional)

Reserve 8 peach slices for garnish. In each of 4 parfait glasses, layer ¼ remaining peaches, some yogurt, ¼ grapes, some yogurt, ¼ pears, some yogurt, ¼ pineapple and remaining yogurt. Top with dollop of whipped topping and cherry, if desired. Garnish each with 2 reserved peach slices. Makes 4 servings.

Per serving: 144 calories; 5 g. protein; 0 g. fat; 4% calories from fat; 1 mg. cholesterol; 32 g. carbohydrates; 62 mg. sodium; 3 g. fiber

Frozen Pineapple Yogurt

2 cups nonfat plain yogurt
1 can (6 ounces) undiluted thawed frozen pineapple juice concentrate
2 teaspoons vanilla extract
Sugar or artificial sweetener to taste (optional)

In small bowl, stir yogurt, juice concentrate and vanilla until well blended. Add sugar or artificial sweetener, if desired. Spoon into shallow metal baking pan; freeze, uncovered, until partially frozen. In large bowl with mixer, beat yogurt mixture until slushy; return to chilled pan. Freeze until firm. To serve, soften in refrigerator 30 to 40 minutes before scooping. Makes 5 servings.

VARIATION

Substitute orange juice concentrate or any other unsweetened fruit juice concentrate for pineapple.

Per serving: 112 calories; 5 g. protein; 0 g. fat; 2% calories from fat; 1 mg. cholesterol; 22 g. carbohydrates; 70 mg. sodium; 0 g. fiber